Diagnosis in Speech-Language Pathology

Singular Textbook Series
Series Editor: M.N. Hegde

DIAGNOSIS
in Speech-Language Pathology

Second Edition

Edited by

J. Bruce Tomblin, Ph.D.

Hughlett L. Morris, Ph.D.

D. C. Spriestersbach, Ph.D.

Assistant to the Editors:

Juanita C. Limas

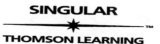

Africa • Australia • Canada • Denmark • Japan • Mexico • New Zealand • Philippines
Puerto Rico • Singapore • Spain • United Kingdom • United States

NOTICE TO THE READER

COPYRIGHT © 2002 Delmar. Singular Publishing Group is an imprint of Delmar, a division of Thomson Learning. Thomson Learning™ is a trademark used herein under license.

Printed in United States of America
    XXX

For more information, contact Singular Publishing Group, 401 West "A" Street, Suite 325 San Diego, CA 92101-7904; or find us on the World Wide Web at http://www.singpub.com

Library of Congress Cataloging-in-Publication Data:
Diagnosis in speech-language pathology / edited by J. Bruce Tomblin,
    Hughlett L. Morris, D.C. Spriestersbach. — 2nd ed.
      p. cm.
    ISBN 0-7693-0050-2 (softcover : alk. paper)
    1. Speech disorders—Diagnosis. I. Tomblin, J. Bruce.
  II. Morris, Hughlett L. III. Spriestersbach, D.C.
    [DNLM: 1. Language Disorders. 2. Speech Disorders. 3. Speech-Language Pathology.
WM 475 D5362 1999]
RC423.D473 1999
616.85'5075—dc21
DNLM/DLC   99-25480
for Library of Congress   CIP

Contents

SECTION III: SOME SPECIAL POPULATIONS   281

Photography by: Rex Bavousett & Jeff Nichols; University of Iowa Photo Service.

Introductory Remarks

This book has a long and, we trust, venerable history. Its beginnings can be traced to the fall of 1939 when Fred Darley and D. C. Spriestersbach were among the crop of new graduate students seeking master's degrees in the Department of Speech and Dramatic Art at the University of Iowa. One of the core courses required of all of them, regardless of their future major emphases, was "Voice and Phonetics" taught by a young, brilliant, dynamic professor, Grant Fairbanks. The course had the characteristic of all of Fairbanks' pedagogy: teaching students by building on meticulous attention to, and mastery of, the basic elements of the subject matter.

That year Fairbanks had numerous handouts that provided drills designed to give proficiency in General American Speech to each member of the class. Each class member was tested to make sure that she or he was able to speak within norms that Fairbanks and his assistants (of whom Spriestersbach ultimately became one) found acceptable. The class materials were soon published by Harper and Brothers in 1940 as *Voice and Articulation Drillbook*.

The experiences in that course and the exposure to the Fairbanks' teaching style left their mark on Darley and Spriestersbach. Ten years later both of them were on the faculty of the University of Iowa Department of Speech Pathology and Audiology (which had separated from the Department of Speech and Dramatic Art in 1956). Darley was teaching a course on the introduction to clinical practice and Spriestersbach was teaching a course on voice and articulation disorders, presumably with a "functional" origin. They found themselves teaching with approaches similar to those of Fairbanks, with emphasis on systematic and thoughtful observation of the client's communicative behavior. In the process, they generated many class exercises which they put into a workbook with tear-out pages for students to use in making their observations. Eventually they decided to turn the workbook into a text. Wendell Johnson supported their plan and agreed to participate as well. The result was the *Diagnostic Manual in Speech Correction*, published by Harper and Row in 1952.

Understanding of normal and disordered communicative behavior grew. The exercise forms, preceded by cryptic "whereas" introductions, became increasingly unsatisfactory. The consequence was the publication of *Diagnostic Methods in Speech Pathology* by Harper and Row in 1963. To be sure, some of the exercise forms were still in the new book, but arrangements were made with Interstate Printers and Publishers, Inc. of Danville, Illinois to supply them on a commercial basis.

The second edition of *Diagnostic Methods* was published by Harper and Row in 1978 by Darley and Spriestersbach with contributions from Charles V. Anderson, Arnold E. Aronson, Margaret C. Byrne, Julia Davis, Hughlett L. Morris, and Dean E. Williams. Its Preface includes the following:

> This is a textbook for students who are learning to be speech and language pathologists. It is designed to give them a philosophy for clinical practice, to teach them how to be efficient observers of oral communicative behavior and of the speech mechanism, and to help them develop skills for arriving at therapy decisions based on differentiations made among the possible etiological implications of the communicative behaviors they observe. . . .
>
> The current edition represents yet another stage in our thinking about the most effective way to teach diagnosis and appraisal. The forms have largely disappeared and the substantive material has been further enlarged. The major change, however, relates to our recognition that the previous editions were concerned primarily with appraisal; little was said about diagnosis. In this edition a major section of the book concerns diagnosis.

We see t' present book not as a revised edition, but as a continuation of the rour earlier books. In the new book, we want to continue the philosophy for diagnosis in speech-language pathology reflected in the earlier ones. That philosophy emphasizes the importance of disciplined, comprehensive descriptions of behavior, using the best tools available; comparing that information with information about the normal population; and bringing these data together with the clinical history information to arrive at hypotheses about diagnoses which can then be rationally tested by therapy in a problem-solving mode.

We want to focus on this philosophy because, in our opinion, a major hazard of diagnosis is the development by the clinician of preferences for specific diagnostic instruments and their continued use based in large part on familiarity with them. Any seasoned practitioner will recognize that likelihood. Here we want to emphasize for the student our preference for a model of diagnosis which is more open-ended. This philosophy leads to a continual search for better descriptors in arriving at an overview of the behavior, at the same time mindful of the cost of professional time. The goal is to arrive at a defensible and workable diagnosis.

The chapters that follow introduce you to the process of diagnosis in speech-language pathology. By design, they are a mixed bag, containing different kinds of discussions from different perspectives. Some are philosophic, intended to help you think about general issues of asking questions, making observations, and interpreting findings, while the chapter on multicultural issues helps place the diagnostic process in terms of societal influences.

Another group of chapters contains discussion of "basic" parameters of oral communication: language, speech production, voice, and fluency. Obviously material in these chapters has some important generic uses. That is, the information is relevant to a variety of complaints.

Another group of chapters is about specific disorders and demonstrates how we must adapt our general principles to fit the needs of the specific client. These discussions, as others, are not intended to be so comprehensive that the reader is now qualified for independent practice with the disorder. Rather, the material offers the beginning student some notion about questions to be asked and perspectives to be taken in approaching the task of diagnosis with that disorder.

Finally, several chapters illustrate differences in the clinical practice of speech-language pathology according to setting: the classroom, the hospital and clinic, and the private and public agency.

Note that the word we use to refer to the consumer of our service changes with setting. In general, a *patient* is examined in a health care setting, but a *client* is provided services in a free-standing speech pathology clinic or in a training clinic. The speech-language pathologist works with *students* or *children* in a school. One author (Kent) even reports that, in programs where she works, services are offered to the *consumer*! We have no preference for any terminology but instead urge the speech-language pathologist to follow the customs of her or his work setting.

By the way, we've tried hard in our language use to indicate that some clients/patients/students/consumers are girls and women and some are boys and men, and that likewise some speech-language pathologists are women and some are men. We think our references to gender are suitably done; forgive us if we missed one or two.

Finally, a word about the contributing authors. This is a University of Iowa book, and all authors have a connection with the university, either as alumnae or present faculty. We're very proud to emphasize this Iowa connection. However, we are prouder still that all these "Iowa-connection" authors are accomplished and dedicated clinical speech-language pathologists who write about clinical diagnosis in practical terms and from extensive clinical experience. No ivory-tower people here! Many thanks to them for agreeing to fit this assignment into their busy schedules.

A very big thanks to the Assistant to the Editors, Juanita C. Limas. She kept us and the contributing authors on track with great efficiency and good humor. We could never have managed without her good work.

We hope that you find the book useful and, better yet, that you find it interesting. Let us know if you have comments.

Preface
to the
Second Edition

In making the revisions for this edition we have been sensitive to critiques of the first edition. These have come from professionals in the field, critical reviews in scholarly journals, and our own evaluations.

Some of our efforts have been directed to clarifying our objectives in writing the book. We have also seen the need in some cases to extend the age ranges of the clients that we are covering, and in the organization of the text. It is our hope that arranging the chapters in sections will provide a logical framework for both students and teachers. Furthermore, there are a few changes in authorship. Because of illness or personal decisions, two authors in the first edition declined to write for this second edition, and so we welcome three new ones. Nevertheless, we continue to define a model for the diagnosis of speech-language pathologies that we think will be useful to beginning students. And in most instances, we have succeeded in doing so in a style that is easy and interesting to follow.

We continue to weigh our judgments about how much students need to know about the several speech-language disorders before thinking about their diagnoses. This is a challenge all professors face with beginning students regardless of specialty, including medicine and dentistry. We know, of course, that there is no final answer to this issue. Perhaps this book will be helpful to each professor as she or he organizes individual courses of study for beginning students.

Finally, this book continues to be a University of Iowa effort. As pointed out above, the first edition was written in 1952 by three Iowa faculty. We continue to follow that tradition, now including master clinicians as well as faculty. The reader, of course, will be the judge of the author selections that we have made.

J.B.T.
H.L.M.
D.C.S.
March 15, 1999
Iowa City, Iowa

Contributors

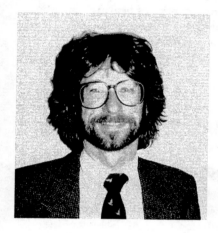

FRANK M. CIRRIN, Ph.D.

Ph.D. 1980, The University of Iowa

Dr. Cirrin is Resource Teacher in the Speech-Language Program, Department of Special Education, Minneapolis Public Schools, in Minneapolis, Minnesota. His current work includes developing classroom-based service delivery models for language intervention, and consulting with school-based collaborative teams to provide special education services for students with language-learning disabilities.

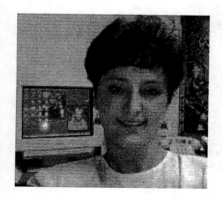

HEATHER M. CLARK, Ph.D.

M.S. 1992, University of North Dakota

Ph.D. 1996, University of Iowa

Dr. Clark is an Assistant Professor in the Department of Language, Reading, and Exceptionalities at Appalachian State University in Boone, North Carolina. Her clinical, teaching, and research interests include peripheral and central motor control for speech production and swallowing, and clinical service delivery in acute care settings.

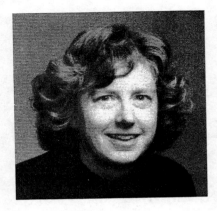

JILL L. ELFENBEIN, Ph.D.

M.A. 1975, University of Iowa

Ph.D. 1986, University of Iowa

Dr. Elfenbein is an Assistant Professor in the Department of Audiology and Speech Sciences at Michigan State University. She is a speech-language pathologist and an audiologist. Her research interests are in the areas of rehabilitative audiology and genetics of hearing loss. She teaches courses in rehabilitative audiology, manual communication, and diagnostic audiology. She also supervises students' practicum experiences.

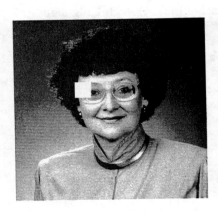

PENELOPE K. HALL, M.A.

M.A. 1967, The University of Iowa

Penelope K. Hall is an Associate Professor in the Department of Speech Pathology and Audiology at the University of Iowa. Her teaching, clinical, and research interests are in the areas of assessment and remediation of speech sound disorders and developmental language disorders, including developmental apraxia of speech.

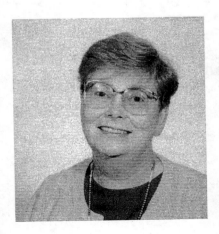

LOUISE KENT, Ph.D.

M.A. 1957, Indiana University

Ph.D. 1966, The University of Iowa

Dr. Kent is a speech-language pathologist in private practice in New Jersey. Her special interests are as an advocate for consumers with mental retardation.

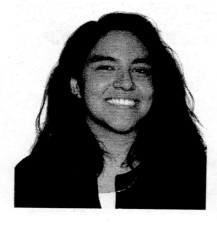

JUANITA C. LIMAS

B.A. 1999, The University of Iowa

Ms. Limas was the Assistant to the Editors during the production of this second edition. She worked as Assistant to the Editors for the first edition of this text as well. She is currently completing studies toward a double major in Biochemistry and Spanish at the University of Iowa.

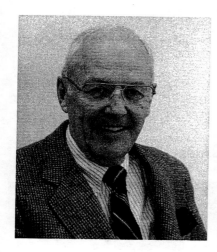

HUGHLETT L. MORRIS, Ph.D.

M.A. 1957, The University of Iowa

Ph.D. 1960, The University of Iowa

Dr. Morris is Professor Emeritus of the Department of Speech Pathology and Audiology and of the Department of Otolaryngology—Head and Neck Surgery, The University of Iowa. His special interests are in cleft palate and related disorders, voice disorders, and speech and voice disorders associated with head and neck cancer. He lives in Tucson, Arizona.

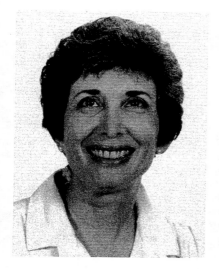

ADRIENNE L. PERLMAN, Ph.D.

Ph.D. 1985, The University of Iowa

Dr. Perlman is an Associate Professor in the Department of Speech and Hearing Science, Adjunct Associate Professor in the Department of Medicine, College of Medicine, and a member of the Bioengineering faculty in the College of Engineering at the University of Illinois at Urbana-Champaign. Her research has been devoted to laryngeal physiology and the study of normal and disordered swallowing. She teaches courses in normal and disordered swallowing, voice disorders, and motor speech disorders.

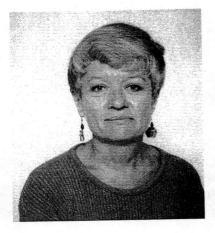

SALLY J. PETERSON-FALZONE, Ph.D.

M.A. 1965, The University of Illinois at Urbana

Ph.D. 1971, The University of Iowa

Dr. Peterson-Falzone is a speech-language pathologist for the Center for Craniofacial Anomalies and a Clinical Professor in the Department of Growth and Development at the University of California-San Francisco. Her special interests are in cleft lip and palate, craniofacial anomalies, and related disorders.

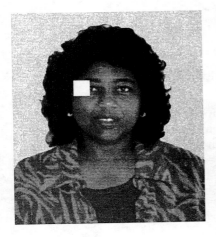

BETTY J. PRICE, M.S.

M.S. 1977, University of Texas at Houston

Ms. Price is a speech language clinician with the Mental Health and Mental Retardation Authority of Harris County, Medical and Consultative Services Department, in Houston, Texas. She specializes in the diagnosis and treatment of communication disorders of adults with developmental disabilities including mental retardation, autism, and hearing impairments. She also provides consultative and continuing education services in these problem areas.

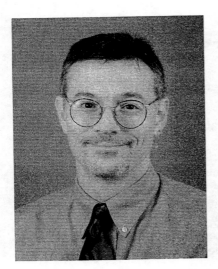

DONALD A. ROBIN, Ph.D.

M.S. 1981, University of Redlands

Ph.D. 1984, Case Western Reserve University

Dr. Robin is a Professor in the Department of Speech Pathology and Audiology at the University of Iowa. His research, teaching, and clinical interests are in neurogenic disorders of speech and language.

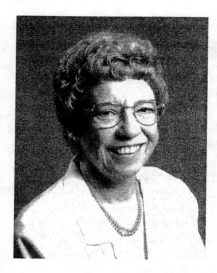

SHIRLEY J. SALMON, Ph.D.

M.A. 1961, The University of Iowa

Ph.D. 1965, The University of Iowa

Dr. Salmon recently retired as a speech pathologist at the Veterans Affairs Medical Center in Kansas City, Missouri. She is Professor Emeritus at the University of Kansas Medical Center in Kansas City, Kansas. Her special interest is in laryngectomee rehabilitation and she continues to write about this topic as well as lecture about various facets of this subject.

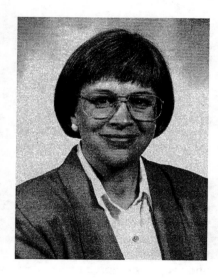

ANN BOSMA SMIT, Ph.D.

M.A. 1969, The University of Iowa

Ph.D. 1980, The University of Maryland

Dr. Smit is an Associate Professor at Kansas State University in Manhattan, Kansas. Her research interests are in developmental speech sound disorders. She teaches and supervises in the areas of phonological disorders and fluency disorders and has taught neuromotor disorders as well.

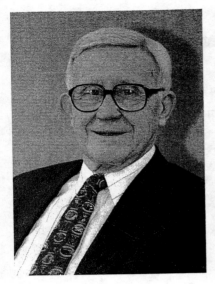

D. C. SPRIESTERSBACH, Ph.D.

M.A. 1940, The University of Iowa

Ph.D. 1948, The University of Iowa

Dr. Spriestersbach is Professor Emeritus at the University of Iowa. He joined the faculty of the Department of Speech Pathology and Audiology in 1948, was appointed Dean of the Graduate College in 1965, Vice President for Educational Development and Research in 1966, and served as Interim President of the University of Iowa in 1981–1982. In speech-language pathology, his major interests are in cleft palate and related disorders and in clinical outcome research. Currently, he is involved in Breakthrough, which develops and markets a system for helping children from prekindergarten through first grade learn to read.

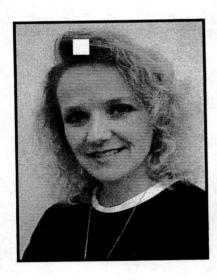

JULIE A. G. STIERWALT, Ph.D.

Ph.D. 1997, The University of Iowa

Dr. Stierwalt is an Assistant Professor in the Department of Communication Sciences and Disorders at Southwest Missouri State University. Her clinical, teaching, and research interests are in the evaluation and treatment of patients with neurogenic and swallowing problems including traumatic brain injury.

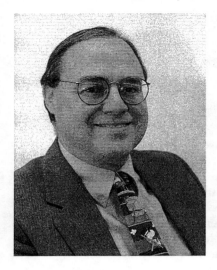

J. BRUCE TOMBLIN, Ph.D.

M.A. 1967, The University of Redlands

Ph.D. 1970, The University of Wisconsin at Madison

Dr. Tomblin is a Professor in the Department of Speech Pathology and Audiology and director of the Child Language Research Center at the University of Iowa. His research interests concern the etiology, diagnosis, and outcomes of developmental language disorders. He teaches courses in developmental language disorders, particularly of the school-age child, and diagnosis.

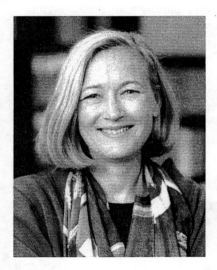

NANCY TYE-MURRAY, Ph.D.

Ph.D. 1984, The University of Iowa

Dr. Tye-Murray is the Richard Silverman Chair and Director of Research at the Central Institute for the Deaf and is a Professor at Washington University. Her teaching and research has focused on speech and language characteristics and rehabilitation of children and adults who have severe and profound hearing loss.

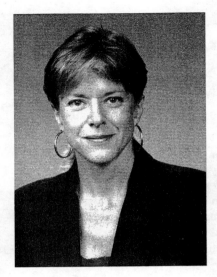

KATHERINE VERDOLINI, Ph.D.

M.A. 1982, Indiana University

Ph.D. 1991, Washington University

Dr. Verdolini is Assistant Professor, Otology and Laryngology, Harvard Medical School; Associate Professor, Communication Sciences and Disorders, MGH Institute of Health Professions; Research Associate, Voice and Speech Lab, Massachusetts Eye and Ear Infirmary; Research Coordinator, Voice/Speech/Swallowing, Beth Israel Deaconess Medical Center and Brigham and Women's Hospital, Boston, Massachusetts. She was formerly Assistant Professor, Department of Speech Pathology and Audiology, The University of Iowa. Her research interests are in voice physiology, skill acquisition in voice, and voice therapy efficacy. She teaches anatomy and physiology of speech and voice disorders as well as maintaining an active clinical practice.

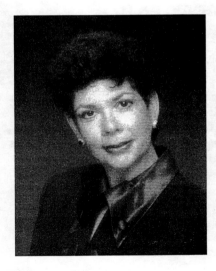

AMY L. WEISS, Ph.D.

M.A. 1976, University of Illinois at Urbana-Champaign

Ph.D. 1983, Purdue University

Dr. Weiss is an Associate Professor in the Department of Speech Pathology and Audiology at the University of Iowa. Her research interests are in language development and disorders of preschool children as well as the language and communication performance of children who stutter. She teaches courses in speech and language disorders, clinical intervention, and multicultural issues in communication disorders. She also supervises in the clinic.

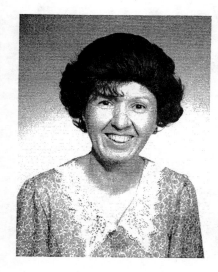

CAROL E. WESTBY, Ph.D.

M.A. 1968, University of Iowa

Ph.D. 1971, University of Iowa

Dr. Westby is a Professor in the Department of Communicative Disorders and Sciences at Wichita State University, Wichita, Kansas and a senior research associate with the Center for Family and Community Partnerships with the University of New Mexico, Albuquerque. Among her special interests are the development of culturally appropriate assessment and intervention programs, infancy through young adulthood; play and narrative development; language/literacy relationships; ethnographic interviewing; and cultural variations in discourse and adult-child interactions.

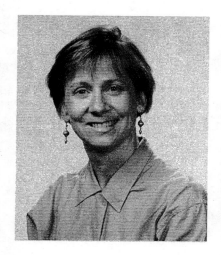

PATRICIA M. ZEBROWSKI, Ph.D.

Ph.D. 1987, Syracuse University

Dr. Zebrowski is an Associate Professor in the Department of Speech Pathology and Audiology at the University of Iowa. Her research interests are in the area of stuttering, with special emphasis on childhood stuttering. She teaches courses in stuttering and intervention and supervises master's level students in diagnostic and therapy practicum with children and adults who stutter.

DEDICATION

We would like to dedicate the second edition of this book,
Diagnosis in Speech-Language Pathology,
to Joan Marie Bodenham Morris
1929–1998

SECTION I

Perspectives

We begin with two chapters containing material that we consider the foundation of diagnosis in speech-language pathology. In the first, Tomblin presents a philosophy of diagnosis in our field that might easily be titled, "basic principles." In the second, Westby reminds us that human communication disorders and their diagnosis must always be viewed within the cultural context.

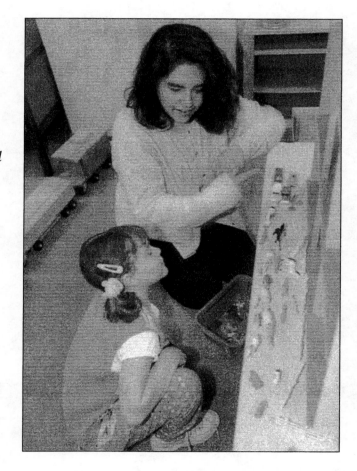

Perspectives on Diagnosis

J. Bruce Tomblin, Ph.D.

PERSPECTIVES ON DIAGNOSIS

If you are like most readers of this book, you are a student preparing for a career in speech-language pathology and/or audiology. For most students, the prospect of beginning work in a clinical field brings on mixed feelings. You are no doubt looking forward to clinical work because you will finally get to apply the information you have learned in the classroom. Furthermore, your practice may actually help someone else. Considerable apprehension may accompany this positive feeling, because speech-language pathology includes many roles and responsibilities that are unfamiliar to you. Few students have had the opportunity to receive services from a speech-language clinician and, unlike the professions of law and medicine, there are no television shows to inspire students and provide examples of the practice of speech-language pathology. You may have observed a speech-language clinician providing services and, if the clinician was skillful, you may have thought: "Will I be able to do that when I'm done with my professional education?" "Am I likely to have the talent to be able to provide clinical services?" And, worst of all, "what if I am no good at being a clinician or find that I don't like this type of work?"

It is very likely that these questions and other similar ones are going through your mind as you begin your professional education. Some of them cannot be addressed until you begin clinical work. Clinical work will require many things from you and only by actually doing the work will you begin to discover if this type of practice is satisfying to you. We want, in this book, to make at least one aspect of the clinical process clearer to you and to reduce some of the uncertainty and mystery about one important aspect of clinical service: diagnosis of speech and language disorders.

THE CLINICAL PROCESS

Speech–language clinicians engage in a variety of activities as they provide clinical services. Some of these activities are concerned with efforts to understand the client's communication problems. These activities are often referred to as diagnosis, or assessment. Other clinical activities include efforts to help modify, minimize, or resolve the communication problems, and these are placed in the category called therapy, intervention, or treatment. Before we consider the assessment process, we need to consider what the clinical process is, in general.

There are a variety of professions that, in one way or another, may be viewed as clinical. Certainly, physicians, dentists, clinical psychologists, and social workers perform clinical acts and their practices are characterized as clinical professions. What is it about the things these professionals do that leads us to refer to their activities as "clinical?" The most obvious commonality is that people go to these professionals to seek help for their personal problems. The clinical act, then, has as its basis a quality of "helping." In all human societies there are some who are given the role of providing assistance, in one way or another, to individuals who are ill, suffering, or unable to cope with the routines of life in the "normal" way. In assuming this role, clinicians accept their client's trust that they will work in the client's best interest in relieving a problem. As a result, societies usually hold these clinicians in high esteem. The clinical process is, as a result, an act of helping and caring for others, while at the same time the clinician cannot become so emotionally involved as to be unable to exercise reasoned judgment. This aspect of the clinical process is one that most students in speech-language pathology and audiology understand and, in fact, it is the one that draws most of them to the profession.

A caring soul and a desire to help, however, are not sufficient to produce a clinician. Part of the social contract between those who seek help and the clinicians who provide it is that the clinician has resources to help the client. In the case of a tribal shaman, this may be the determination of the nature of the person's problem, the determination of the cause of the malady based on cultural lore, and the administration of an incantation or provision of herbs to remedy the problem. In such a case, the shaman is applying a body of knowl-

Based on this definition, can you think of other professions that would also be clinical?

edge to the problem being presented and, based on this knowledge, acting to help the affected person. Although we may view our clinical work as being more sophisticated than the work of a native healer, the speech-language clinician also is expected to fulfill a similar role: as a thoughtful problem solver who brings current understanding of communication disorders to bear on the problems of the client.

Problem solving is a major part of the clinician's activities. Beginning student clinicians often observe speech-language clinicians performing therapy or diagnostics, and what they see is the clinician doing things. It may be eliciting a speech sound from a child, instructing a person in better use of the voice, or administering a language test. Obviously, clinical work involves doing things and it is very logical for students to conclude that what they need to learn is how to do these things, and that if they learn about enough of these things they will also be capable clinicians. In fact, nearly all beginning clinicians, when assigned their first client, will ask themselves, "What am I going to do with this person?" Unfortunately, this is the wrong question, because it focuses your attention on doing something rather than the process of problem solving. Instead of asking what do I do, you must focus on the nature of the problem to be solved and the information you need to solve it. Once you have gotten to the point of knowing what information you need, the question of what you need to do will often become obvious. What you ultimately end up doing clinically should be, therefore, a logical part of the overall problem-solving process.

For the experienced clinician, the route between the problems presented by the client and the set of needed actions often requires little deliberation. Consequently, to the experienced clinician the problem-solving process may seem transparent or automatic. If you watch or even talk with an accomplished clinician, it may appear as though there is simply an obvious action for each clinical situation. For the beginning student or the experienced clinician with a difficult case, the problem-solving procedure is likely to be more difficult.

Let's examine this process by considering a situation in which a parent has come to you with a child whose speech is difficult to understand. How can we approach the problem-solving process in such a way that what we need to do becomes a product of that process? We may start by beginning to frame a series of questions that we need to answer, such as, "does the child have a communication disorder?" If so, "what aspects of communication are contributing to this problem?" Also, "are there factors that can be identified that are contributing to or complicating this problem?"

Having asked these questions, we can then begin to consider what information we need to answer them. For example, to answer the first question, "does the child have a communication problem," you need to know how old the child is—information you are likely to get by asking the child's mother. Obviously, we would interpret such a complaint differently if the child were 2 years old rather than 6 years old. In addition to the child's age, you will also want to hear the child speak. After obtaining the information you need to answer the initial

> Good clinical work requires that you think about the problems you need to solve before you act.

questions, you will need to interpret the information using professional guidelines and standards to arrive at a conclusion.

The steps we just went through are depicted in Figure 1–1. We see that the first step is to determine what questions we should ask. Next, we establish what information is needed for us to answer the question. After this, we can decide how to go about getting this information, that is, what we need to do. Notice that the question of what you are going to do becomes much easier to answer when it is placed in the framework of the general problem-solving process.

Once we have determined what we are going to do and, as a result, have gathered the information we needed, we are not done with this process. We still have to interpret the information in relation to the problem we are attempting to solve. This interpretation process is often the area where clinicians differ the most. As you develop as a clinician, you will acquire knowledge, beliefs, and attitudes that will determine your clinical interpretations of the information you have obtained. Therefore, these beliefs and attitudes will lead to your decision that a child is stuttering or that a teenager has a hoarse voice or that an aphasic should be seen for language therapy. I will term this collection of knowledge, beliefs, and attitudes *clinical standards*. Some believe this judgment process is the intangible quality that makes the clinical process an art and makes some clinicians better clinical artists than others.

Some believe that clinical arts cannot be taught, but only learned by extensive experience. If much of this is a definable judgment process, then it would seem that we should be able to teach it.

There is no doubt that, as one gains experience, this process of making clinical judgments becomes easier and probably more often correct. It is also true that, as our profession matures, these intangible notions contained in the mind of the master clinician can be made explicit and taught to beginning student clinicians. Much of what you will read in this book is just this sort of information. You will be reading about the kinds of decisions that confront the clinician in the diagnostic phase of clinical practice. Additionally, the kinds of information you need to obtain to address these questions are presented, as well as the ways in which you can gather this information. Finally, interpretation of the information gathered to answer these diagnostic questions will be covered.

Steps to Clinical Problem Solving

1. Establish the clinical question.

2. Determine the information needed to answer the question.

3. Determine how to obtain this information.

4. Gather the information.

5. Interpret the information using clinical standards.

6. Answer the question.

Figure 1–1. The clinical problem-solving process.

THE DIAGNOSTIC PROCESS—AN OVERVIEW

I have just pointed out that the clinical process involves solving problems. That aspect of clinical work viewed as diagnosis address- es a set of common questions or problems with the objective of gain- ing an understanding of the client's communication disorder. Thus, *diagnosis is the clinical process concerned with understanding the client's communication disorder.*

This sounds rather simple, but actually understanding the client's communication problems involves multiple factors that go well beyond a characterization of a client's communication performance. Because of this complexity, a full understanding of a given commu- nication problem is rarely attained; rather, this is a goal we work toward. Typically, this diagnostic process is the focal point of our clinical activities when we first begin to see a client. Obviously, any treatment efforts will be influenced by our understanding of the communication disorder. Rarely is a full understanding of a problem arrived at before we initiate treatment. In fact, valuable information about the communication problem is often obtained during the treat- ment process, and consequently we need to reassess its status throughout treatment. Therefore, the diagnostic process is an ongo- ing aspect of the total clinical management process.

ASPECTS OF UNDERSTANDING A COMMUNICATION DISORDER

In other chapters you will be learning about what it is you need to know about specific types of communication disorders. In this sec- tion we will consider some basic questions that guide our diagnosis of most communication disorders.

Determination of the Complaint

The first question often confronting the clinician in the diagnostic process deals with determining what has led the person to be seen by the clinician. Unlike medicine or dentistry, few people seek out the speech-language clinician just to have a checkup to see that their communication skills are still fine. When people go to a speech-lan- guage clinician, they usually are seen because either they are con- cerned about their communication performance or someone else is concerned with their performance. The first question to be answered, therefore, often has to do with discovering what has caused the per- son to come to you for a diagnostic evaluation.

As a part of this question, we need to determine who is con- cerned about the person's communication performance and why they are concerned. In some instances, the client initiates the clinical contact and it must be determined what motivated the client to seek help. At other times the client is referred to the speech-language clinician by another professional, such as a physician or a teacher, because of concerns about the person's communication performance. The teacher may be concerned because a child is having difficulty with classroom learning activities and suspects that the child's language abilities are influencing the student's poor performance. The physician may be concerned because a patient has been having recurrent hoarseness and believes this results from the way the patient uses her or his voice. It is also common to have clients referred by family members—often parents or a spouse—because of concern about a child or spouse's communication.

In such cases, we find ourselves having to address the concerns of the person who referred the client to us, as well as the concerns of the client, and we cannot always assume that these concerns are identical. An adolescent who stutters, referred to the speech-language clinician by a concerned teacher, may not view her or his stuttering as a problem. This certainly changes the nature of the problem we are dealing with and what it is that we need to understand. The key concept is that you must identify who is concerned and why they are concerned. It is very easy in a clinical setting to quickly focus on the issues that you think are important. Regardless of how important these issues are, if you do not address the concerns of the client and of those who have initiated the referral, your clinical efforts will fail because you haven't addressed the problem that originally brought the client to you.

In your clinical practice you will continually need to help teachers, physicians, and others know when and how to refer to you.

Determining the Existence of a Communication Disorder

Whether the client is self-referred or referred by someone else, one of the questions we ask early in the diagnostic process is: "Does the client have a communication disorder and, if so, what aspects of communication are affected?" Usually, by the time we have addressed the first question concerning the complaint, we have some idea of the areas of communication that are likely to be contributing to the communication problem. If the complaint is linked to difficulties in being understood, we know that we need to obtain information about those aspects of the client's speech sound production and expressive language skills, but we may need to consider who the listeners are and if they may be a part of the problem. If the complaint is concerned with stuttering, we will look at the client's patterns of fluency and feelings about speech. These examples should convince you that the complaint directs our attention to obtaining sufficient information to determine if the person actually has a problem with that aspect of communication described in the complaint. Although we usually focus on those aspects of communication raised by the complaint, the cautious clinician will observe, at least informally, the person's competency across all domains of communication. A parent may be concerned about a child's fluency, but you may also observe that the child is showing poor language development. The questions that bring the client to you must be addressed in your evaluation, but they should not limit your observations and inquiry into the client's overall communication status. A great deal of what you will learn about the diagnosis of communication disorders will concern this basic issue of how you can observe, describe, measure, and analyze the speech and language behaviors of your clients. You need to understand that the information obtained from your use of these tools will be used to help you address this question.

Earlier, we saw that information obtained in an evaluation needs to be interpreted by the clinician based on a set of clinical standards. Learning how to observe, measure, and describe your client's communication behaviors is not enough to answer the question "does this person have a communication disorder and, if so, what aspects are affected?" In particular, in determining if a client has a communication disorder, we need to consider what our clinical standards are for the determination of a communication disorder so that we can apply these standards to the information we have about the client's communication status.

Long ago Lee Edward Travis proposed that a "speech or voice defect may be defined as an unusually conspicuous deviation in the speech pattern of an individual which is incapable of bringing about an adequate social response and which by the same token constitutes a maladjustment to his environment" (Travis, 1931, p. 36). One of his students, Charles Van Riper, later stated that "speech is defective when it is conspicuous, unintelligible or unpleasant" (Van Riper, 1963, p. 16). Although we have expanded the scope of our field to incorporate more aspects of communication than speech, these definitions provide a good starting point for considering what our standards for diagnosing a communication problem should be.

Each of these definitions recognizes that communication is an essential social tool. As such, there is a communication disorder when a person's communication performance frequently fails to accomplish the social functions needed or the manner in which the person does communicate is viewed negatively by either the speaker or the audience. When you state that a person has a communication disorder, you are making a claim about the likelihood that the client will face difficulties because we all are required by society to accomplish a vast number of communication acts during our lives. This perspective on the definition of a communication disorder emphasizes that it is not solely an attribute of the client, and it is not just the behavior of the client, but rather *it is a relationship between the client and the person's current and future audiences.* I believe that we should include the client as one of these audiences, because the client is often the individual most unhappy with her or his communication and is always a witness to it. Audiences, including the client, have social values about communication and about variations in human behavior. The audiences will naturally apply these

Lee Edward Travis is viewed by many as the founder of American speech-language pathology. Van Riper was one of his most well known students.

values to their communicative partners. As a clinician, you must develop an understanding of the uses of communication in a client's community and the values a given society places on communication and differences in communication performance. This will be easier if the client's social system is the same as yours. But if it is not, then you must try to understand the client's social system and make your clinical decisions in accord with the client's culture.

The ideas we have just discussed can be helpful in understanding the meaning of some terms used to refer to different aspects of health problems. These terms are "impairment," "disability," and "handicap" and you will find them used in some of the following chapters. When used in reference to a communication disorder *impairment* refers to disruptions in the basic biological and psychological systems that are necessary for communication. The person who has difficulties with speech sound production because of a cleft palate has a speech problem because of an impairment in the palate. A *disability* refers to the functions disrupted by the impairment. Therefore, the speech production difficulties arising from the cleft palate constitute a disability. The term *handicap* refers to the limitations in the fulfillment of social and cultural functions that result from impairments and disabilities. You can appreciate the difference between disability and handicap by thinking about a person who has very limited speech capability. When provided with a communication device that allows the person to use a computer to express himself, the person may have less of a communication handicap even though the speech disability has not been altered and the basic impairment has not been altered.

Here we see again that social values play a key role in determining when we say clients have a communication disorder. That is, when clients are handicapped by their communication skills we decide that they have a particular disability, namely a communication disorder. We then attempt to explain why they have this communication disorder by looking for impairments in the basic systems involved in communication. The important thing to notice here is that when we say a person has a communication disorder we are making a statement about a relationship between the person's communication behavior and problems they may face in their life because of their communication skills. Your decision that a client has a communication disorder will involve your judgment of the likely consequences of the interactions between the client's communication skills and the social context in which they will function. If you believe the client is or will face social penalties, then you are justified in concluding that a communication disorder exists. The very fact that the client is sufficiently concerned to come to you is strong evidence that a problem exists.

The concepts we have discussed provide you with a general basis for developing your standards for the determination that a communication disorder exists. Once you have determined that a person presents a communication disorder, it will be necessary for you to begin to pose more questions to learn more about the client's communication disorder.

Cultures differ on how individual differences are viewed. For more information, see Chapter 2.

Notice that I did not give you a specific standard to use for the determination of a communication disorder. That's because the standards differ for different clients and different cultures.

Determining Client and Family Reactions and Attitudes to the Disorder

Communication is a fundamental aspect of being human. A limitation in this ability can lead to considerable social and emotional reactions by the client, the client's family, and friends of the client. These social and emotional responses often can be the most important aspect of the communication problem. Also, as you might expect, you will find that people respond differently to a communication disorder. For some clients, very subtle communication difficulties may provoke considerable concern in a parent or spouse and, yet, in other cases clients with rather striking difficulties may have relatives who are less concerned. Whether you view either response as under- or overreactions, it is very likely that any responses to your client's communication will influence the nature and success of your clinical management. Knowing about the variety of responses and including this information is necessary for a full understanding of a client's communication problem.

Identifying Associated Problems

Often, a communication problem occurs in the context of other problems. The child with a developmental disability such as cerebral palsy is very likely to have problems with feeding and ambulation, and the adult stroke patient may have problems with vision, as well as use of the right arm. Such concomitant problems can directly affect the way you will carry out your assessment and the way you will interpret some of the person's performance. For instance, a paralysis of the right arm of a person with aphasia may influence his performance on some assessment procedures requiring limb movement. So if this patient was previously right-handed, slow responses or even inaccurate responses may be due to the need to use the left hand rather than evidence of a language problem. Paralysis may be more troublesome for some patients than the communication problem that also resulted from the stroke. The relative importance of the communication impairment for such a person may be less than for a person who places a high value on communication. Gathering such information is important in planning a program of rehabilitation combined with your judgment of the extent that the communication problem handicaps the individual. This situation demonstrates that understanding the client's communication problem requires that you place the person's communication in the context of the client's needs.

See Chapter 11 for more on this topic in the context of acquired aphasia.

Determining Factors Causing or Exacerbating the Problem

Identifying the cause of something is usually considered an essential part of understanding it. Our ability to determine the cause of a communication disorder varies considerably across different types of disorders. You will also find that the importance of this decision in the clinical management of the client will vary.

A person with a chronically hoarse voice presents us with a situation in which determining the cause is very important. Often, an early sign of cancer of the larynx is hoarseness and, so, we must ensure that this causal factor can be determined and at least ruled out. If cancer is ruled out, as it often is, we may then hypothesize that vocal abuse may be the cause and use this causal hypothesis to guide our treatment.

There are other communication problems, such as developmental phonological problems, for which there are usually no known explanations. Even in dealing with these problems, however, it is important that you rule out the presence of hearing impairment, which could certainly cause a phonological problem. Once hearing impairment is ruled out, we are likely to proceed with a treatment approach that promotes phonological learning. In such a situation we do not know why the child has difficulty learning the sound system, but at least we can hypothesize that learning is at the root of the problem and that improved learning will remedy it.

These examples demonstrate that for all forms of communication disorders we will be concerned with determining the possible causes of the problem. In some instances, the cause of the problem can be treated, such as cancer of the larynx or hearing loss. In the best of cases such treatments of causes will lead to a resolution of the communication problem as well. In other cases, such as a child with hearing impairment and a phonological problem, the treatment of the hearing impairment allows the phonological treatment to be more successful. In other instances, all we can do is rule out causal factors but even these negative findings are important. Often the client or family of the client will have developed beliefs about why the problem exists and such beliefs can generate unwarranted apprehension and, in some instances, blame. Addressing the causes and ruling out those that are groundless helps the client. Ruling out causal factors can also serve the clinician. As we will see in the next section, the course of the problem will frequently be different depending on the presence or absence of certain contributing factors.

Determining the Course of the Problem (Prognosis)

A basic property of humans is that we are always changing. You are capable of accomplishing different things today than you were a few years ago. It should come as no surprise that most communication problems change over time. For many, this change is toward improved communication skills. We often find this in children who, despite limited communication abilities, show gradual developmental growth. Likewise, the language skills of an aphasic person will usually improve subsequent to the initial brain injury. Other communication problems may not be as predictable. The communication of a preschool child who stutters may improve or may become worse. As you study in this field, you will find that the prognosis for various types of communication disorders will depend on an array of factors, such as the client's age, the severity of the problem, and the cause(s) of the problem, to name some obvious considerations. You will also find that the crystal ball gazing required for developing prognoses is difficult but you won't be able to avoid this process. For the client and the family of the client this is *very* important. They usually know how the client is doing now. What they want to know is: "Will he get better?" If so, "How much better and how soon?"

There are many pieces of information that will go into your decision making concerning prognosis. In later chapters you will find that prognosis is often influenced by characteristics of the speech and language performance of the client, the causal factors affecting these communication behaviors, and the way in which the client and family react to the problem. Note that all of this information relates to decisions we have just talked about.

DETERMINING TREATMENT ALTERNATIVES

Earlier, I said that some clinical activities are focused on understanding the client's communication problem (diagnosis) and that other activities are concerned with efforts to modify the communication problem (therapy) and that these two domains of clinical activity are closely related to each other.

A basic issue concerning treatment deals with whether or not initiating treatment or continuing treatment is warranted. Either can be one of the most difficult decisions you will face and, unfortunately, you will often lack a solid foundation for making such decisions. To make a decision to begin or continue treatment you will need to consider previous questions we have posed, that is, what is the prognosis for the problem, and in particular, will the outcome be improved if the person is provided with some form of treatment? Treatment can only be justified if the person will be better off for having had it. Likewise, treatment should be continued for only so long as you believe that the client will be better off for having received it. This leads us to want information about the client and the nature of the problem that will help us predict the client's future status when given a particular treatment as opposed to no treatment or as opposed to a different type of treatment.

In chapters that follow, you will be provided with information to help you determine treatment alternatives. At this point, I hope you have begun to see that diagnosis is, to a great degree, a thinking, problem-solving process. There are many questions that you will need to ask and with each question there are many procedures you may need to employ to address these questions. Your task at this

Can you think of any ethical reasons why you might continue treatment when you have no reason to expect improvement?

point is to begin learning what questions you need to ask and what information you need to obtain to answer these questions.

MODELS OF DIAGNOSIS

The diagnostic process has been characterized as a decision-making process aimed at developing an understanding of the communication impairment. You will find that clinicians will vary in their views about what they think is required to understand a problem and, as a result, they conduct the decision-making process in different ways. Often, a given orientation will be influenced by the educational background of the clinician, as well as the work setting in which the person is employed. We will consider three different orientations to diagnosis that exemplify contrasting ways in which communication disorders can be understood through the diagnostic process.

The Medical Model

All of us at one time or another go to a physician because we are not feeling well. The doctor will ask some questions and make some observations, such as looking in our throat. After making these observations, we may be told that we have a particular illness, such as strep throat, and as a result, we are given a prescription for an antibiotic. This transaction exemplifies a medical approach to diagnosis. This orientation emphasizes the classification of symptoms into a disease category that often has a particular cause. Thus, the objective in medical diagnosis is on classification and explanation. Once the diagnosis is made, a physician can then turn to knowledge about the disease to make decisions about its course and treatment outcomes. In this orientation, the physician is interested in the symptoms because they provide information about the type of the illness or disease which has a particular cause. It is assumed that the problems the patient presents can be tied to one or more disease categories. Also, it is often assumed that the disease is something that is internal to the patient and that its nature and cause can be determined by examining the patient. Finally, notice that within this approach the treatment is often predicated on knowing the disease type, and, when possible, the treatment is focused on the cause of the disease. You should understand that I am describing this medical approach to diagnosis in its classic form. Often a physician treats the symptoms with a tentative treatment regimen, not fully understanding what is causing the symptoms, but this usually occurs because a traditional diagnosis cannot be made.

If you are working in a medical setting, you will find that your fellow health practitioners will assume that you are using this model. In many instances, however, the problems we are dealing with in speech-language pathology may not fit well into this framework. Some of the types of communication problems will not be the product of a disease process. In such cases, we may need to consider an orientation to the diagnostic process where categorization of problems and identification of causes are not considered to be crucial to our diagnosis and decisions about treatment.

Behavioral Model

Many clients with communication disorders are not seen in a medical setting. Neither they, nor their families, view their problem as a sickness. The majority of clients who receive speech-language services are children or adolescents in school or preschool settings. The problems they have may be viewed as learning or developmental problems and, in many instances, we do not know why they are having these problems or, if we do know, there is little that can be done to resolve the cause. Because of the educational nature of the service setting and the developmental nature of the problems confronted in these settings, those working in educational settings tend to employ an orientation to assessment that is often referred to as a behavioral approach.

Within the behavioral approach, the primary interest is in characterizing the client's performance in tasks that are viewed as important for educational or social success. The focus of this approach is on describing the child's performance on relevant tasks, rather than on identifying certain behaviors that are suggestive of a particular disease. Because the causes of these problems are usually difficult to determine and even more difficult to change, this approach focuses on conditions that may lead to improved communication performance even if these factors were not involved in the cause of the problem. For instance, a clinician may decide that a 4-year-old child with a language problem will be helped if the parents spend more time reading bedtime stories, even though the clinician does not believe that the absence of bedtime stories contributed to the child's language problem. Thus, we see that the clinician using this approach is interested in finding ways to change the child's behavior, often by using educational or behavioral models to encourage change.

Systems Model

The two models we have considered so far assume that to learn about a problem we must look carefully at the client and learn about the person's behavior and possibly factors within the person that led to the communication problem. That is, we believe that the problem lies in or with the client. In contrast, some argue that an adequate account of a communication problem requires that we look at the family and cultural context within which the person lives. This view leads the clinician to include the parents, spouse, and/or teacher of the client in the diagnostic process to learn about the dynamics of the communication problem. A good example of this approach can be found in Chapter 10, which describes the assessment of children in school environments. As you will see, those using this approach often observe the client in a natural context. Accordingly, rather than performing the assessment in the clinician's office or examination room, the clinician will observe the client at home or in the classroom. Furthermore, the clinician will seek to learn which contexts and interactions seem to promote better communication and which seem to impede communication success. The communication problem, in this case, is seen as a mismatch between the client and the environment. As you can see this approach shares features of the behavioral approach in that it focuses on describing what the person does in natural settings. The systems approach places an equal emphasis on the environment and the client and assumes the problem lies in the mismatch or interaction between these, rather than with the client alone as is seen with the behavioral approach.

The three models presented are not the only approaches you will encounter in your career, but these three show us that as clinicians we adopt general philosophies about what we think is important in our attempt to understand the nature of a communication problem. It is difficult to argue that one of these models is better than the others. Each provides a different view of the problem and, in fact, if you are going to be a thoughtful clinician, you should be able to adopt all or part of each model, depending on the needs of particular clients. For instance, the acceptance of a behavioral orientation should not lead you to assume that you can simply ignore assessment questions that are associated more with the medical approach, such as etiology and prognosis. Likewise, the clinician using the medical model will sometimes deviate from the standard medical model and treat the symptoms in a way that is similar to the behavioral model. All clinicians should be able to move from one model to another and sometimes combine approaches. In this way our understanding of the communication disorder is enriched and, hopefully, we are provided with more insight into the problem.

METHODS FOR OBTAINING INFORMATION

It should be very clear by now that the assessment of communication disorders requires the clinician to obtain a variety of types of information and that this information gathering is conducted for a variety of purposes. The clinician has a wide range of methods of assessment from which to choose to obtain information. The most prominent of these assessment methods are discussed in following chapters and you will see that these methods usually fall into one of the following five categories.

Interviews

A very common diagnostic method is by some form of interview. The primary example is the clinical history (Chapter 3). In an interview the clinician usually poses questions to an informant. The questions are used to obtain information to help make some of the basic diagnostic decisions. The informant is often the client with a communication problem; however, it is also common for us to interview parents, spouses, teachers, or even employers. No doubt, the most common type of information obtained by means of interview has to do with the basic complaint. That is, early in the diagnostic process you need to hear why the client is coming to you. Along with this, you will probably obtain a basic description of the communication problem through an interview.

See Chapter 3 with respect to an in-depth discussion of interviewing.

Some interviews are unstructured in that the questions asked are generated by the clinician "on the spot" and are driven by the clinician's problem-solving goals. In other instances, the clinician may administer a structured interview by following a script, systematically gathering information regardless of the particular client and clinical situation. It is not at all uncommon for clinicians to develop their own structured interview tool, particularly to collect information on the history of the communication problem.

Written Questionnaires

The use of a written questionnaire is another method that is similar to the structured interview. There is a wide variety of questionnaires. Many are generated by clinicians for their own use; others are available from commercial sources. The items in these questionnaires may require that the informant respond to yes-no type questions and others may ask for open-ended responses that allow the client to provide input. The information obtained from questionnaires often covers background information about the client and the history of the client's problem, but the forms may also allow for information gathering about the client's feelings about the communication disorder and/or the communication settings that are most troubling to the client. The informant may also be someone other than the client. Through questionnaires, parents can provide developmental history, teachers can provide systematic information on children's school performance, and nurses and other care givers can provide insight into how a patient is communicating.

You can see that questionnaires are handy tools. They can provide you with useful information that may be difficult to obtain in other ways. Also, you can use them to obtain information efficiently and inexpensively because you don't need to be involved in the information collection. Efficiency is important because, as a professional clinician, your time has to be paid for by someone. As you consider your diagnostic procedures, you will have to consider the cost involved in obtaining the information you seek and try to find ways to reduce it.

Standardized Tests

The standardized test is one of the most common assessment tools used by clinicians. A standardized test is usually designed to measure a client's performance in one or more domains, such as phonological ability or sentence comprehension. Some tests are developed to measure some presumed individual trait such as intelligence. Usually the authors of such tests assume that the *trait* being measured is an enduring characteristic of the person similar to hair color. Traits of communication may include the client's ability to understand words and sentences or the client's word retrieval ability. These trait-oriented tests, therefore, test some hypothetical enduring property of the client.

In contrast to these trait-oriented tests, there are tests designed to characterize or describe a person's speech and language behavior, such as the rate of certain types of speech disfluencies. These tests are designed to tell the clinician if and how much the client does of something and, thus, provide information on the characteristics of the client's communicative performance. Usually no effort is made to use these measures as evidence of some underlying trait.

The important point to be understood here is that tests are designed for different purposes. The people who develop the tests should be very clear about a test's purposes and should provide you with evidence that the tests measure what they are purported to measure. Later we will see that this property of a test is called its validity. As a clinician, you must determine if the test will provide you with appropriate information to help you address the clinical problem confronting you.

I said earlier that there is a variety of types of tests. For a test to be considered a *standardized* test, it must be constructed to ensure that whatever is being measured is not influenced by the person administering and interpreting the test. That is, we want the measurement procedure to be uniform across examiners. Written directions must clearly outline what the examiner says and does during the testing, including "scripts" for the instructions to the client. Also, the stimuli used to elicit the client's behavior must be given and, finally, explicit rules for scoring the client's responses must be provided. By standardizing the method of a test, it should be possible to compare the results of one test administration with another. As I show you later, this allows us to compare a client's test performance with the same client's earlier performance, or with the performance of some normative group, or with some established standards for performance on a given test. Standardization allows us to assume that differences in performance are based on differences in the client's ability or trait status rather than differences in the test circumstances.

Some other examples of traits measured by tests are aptitude for music, or college performance.

The value of standardized tests as tools for the assessment of communication performance has been debated for many years. Often, clinicians believe that, by being so structured, standardized tests destroy the fundamental social-interactive quality of communication. Many of the tests available to us attempt to isolate and measure particular aspects of communication such as expressive grammatical ability, but in so doing strip away the pragmatic and semantic dimensions of language that naturally interact with the grammatic skill in which we are interested. As a result, the performance sampled by standardized tests of communication is usually less "natural." Better and more thoughtful test construction may solve some of these problems; nevertheless, we also must recognize that the price to be paid for replicable and objective measures is a restriction on some of the things that the clinician can measure. Standardized tests are likely to be valuable tools for you to use, but they need not be the only tools you use. As I have been saying throughout this chapter, your decision to use a standardized test should be dictated by the clinical problem you are trying to solve. In many instances the criticisms of standardized tests have more to do with the inappropriate use of tests than with the inadequacy of standardized testing per se.

In quantum physics, it has been found that the act of observing atomic particles changes their character. Likewise, it seems difficult to measure communication performance precisely without disrupting it in some way.

Observation

The standardized testing method of assessment attempts to measure a person's performance on explicitly defined tasks. The advantage of this assessment method is that, in theory, the measures are replicable. The disadvantage is that the things being measured are in an unnatural context and, therefore, we are often left wondering how the person performs in the "real world," or at least in settings that are like the real world. In some assessment situations, the clinician may want to change a task to see how the variation influences the client's performance—something you are not supposed to do within strict standardized testing situations.

To meet the needs for naturalness and flexibility, the clinician often turns to observation. The clinician may observe the characteristics of a person's voice, fluency, or language during a conversation. During such an activity the clinician may notice a relationship between his or her own speaking rate and the rate of disfluencies by the client. Having noted this, she or he could be in a position of manipulating her or his own rate systematically while continuing to track the client's disfluencies.

The observation of communication performance is certainly a vital and useful assessment method. However, for this method to be useful the clinician must know what to observe. To do this you need to have developed a general framework for describing the various dimensions of communication. You have already begun to do this by learning about the nature of normal and disordered communication. As you gain experience, you will refine this scheme. In other chapters you will also be given some protocols to provide you with schemes to observe systematically a variety of the client's characteristics, including such things as the client's oral mechanism and various aspects of his or her language, as well as properties of his or her voice and fluency.

Instrumented Observation

There are a number of aspects of speech and swallowing that are difficult to observe without the aid of instruments. For these circumstances, technological advances have provided the clinician with an ever-increasing array of tools to aid in observation and measurement of these physical systems. The acoustic properties of voice and speech can be obtained from a computer equipped to analyze acoustic data. Through the use of a fiber optic tube, clinicians can look directly at the vocal folds. Also, in association with a radiologist, the clinician can use x-ray images to observe the actions of the oral mechanism during swallowing. With such technology, the clinician can make very detailed observations and measurements. Whereas clinicians were denied such precision in the past, now you will be faced with having to determine which of the measures will be useful in your clinical problem solving. Otherwise, you will spend a great deal of your time and the client's time and money gathering information of limited use. As in all fields, as we obtain new technology we have to learn to use it appropriately.

BASIC CONCEPTS OF CLINICAL MEASUREMENT

So far we have talked about the various ways by which we can obtain diagnostic information, that is, the different measurement methods. You can see that there are a wide variety of tools available to you and you must learn to select the measurement methods that will be accurate and meaningful, because your clinical decisions depend on the data obtained from them. To make selections wisely, you will need to know how to interpret the accuracy and meaningfulness of a clinical measure. But before we discuss this, we need to talk briefly about the categories of measurement scales used, because the type of measurement scale will influence how we can describe the accuracy and meaningfulness of our measure.

Measurement Scales

Sometimes the measure you use allows you to represent your observation in terms of a category, or name, such as hoarseness and, therefore, a category measure can be represented as either being present or absent. This type of measurement scale is a *nominal scale*. At other times, the measure may be in the form of a scale having to do with more or less of something such as with a judgment of the severity of stuttering. With such a scale you might have possible values ranging from 1 to 7, in which a value of 4 would be viewed as greater than 2, but we may not be able to justify saying that a severity of 4 is twice as severe as a severity of 2. This form of measurement is termed *ordinal* because there is order or ranking information contained in the measure. Finally, we also have measures that employ numbers in their ordinary sense in that the numbers represent counts of the number or magnitude of something. For example, we may measure the rate a person can repeat a syllable over the span of 10 seconds. The person who produces 30 syllables is speaking twice as fast as the person who only produces 15 syllables. This type of measurement scale is usually referred to as a *ratio scale*. You can see that there are various ways in which the measures you make can be represented, ranging from a nominal system to one that involves true counting. Now we can turn to the ways in which we can describe the accuracy and meaningfulness of our measures.

> A nominal scale employs categories that have names as values. Thus, "stuttered" and "fluent" are nominal values in a scale of speech fluency.

Reliability

Regardless of the method of measurement you employ, there is always the likelihood of measurement error. One type of measurement error reflects variability between repeated administrations of a test or observation. Even when we use the same test and give the test under apparently identical circumstances, we will usually obtain somewhat different results. Maybe the difference is slight in absolute terms, but nevertheless is real. The property of a test or measure having to do with its replicability is termed *reliability* and it is important for a clinician to know something about the reliability of the measures obtained. If a test is not very reliable, the clinician needs to be cautious about interpreting the results.

The reliability of a measure can be influenced by several factors. Some portion of the variability can be a product of the behavior of the client. On one administration the examinee may have been more attentive or less fatigued than during another examination session. Also, measurement error can be introduced by the procedure by which the measurement is obtained. For instance, a clinician may be interested in the fundamental frequency of a speaker's voice and use electronic equipment to obtain this information. If a different microphone is used for separate sessions, there may be a slight variation in the fundamental frequency even though the speaker may have actually produced the same acoustic signal during both sessions.

Many of the factors that influence the reliability of a measure are random or at least not systematically associated with the measurement process. Sometimes error will cause a measure to be too small and at other times the error will cause the measure to be too large. This points to a way to improve the reliability of a measure. If you repeat the measure several times, the errors will tend to cancel each other out. As you can see, the more measures you take, the more stable (or less variable) your overall measure will be. Therefore, if you are interested in a child's grammatical ability and you measure this by means of the average number of words in the child's utterances, you will have a more reliable measure if you compute this measure of grammatical ability on 100 utterances than if you compute it on 50 utterances. Likewise, all other things being equal, longer tests are more reliable than shorter tests. It is also true that longer tests and repeated administrations of a measure take more time than shorter tests and single administrations. For the clinician, this often means balancing the need for greater reliability against the cost of conducting additional measures.

Ways of Describing Reliability

The reliability of a clinical measure is often provided to you by those who have developed the tool. Many of the clinical measures you will be using are commercial products that cost quite a bit of money. Part of the publisher's or manufacturer's justification for the price of the tool is the cost associated with determining its reliability. As an educated consumer, you need to require that the supplier and developer of a tool provide information concerning its reliability. You will need to be able to read the manual and understand and evaluate the information provided on reliability.

You will find that there are different types of reliability indices reported for particular instruments. Remember that earlier I talked about the fact that we could measure things with different measurement scales? Such information is used in describing reliability. The type of measurement scale employed influences the way the test developer reports reliability.

Often the reliability of our clinical measures is based on normal speakers. Do you think this creates a problem when we use the tools on speakers with communication disorders?

Agreement

If the instrument uses a nominal scale for measuring aspects such as the presence or absence of a moment of stuttering, then the reliability of the measure is in the form of a measure of agreement. Let's assume that a clinician reviews a videotape and tallies the occurrences of stuttering and then repeats this observation of this videotape again the next day. Table 1–1 displays the results of our hypothetical clinician. Notice that the clinician wasn't always consistent in these judgments. This inconsistency can be represented by rate of agreement. There are several ways that this agreement can be computed. The generally accepted method uses the formula in Figure 1–2. Using this method, our clinician achieved a 71% agreement. Since both sets of observations were performed by the same clinician, this is an *intrajudge* (within judge) *agreement* measure. If, in our

Table 1–1. Decisions made by a clinician regarding instances of stuttering during two different listening sessions of a videotape.

Listening Session	Word 1	Word 2	Word 3	Word 4	Word 5	Word 6	Word 7
1	Yes	No	No	Yes	No	Yes	No
2	Yes	Yes	No	Yes	No	No	No
	Agree	Disagree	Agree	Agree	Agree	Disagree	Agree

% Agreement = (Agreements/Agreements+Disagreements) × 100

Figure 1–2. Formula for computing percent agreement.

example, the second set of observations had been performed by another observer, this measure would have been a measure of *inter-judge* (between judge) *agreement*.

Stability

In many measurement situations the scale used will involve a test score or a physical measure, such as a person's fundamental frequency. Earlier, we described this type of scaling as a ratio scale. In this case the reliability measure should reflect the *stability* of the measure or score. Let's assume that we administered a vocabulary test to a group of children twice. This would allow us to determine the *test-retest* reliability of the measure. We could look at the stability of the scores by plotting each child's scores. Data like these are contained in Figure 1–3. Each child's score on the first administration is plotted on the horizontal axis and the second score is plotted on the vertical axis. Given perfect reliability, the scores should line up on the diagonal. You can see that they do not. The extent to which the scores deviate from the diagonal reflects the unreliability of the test. If you have had a basic course in statistics, you know that we can measure the correspondence between two such sets of measures by calculating a correlation coefficient. A common correlation coefficient used for this purpose is the Pearson Product Moment (r). In our example the test-retest reliability coefficient is .93. Some believe that a test should have a test-retest reliability coefficient of .90 or greater (Salvia & Yessldyke, 1991) for it to be used with confidence.

Internal Consistency

So far we have considered test-retest reliability. In many cases, a score will consist of several items combined to measure a trait such as vocabulary level. The test developer can obtain a measure of reli-

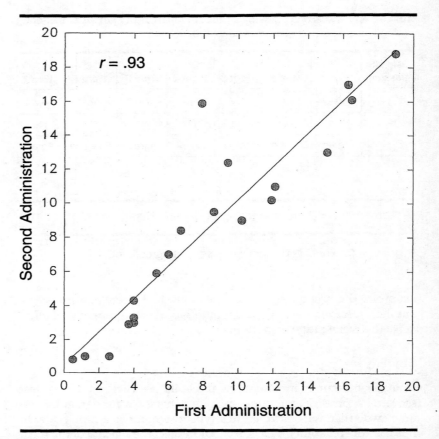

Figure 1–3. These data are hypothetical scores from two administrations of a test to the same individuals. Notice that the scores don't change much and thus the correlation (.93) shown by the straight line is high.

ability by comparing the scores obtained on one-half of the test, for instance the odd items, with those obtained on the other half, that is the even items. This type of reliability is called *split-half reliability* and reflects the internal consistency of the test in contrast with the test's stability reflected in the test-retest reliability.

Validity

The validity of a measure refers to how accurately the measurement tool measures the characteristic in which we are interested. Validity provides us with information about what the measurement means and, therefore, what conclusions can be made from the measure. In a sense then, validity is concerned with the truthfulness of the measure. For instance, there may be several ways to obtain a measure of a speaker's fundamental frequency. If these measures provide conflicting results, which, do you believe, is the most truthful index of fundamental frequency?

It shouldn't surprise you that a concept dealing with meaning and truth is not clear–cut. Although some people will make a blanket claim that a certain clinical measure is valid, in fact it is always necessary to specify the measurement purpose when discussing validity. A given measure can have strong validity for some purposes and poor validity for other purposes. The *Peabody Picture Vocabulary Test-R* (PPVT-R) originally was designed to be used as an intelligence measure. Over the years, psychologists have found that it is not a particularly good measure of intelligence, because it depends on only one skill. Hence, it is not regarded as a valid intelligence measure. In contrast the PPVT-R is viewed as a valid measure of receptive vocabulary. This demonstrates that, as a clinician, you are responsible for learning about the issues of validity associated with the measures you use.

To evaluate the validity of a new measure, we must have some external standard of truth. Then we can compare our new measure with this standard. There are three common types of external standards used by test developers to establish validity resulting, therefore, in three types of validity indices. The first type of validity is *concurrent validity*. To establish this type of validity a new or untested measure is compared with another measure that is widely regarded as accurately measuring the same property. The Stanford–Binet Intelligence Scale has served as a standard against which many newer intelligence tests have been validated and thus shown to have concurrent validity with the Stanford–Binet.

In other situations a test developer may want to show that the measure can be used to make predictions about a person's likely performance in some other place or time or maybe at another type of task. This type of validity is called *predictive validity*. A speech-language pathologist may develop a listening task that will predict how well a child will understand classroom instructions. This requires a predictive validity type of interpretation and, therefore, the measure needs to be compared with an acceptable measure of classroom comprehension to determine its predictive validity.

There is one other common form of validity. Often our measures have to do with some hypothetical trait or attribute that we believe underlies a person's performance. In our clinical practice we may use many hypothetical constructs such as short-term memory, anxiety, or linguistic competence. These are usually things about a person that can not be directly observed, and it is possible that the thing being measured may not actually exist. When we think we are measuring such a construct, our measurement instruments need to demonstrate *construct validity*. An example may help you get a sense of what construct validity involves. Let's assume that we want to develop a measure of English grammatical competence. First we need a theory about the nature of grammatical knowledge; there-

Validity is dependent on the reliability of a measure. Why do you think this is so?

fore, we need a grammatical theory. Next, based on our theory we will need to make some predictions about how people may differ with respect to this knowledge and who is likely to show these differences. For example, we may expect children to have a different knowledge than adults. Also, the theory needs to predict how this construct should be displayed within a person's grammatical performance. Therefore, we may expect to see evidence of grammatical knowledge in listening, speaking, and maybe judgments about the grammaticality of sentences. With this theory in mind we must develop tasks that will measure this construct in the most straightforward manner in order that differences in people's performance is likely to be due to their differences in grammatical knowledge and not other extraneous factors. Finally, research will be needed to show that our test of grammar does appear to be consistent with the predictions of the theory and that persons who are likely to have differences in grammatical knowledge do indeed differ on our test. Moreover, we would expect that their performance on our test correlates well with other indices of their grammatical knowledge.

As you can see, construct validity is most difficult to achieve. First, it requires that your measurements be based upon a theory. Then the test must be developed in a way that is consistent with the theory. Finally, there must be considerable supporting research demonstrating that the test does conform to the predictions of the theory. Because of the complexity of this process, the construct validity of a test may gradually be documented over time.

Diagnostic Accuracy

Our attention so far has been directed toward the measurement tools we use in the assessment process. These clinical tools that provide us with measures of speech, language, or swallowing do not make decisions; that is what the clinician does. In order to do this, recall that the clinician must bring a set of interpretive standards to bear on the information gathered in making decisions. The measures used by the clinician might be highly reliable and very valid, but if the standards used to interpret these measures are poor, the clinical decision will be poor. Therefore, not only is it possible for us to evaluate the accuracy of the measurement process, it is also possible to evaluate the accuracy of the whole diagnostic process involving both the instruments and the diagnostic standards used by a clinician to arrive at a final decision.

The notion of diagnostic accuracy is very similar to that of measurement validity, in that it deals with the correctness of the clinical decision. Just as we needed some standard of truth for establishing validity, we also need one for diagnostic accuracy. This standard is referred to as the "gold standard" because, whatever it is, it is assumed to be the truth against which clinical decisions are measured. In medicine, a gold standard can often be a laboratory test or an autopsy performed by a pathologist. The results of such extensive examinations are then compared with the clinical diagnosis made by a physician. We must realize that gold standards often are not perfect, but rather represent the best that can be done at a given time.

Once a gold standard has been established, we can compare clinical decisions with it to judge how accurate these decisions are. Let's assume we screen by observation for hoarseness in a group of children and then perform a more in–depth examination that determines their true hoarseness status. The results of such a hypothetical clinical study are displayed in Figure 1–4. We can see that the screening decisions did not always agree with the gold standard of the in–depth study. Of those children who were thought to be hoarse from the initial screening, 20 (25%) turned out to have normal voices, meaning the screening decision had a false positive rate of 25%. Also, there were 9 children (3%) who were thought to have normal voices but were found to be hoarse. Accordingly, the screening test had a *false negative rate* of 3%.

The terms "positive" and "negative" are a little confusing here. A positive decision is one that says the person has the clinical condition, thus positive usually means bad because it indicates a clinical condition. A negative decision, on the other hand, is construed to be good, because it represents an absence of the clinical condition. Clinicians want to have low false positive and false negative rates. No one likes making mistakes, but how can you reduce your mistakes? One way you can lower both of these error rates is by using better measurement tools. But if you can't change your measurement instruments, the only thing you can change is the diagnostic standard you are using.

In the voice diagnosis example we have been talking about, you might believe that you are diagnosing too many children with normal voices as having hoarse voices. In such a case, you will want to reduce your false positive rate. The way you can do this is by becom-

When making clinical decisions we have to decide what kind of error is the worst to make—saying someone is okay when they are not, or saying they have a problem when they don't have one.

		Gold Standard Diagnosis			
		Hoarse	Normal	Total Diagnosed	Error Rate
Clinical Diagnosis	Hoarse	60	20	80	False Positive 20/89=.25
	Normal	9	291	300	False Negative 9/300=.03

Figure 1–4. Diagnostic accuracy of hoarseness.

ing more reluctant to say a child has a hoarse voice. As a result, some of those cases that were marginal, but considered to be hoarse during the earlier screening example, now will be judged as normal. Unfortunately, this change in your standard will probably also have an impact on your false negative rate and it won't be a good change. By becoming more stringent in your determination of hoarseness, you will have a greater tendency to say a child has a normal voice and therefore you will increase your false negative rate—saying a child is normal when actually the child is hoarse. That is, when you change your diagnostic standard to reduce one type of error, you will usually increase the other type of error.

The major point is that the accuracy of our clinical decisions can be evaluated. By studying our decisions we can begin to learn where errors are coming from and we can discover ways to reduce errors. Remember, the way to become better clinicians is by making better, more accurate decisions. As our measures improve and our standards for making decisions improve, our clinical effectiveness will improve.

APPROACHES TO MEASUREMENT INTERPRETATION

So far, what we have talked about are rather abstract ideas impacting the quality of our clinical measures. How do clinicians actually interpret the data they obtain from their clinical observations to arrive at conclusions about the performance of their clients?

The specific approaches and standards used to make diagnostic decisions will be detailed in the other chapters. You will find that most of the approaches for interpretation of clinical information can be placed within three general categories: (1) norm-referenced interpretations, (2) criterion-referenced interpretations, and (3) client-referenced interpretations.

Norm-referenced Interpretation

One common way that we can interpret measures we obtain is by comparing the client's performance to some other group of individuals, sometimes called the normative group. Often the normative group is a representative sample of individuals who are of the same age and possibly same sex as the client. There are two ways we can compare a client's performance to a normative group—standard scores and equivalent scores.

Standard Scores

For norm-referenced measures, the standard score approach evaluates the client's placement within the normative group. To understand

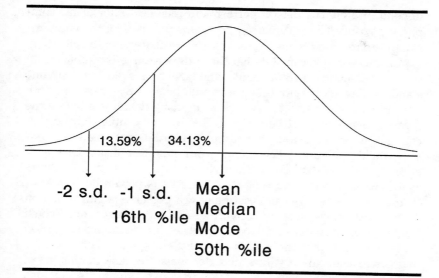

13.59%   34.13%

-2 s.d. -1 s.d.   Mean
        16th %ile Median
                   Mode
                   50th %ile

Figure 1–5. The normal curve and the terms used to identify the location of a score on this curve.

this, we need to review some basic characteristics of the *normal distribution*. Figure 1–5 depicts such a distribution. This distribution is no doubt familiar to you. Along the horizonal axis we can have a range of scores or values of a measure. On the vertical axis is the number of people receiving a particular score. You can see that there is a concentration of people toward the middle and then a rapid decrease in the number of individuals as you move away from the middle of the distribution in either direction. If we divide the group up into the upper half of the distribution and the lower half, the dividing line represents the *median* score for the group. This would also be the 50th percentile. We can also compute the average score for the group. This *mean* value will also be near the center of the distribution and, for truly normally distributed data, the median and the mean will be the same. The extent to which scores deviate away from the mean is represented by the standard deviation. For scores with a normal distribution, 34.13% of the scores will fall within 1 *standard deviation* above the mean and 34.13% will fall within 1 standard deviation below the mean. These statistical descriptors for characterizing the middle of the distribution and then the location of a score's distance from the middle of the distribution allow us to describe where our client stands in this distribution, using scales based on the normal distribution.

A very common scale based on the normal distribution is the percentile scale. Percentile should not be confused with the percentage correct on a test. Your client could get 65% of the items correct on a test and yet be at the 10th percentile. The client's percentile score will depend on how the person performs in relation to her or his comparison group. The 10th percentile means that 90% of the comparison group received higher values on the measure than the client.

You can see in Figure 1–5 that the 50th percentile is equivalent to the median and the mean. People who have scores placing them one standard deviation below the mean will be slightly below the 16th percentile. If the person's score is 2 standard deviations below the mean, the person will be close to the 2nd percentile. Notice that changes in percentile and changes in standard deviation are not consistent with each other. The change from the mean (0 standard deviations) to −1 standard deviation involves 34 percentile points whereas the change from −1 to −2 only represents 14 percentile points.

You can see that we can describe how a person has performed on a norm–referenced test by converting the actual test score, which might be the number of correct responses, into standard deviation units. Standard deviation units are a little awkward because they may involve negative values and decimals. Because of this, most norm-referenced measures allow you to convert the test score, also called the raw score, into a *standard score* that does not have a negative number or decimals. The intelligence quotient (IQ) is an example of a standard score. When a test is developed, a number is established that will represent the mean. In the case of IQ, the number representing the mean is 100. Also, a value is given to represent the standard deviation for the standard scores, which in the case of most IQ tests is 15. The test publisher will usually provide you with tables that allow you to convert the raw score into standard score units. Further, there are likely to be different tables for different age groups and, therefore, you can select the group that best matches your client. Once you know what the standard score equivalent is for your client's raw score, you can use your knowledge about what the mean and standard deviation is for this standard score in order to determine where on the normal distribution the client's score will fall.

Another standard score system is used with the SAT and GREs. For these tests, the mean is 500 and the standard deviation is 100.

Equivalent Scores

So far we have been talking about interpreting measures by comparing an individual to a group by describing where a person falls in the normal distribution of the group. It is also possible to interpret the score by identifying the group of individuals that are most likely to achieve a given score. Let's assume that a client obtains a score of 25 on a vocabulary test. Because children's vocabulary improves with age, we could then ask what age group is most likely to obtain this score. Our client may be 4 years old, but we may find that the obtained score is typical of 3-year-old children. Equivalent scores usually represent the group that has a median score equal to a given raw score. Therefore, we might put in a diagnostic report that the child's vocabulary age is 3 years, meaning that our 4-year-old is like the median 3-year-old with respect to vocabulary. This is an example of an age–equivalent score, but you will also find grade-equivalent scores. Parents find age- and grade-equivalent scores easy to understand and, because of this, many clinicians employ equivalence scoring. We have to be cautious about how we interpret the equivalent scores, however. With these scores, we have no idea whether differences in equivalent scores are unusual or common in the general population, and often uncommonly low performance is taken as a sign of a problem. For instance, returning to our example, although we know our 4-year-old obtained a vocabulary score similar to the typical 3-year-old, we don't know how unusual this is. It may turn out that our vocabulary score of 25 places the child at the 40th percentile for 4-year-olds and, therefore, this score is not particularly discrepant for all 4-year-olds. On the other hand, this score could place the child at -2 standard deviations and therefore be unusual for a 4-year-old. It is because of this problem with equivalent scores that clinicians are being discouraged from using them.

Criterion-referenced Interpretation

Norm-referenced interpretation of measurement information makes the measurement interpretation meaningful by comparing the client's performance with some group of other individuals. There are some decisions, nevertheless, that do not call for this type of interpretation. For instance, you may be working with a patient who has a swallowing disorder that results in the aspiration of material into the lungs during swallowing. It is not important how this person's swallowing behavior compares with a group of adults. Instead, you are interested in whether there is significant aspiration. In such a case you need a standard defining unacceptable aspiration which may be based on data about the likelihood of respiratory complications. Clinical standards such as these are sometimes referred to as criterion-referenced standards. That is, there is some level of performance that can be viewed as minimal for it to be acceptable. What is acceptable may be determined by a group of experts; or, as in the case of our swallowing problem, there may be evidence that undesirable outcomes become common below or above some level of performance. You should be able to see that criterion-referenced interpretation often involves a qualitative evaluation of the performance having to do with "good–bad" or at least "acceptable–unacceptable," whereas, a norm-referenced interpretation brings with it more of a quantitative meaning having to do with "common–uncommon," "typical–unusual" or "high–average–low." The two can be combined in some instances since "unusual" or "low" levels of performance may often also be associated with unacceptable or undesirable outcomes.

Client-referenced Interpretation

So far we have talked about ways of interpreting a client's performance by comparing the measures we have obtained with similar measures obtained on another group of individuals or against some criterion-based standard of performance. There are times that neither of these two approaches serve the decisions we need to make. Instead, we may be more interested in comparing a client's performance in one area of communication at two or more points in time, or with some other area of communication performance. In fact this type of comparison may be the most common form of clinical interpretation. We frequently do this as we track the client's progress in therapy by comparing levels of performance at different points in time. In many settings it is necessary to be able to document that in association with clinical intervention there is improvement and this requires that we obtain repeated measures of the same or very similar behavior from the client across the treatment period.

Sometimes the questions we are addressing call for comparing the client's results on two or more different tasks or different types of behavior. When evaluating a person with an aphasia, clinicians will often compare the client's ability to understand with her or his ability to express words and sentences. Thus, a profile may be formed with some areas showing deficits and other areas showing little impairment. Client-referenced interpretations that involve either the same type of measures at different times or different types of measures obtained during the same examining session will be covered in other chapters.

SUMMARY

In this chapter you have been introduced to the process of diagnosis. We have seen that it is a problem-solving task requiring the clinician to set up the problem, gather data, interpret the data, and arrive at conclusions. The objective of the diagnostic process is to develop an understanding of the multiple dimensions of a client's problem. In so doing, the clinician employs a wide range of skills and knowledge having to do with ways of evaluating measurement methods, as well as the interpretation of the information obtained from these methods. Thus, although the diagnostic process does involve actions that we have described as measurement, these actions all must serve the specific problem-solving purposes you require to best help your client.

REFERENCES

Travis, L. E. (1931). *Speech pathology*. New York: Appleton-Century Co.

Van Riper, C. (1963). *Speech correction*. Englewood Cliffs, NJ: Prentice-Hall.

Salvia, J., & Yessldyke, J. (1991). *Assessment*. Boston: Houghton Mifflin Co.

RECOMMENDED READINGS

Bellack, A., & Hersen, M. (Eds.). (1988). *Behavioral assessment: A practical handbook*. Boston: Allyn & Bacon.

McCauley, R. J., & Swisher, L. (1984). Use and misuse of norm-referenced tests in clinical assessment: A hypothetical case. *The Journal of Speech and Hearing Disorders, 49*, 338–348.

Nunnally, J. (1972). *Educational measurement and evaluation*. New York: McGraw-Hill.

Multicultural Issues in Speech and Language Assessment

Carol E. Westby, Ph.D.

A man's home is his castle. (English)
Mi casa, su casa. (Spanish)

The squeaky wheel gets the grease. (American)
The duck that quacks loudest gets shot. (Chinese)

Take care of Number One. (American)
The group always comes first. (many traditional cultures)

Appropriate assessment and treatment of culturally/linguistically diverse clients require an understanding of their culture. What does it mean to understand a culture? Numerous misconceptions of culture exist. It is often equated with art, music, food, and holiday celebrations, or with the language one speaks. Such a view of culture results in the belief that understanding another culture can be accomplished simply by participating in its celebrations and learning the language.

Describe your family's culture. How does your family's culture differ from the family culture of some of your friends?

But culture involves more than the things people make and use. It also includes how people interact with one another and their beliefs and values. The statements at the beginning of this chapter represent contrasting values that affect persons' interactions.

Being bilingual is often equated with being bicultural, but a bilingual person is not necessarily bicultural. If we do not recognize a person's values, beliefs, and patterns of interaction, being bilingual will not insure effective communication. In fact, some of our most serious miscommunications may occur when we are speaking the same language.

Gary Larson, author of the *Far Side* cartoons, mistakenly assumed that being bilingual results in effective communication. In one cartoon he depicts a man attempting to talk with a duck. The man tries, "Sprechen sie Deutsch?" and gets no response. Next he tries, "Habla español?" and still he receives no response. He then tries, "Parlez vous français?" The duck continues to stare at him. Finally the man looks at the duck and says, "Quack?" The duck responds with "Quack!" and the man and the duck continue their conversation. The caption reads "It's nice to have someone who understands me."

Now, I had a pet duck, Mocha, and I learned that speaking quack was not sufficient for effective communication with a duck. I speak quack. I knew that a loud, prolonged "muck muck muck" meant, "You've left me outside, and I want in." I knew that a soft, short, quick series of "muck, muck, muck" meant, "I've just seen a big, black New Mexican cockroach"—which are the chocolate chips of the duck world. Despite being bilingual in English and Quack, I was not able to avoid miscommunication problems with Mocha.

We bought Mocha shortly after he hatched from his egg at the feed store. He quickly imprinted on my husband and for several months followed him everywhere. Eventually, he began to show an interest in me. He would nibble at my ankles and stretch and bob his neck. Because he looked uncomfortable as he did this, I thought that he had a sore throat or something in his throat. I took him to the vet. It cost me $15 to learn that this duck was a drake, he was going through his second imprinting, and his head bobbing meant he was propositioning me to be his mate.

You can see that an adequate evaluation of Mocha's behavior required an understanding of duck culture. I cannot assume that what I know to be true of humans is true for ducks. Otherwise, I might have treated Mocha's normal behaviors as pathological and sought unnecessary and inappropriate treatment.

THE NEED FOR UNDERSTANDING CULTURAL/LINGUISTIC DIVERSITY

I do not believe that Mocha suffered from my lack of knowledge of duck culture. Inadequate understanding of human cultural/linguistic diversity can, however, harm persons. Culturally/linguistically different clients have frequently been inappropriately placed in special

Not counting Native American languages, school distri · · in the United States have identified more than 100 languages from more than 120 countries.

Can you think of a situation in which you experienced a major miscommunication with someone with whom you were speaking even though the two of you were speaking the same language?

education classes; treatment approaches have been used that violate client values and beliefs; and true speech, language, and hearing problems have sometimes not been identified.

Changing Population Demographics

Changing demographics are resulting in significant changes in the types of clients being served by speech-language pathologists and audiologists. According to the 1990 U.S. Census, which admittedly undercounted people of color, the so-called minority population of the United States exceeds 60 million. One American in four already defines himself or herself as Hispanic, African American, Asian American, Pacific Islander, or Native American. Before 1965, the majority of immigrants to the United States came from Europe. Since that time, however, the majority of immigrants have been from diverse cultures in Asia and Latin America. By 2007, Hispanics will become the largest minority group. Although the total number of Asians is smaller than Hispanics and African Americans, Asians are the most rapidly growing minority group. Several states already have a third or more of their populations from nondominant cultural groups and many large cities are more than 50% minority. By 2010, one third of the American people will be people of color and by 2056, White Americans will be a minority group.

Between 1980 and 1990 there was a nearly 40% increase in the numbers of persons whose home language was not English. Speakers of Asian languages increased between 109% to 165%; Spanish speakers increased by 56%. In 1990, limited-English proficient students included 24.4% of students in kindergarten to Grade 3, 16.3% in Grades 4 through 8, and 12.9% in Grades 9 through 12. The implication is that whether you identify yourself with the Euro-American culture or with a so-called minority culture, many of your clients will come from a culture different from your own. Traditionally, there were few minorities in the Midwest, but this is changing as Hispanics and Asians have found jobs in rural communities. For example, now more than half the population of Garden City, Kansas, is Hispanic or Asian. The American Speech-Language-Hearing Association estimates that 10% of the U.S. population has a disorder of speech, hearing, or language. If the prevalence of communication disorders among minority groups is consistent with that for the general population, it is estimated that 6.2 million culturally/linguistically diverse Americans have communication disorders in this country (Battle, 1998).

This chapter is intended to familiarize you with the issues and considerations you will encounter in assessing speech and language abilities of individuals from culturally/linguistically diverse backgrounds. The discussion in Chapter 6 (Weiss, Tomblin, and Robin) is specifically relevant since a major issue in thinking about multicultural diversity and communication disorders is that of English as a second language. Specifically, I focus here on the reasons

It is estimated that in certain categories of special education individuals from culturally/linguistically different populations are overrepresented by as much as 60–80%.

Presently, less than 5% of members of the American Speech-Language-Hearing Association are from Asian, Hispanic, African American, or Native American backgrounds.

why it is so very difficult to conduct valid and reliable speech and language assessments of such clients and some ideas for dealing with those difficulties.

Speech–Language–Hearing Disorders in Diverse Ethnic/Racial Groups

While persons from nonmainstream American backgrounds generally have the same types of communication disorders as those in the dominant culture, the frequency and causes of particular conditions may vary. Native American populations have a higher incidence of otitis media, or middle ear infections, than other racial/ethnic groups (Downs, 1985). These infections occur earlier and are more frequent. Otitis media is associated with mild, intermittent hearing loss, and, in some circumstances, may result in delayed speech and language skills. White adults are more likely to experience significant hearing loss associated with aging than are Black adults (Post, 1964). Native American and Asian populations exhibit a higher incidence of oral facial anomalies such as cleft lip and palate (Vanderas, 1987). There are distinct differences in frequency of occurrence of cleft lip and palate among skin color groups, with clefts less frequent in darkly pigmented skin colors and more frequent in lightly pigmented skin colors (McWilliams, Morris, & Shelton, 1990). African American populations are at greater risk for high blood pressure, which increases their risk for strokes that can affect their speech and language (Spector, 1985). Persons of African and Mediterranean descent are more likely than other populations to carry a gene for sickle cell anemia. This genetic condition causes the red blood cells to be abnormally curved. These deformed cells tend to clump together, blocking blood vessels, and causing strokes. Strokes can occur in all parts of the body, including the blood vessels in the inner ear and brain, thus causing hearing loss and speech, language, and cognitive disabilities (Scott, 1985).

Lead poisoning is also known to cause decreased cognitive abilities and associated speech and language delays. Individuals from low socioeconomic urban environments are at greater risk for lead poisoning than middle class individuals from suburban or rural areas because of lead-based paints in old buildings or exposure to lead fumes from vehicle exhaust or factories. Even when socioeconomic levels and environment are held constant, persons of color appear to have a higher incidence of lead poisoning than White persons (Mayfield, 1985).

Cultural Attitudes Toward Disabilities

What people do about speech, language, and hearing disorders is related to their beliefs about what is a disability. Professionals from mainstream American culture generally regard hearing loss and

Knowledge about ethnic/ racial differences in prevalence of communication disorders is critical in counseling families about possible causes of communication disorders and risk of communication disorders in other family members.

speech-language delays and disorders as potential and significant disabilities. Consequently, they are likely to recommend medical treatment for otitis media, hearing aids for sensorineural hearing loss, and therapy for speech-language delays and disorders. In taciturn cultures and cultures where children are to be seen and not heard, families may not recognize the hearing or speech-language disorders that concern mainstream professionals. Mainstream culture places a high value on communication skills. Adults encourage children to ask and answer questions and to tell stories. Once a child walks, parents focus on a child's talking. If a mainstream child is not talking by age 18 months or 2 years, parents express concern. In contrast, many nonmainstream cultures do not place a high value on verbal children. Crago (1988), in a study of Inuit children, reports being intrigued with a young Inuit child who was more verbal than other children. She viewed the child as highly capable. When she questioned adults about this child, however, she gained a different perspective. They reported that they too were concerned about the child—because he didn't know when to keep quiet!

In order to understand peoples' responses to communicative disorders, you must understand what they value. Table 2–1 summarizes the dimensions of cultural value-orientation systems (Sue & Sue, 1990). Cultures differ in how they perceive time; some emphasize history and tradition, some the here and now, and some the distant future. Cultures also differ in their attitudes toward activity. Some value active doing, others simply value a person's existence, while others focus on being-in-becoming in which one develops one's inner self. Most of the world's cultures differ along a dimension of individualism to collectivism. In individualistic cultures, "I" is most important; in collectivistic cultures (both lineal/hierarchical and collateral/equal) the group is most important. Cultures also have differing views of their relationship to nature, from being masters of nature, to living in harmony with nature, to being subjugated by nature.

Persons in the mainstream American culture tend to look toward the future. They focus on being active and demonstrating their accomplishments. Who they are and what they are worth are dependent upon what they do. Children are socialized to be independent. They are rewarded for accomplishments they achieve on their own. People are viewed as having power over nature. As adults, persons are responsible for mastering circumstances that arise. With this value system, mainstream families tend to think about the significance of a disability for the future. They may ask, "When will she learn to talk?" "Will therapy correct the problem?" or "When can he return to his teaching position?" They express concern regarding what persons cannot do, what they will be able to do, and when they will be able to do it. Parents, spouses, or clients take responsibility for alleviating the disability. Persons with these mainstream values seek treatment for speech-language-hearing disabilities and are coparticipants in their therapy.

Think about your family. What are their value orientations with respect to time, human activity, social relations, and relationship with nature?

Table 2–1. Value orientation model.

Dimensions	Value Orientation		
1. *Time focus* What is the temporary focus of human life?	*Past* The past is important. Learn from history.	*Present* The present moment is everything. Don't worry about tomorrow.	*Future* Plan for the future. Sacrifice today for a better tomorrow.
2. *Human Activity* What is the modality of human activity?	*Being* It's enough just to be.	*Being and In-Becoming* Our purpose in life is to develop our inner self.	*Doing* Be active. Work hard and your efforts will be rewarded.
3. *Social Relations* How are human relationships defined?	*Lineal* Relationships are vertical. There are leaders and followers in this world.	*Collateral* We should consult with friends/families when problems arise.	*Individualistic* Individual autonomy is important. We control our own destiny.
4. *People/Nature Relationship* What is the relationship of people to nature?	*Subjugation to Nature* Life is largely determined by eternal forces (God, fate, genetics, etc.).	*Harmony with Nature* People and nature co-exist in harmony.	*Mastery over Nature* Our challenge is to conquer and control nature.

Source: From Sue, D. W., & Sue, D. (1990). *Counseling the culturally different: Theory and practice*, p. 139. New York: John Wiley, reprinted with permission.

In nonmainstream families, adults are primary caregivers for young children and older siblings are primary socializers who may be candidates for training to carry out therapeutic activities with a younger brother or sister.

Many nonmainstream American cultures focus on the present and value the past. Persons are valued simply for their existence or being, not for what they can do. Persons are interdependent, not independent. Families may consist not only of children and parents, but also of grandparents, aunts, uncles, cousins, and even nonrelated friends. People believe that they cannot affect nature and what happens to them; they may attempt to live in harmony with events in the world as it is or they may believe there is nothing they can do about their circumstances. In these nonmainstream cultures, people generally have a greater tolerance for variation; they may feel less need to "fix things" and focus instead on learning how to accept and cope with their circumstances. Families may recognize that a family member is different, but accept that difference as being who the person is. As an Hispanic mother said when enrolling her non-speaking child in kindergarten, "Luis is my quiet one." She was aware that Luis did not talk much, but she accepted his quietness as just being Luis. Because of such outlooks, persons from cultures with nonmainstream values may be less likely to seek out evaluation and treatment services. When they do become involved, it is important to include the extended family in decisions.

Even when a speech, language, or hearing problem is recognized, nonmainstream families may not approach treatment in the expected way. Mainstream professionals generally believe that a physician or certified therapist should be immediately consulted to perform necessary surgery or treatment when a handicapping condition is diagnosed. In contrast, Native American families may need to consult a medicine man before having their child treated for otitis media. Asians may consult an herbalist. Hispanics may employ the services of a "curandero" (healer) before or while they are receiving mainstream therapies.

NO SUCH THING AS CULTURE-FREE TESTING

When you work with nonmainstream American cultures you may need to spend time laying the groundwork for referral for evaluation and intervention services. Evaluation may involve testing with standardized tests that have norms as well as activities presented in a standardized manner but for which there are no norms (such as narrative language sampling). Evaluation may also involve observation in a naturalistic environment in which the client performs familiar activities in a familiar setting. Or the client may be tested on a task, then taught the task, then tested again (How quickly does she or he learn?).

The issue of "testing" is a complicated matter. Traditional evaluation often emphasizes administration of standardized, normed tests and testlike activities. Professionals who evaluate bilingual and culturally different clients frequently ask me, "What tests should I use?" Or they tell me, "As long as I test in the client's dominant language or use nonverbal tests, the client's language background is not an issue." Such questions and statements reflect the fallacious assumption that there are valid tests for culturally different persons. You need to understand why there are no valid tests for culturally/linguistically diverse populations.

Because the act of testing is itself culturally biased, testing in the native language or using nonverbal tests are not adequate solutions to the problems of assessing culturally different or limited-English-proficient individuals. Testing involves the presentation of tasks out of a usual context and structured interactions with an adult (the clinician) that are unfamiliar to persons from many cultures. As a consequence, there can be no valid tests for culturally different clients regardless of the content and language of the tests. To understand the issues in assessing culturally different clients, you must understand how the behavioral interactions and language requirements of the testing culture differ from the culture of the clients being assessed.

Persons raised in societies with many rectangular objects (e.g., square houses) are more likely than persons raised in societies without rectangular objects (e.g., round or octagonal houses) to perceive the top horizontal segment line as shorter than the bottom horizontal segment line even though they are equal in length.

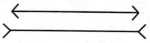

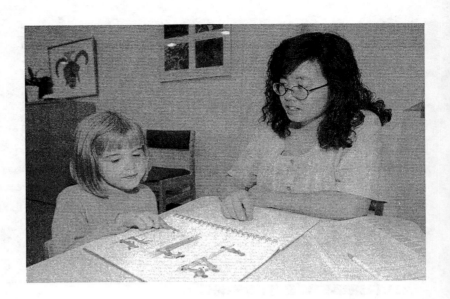

Nonverbal Aspects of the Testing Culture

Perception and Use of Time

In mainstream society, time is monochronic where things are accomplished one-at-a-time in a linear fashion. In many nonmainstream societies, time is polychronic where many activities take place simultaneously and schedules are invisible.

In the testing culture, we are apt to view testing as a time-bound activity (Tuesday, September 2, 10:00–12:00). Subtests within the assessment are also time-bound. One activity is completed before moving on to the next. There is no going back, even if the client later realizes the answer to an earlier question. Time is part of what's being tested: the faster the better. To appear intelligent, clients must perform quickly within the given time limits. Native American, Latin, and Middle Eastern cultures are less bound to this view of time. In these cultures, activities are done "when the time is right" and need not be started and completed within a specified time frame. Culturally different persons may not respond to efforts to have them complete a task as quickly as possible, either because they do not view speed as critical, or because they have not previously had to manage time in the way demanded by testing.

Learning and Displaying Learning

Beliefs about how learning occurs vary in different cultures. In mainstream American culture, adults assume that for learning to occur children must be explicitly taught with words. In many African American, Hispanic, and Native American cultures learning more often occurs by observing others. Children are encouraged by adults to "watch me." Adults may seldom give verbal explanations. Children watch until they can do the task. They may watch for many months or years before they are expected to do the task, and they may not attempt the task until they are certain they have mastered it. Children from nonmainstream cultures may expect you to show them how to do the tasks, and few standardized tests permit this. Clients who are used to having tasks demonstrated for them may lack strategies for trial and error learning. They may be hesitant to attempt unfamiliar tasks of the type that you present in testing situations, even if they understand the words of the language and the instructions of the test.

Group Versus Individual Orientation

Mainstream American culture values and encourages individual achievement. From infancy, children are encouraged to display their abilities and the child who displays the best skills is publicly rewarded. In contrast, in a number of cultures, a high value is placed on being part of the group and not appearing better than others in the group. In these cultures, showing how well one can do, as required by tests, is socially inappropriate, and persons may be hesitant to perform if they feel their performance will separate them from their peers. Also in such cultures, children may not be expected to perform a new, unfamiliar task alone. Children expect assistance from peers and readily give assistance to peers.

Verbal Aspects of the Testing Culture

Language differences complicate any testing—and the differences involve not only the dialect or language that is spoken but also the functions of language, the content of the language, and the way the language is organized for the various functions and content in the test situation.

Language Function

Testing often involves questioning. Cultures vary in terms of who asks questions, the types of questions that are asked, and the reasons they are asked. In all cultures people generally ask genuine questions when they need information. Adults from mainstream American culture, however, also engage in much pseudoquestioning (asking questions to which they know the answers). They do this from the time children begin to talk. They ask "What's this?" while looking at a picture book. Mainstream children know that the adults asking the questions know the answers and they recognize these pseudoquestions as requests to perform.

Some cultural groups rarely ask pseudoquestions. Native American children are unlikely to answer a question if they think the adult should know the answer. To do so would be insulting because it would suggest that the adult does not know. Heath (1982) noted that members of a Black community in the Carolina Piedmont

---

Verbal approaches to learning tend to result in field-independent learners who are good at perceiving discrete parts and abstract analytical thought. Watching approaches to learning tend to result in field-dependent learners who are good at global perception and sensitive to the social environment.

How could you encourage and reinforce good performance in children from a group-oriented culture?

Asking "What's that?" may get children to label, while asking them "What's that like?" may get them to give an analogy.

seldom asked pseudoquestions. When pseudoquestions were asked, they were usually asked by an adult following some transgression by the child, for example, "Who ate the last piece of cake?" A pseudoquestion signaled to children that they were in trouble. They could leave the scene quickly, they could produce a highly creative response/excuse that might distract the adult from punishing them for the transgression, or they could claim no responsibility for the act. At a workshop I conducted in Mississippi, a psychologist commented that she frequently received the responses, "I didn't do it!" or "Not me!" when she asked the question, "Who discovered America?" on the Wechsler Intelligence Scale—Revised. These students believed they were being accused of a bad deed.

Questioning is inherent in the testing process. If clients are not familiar with the ways questions are used in testing, any test you give will be culturally biased regardless of the language you use and the specific content of the items.

Language Content—Where Is the Meaning?

In everyday conversation, speakers and listeners rely heavily on the context to communicate the meaning of the message. Much testing, however, presents tasks without any context. Persons are expected to follow instructions in which there are no contextual cues as to the appropriate response ("Touch the blue square to the yellow circle after you pick up the red circle."). They are expected to be able to reason from the words, even if they are unfamiliar with the content. Clients who expect to look to the context for meaning and not the words alone will not perform well on decontextualized test items. Many will attempt to make sense of the items by personalizing them or searching the environment for cues. This results in responses such as "I got one at home," or "Where is it?" when you ask them to define words such as coat or bird; or in responses based on their own experiences that are judged as associative or illogical.

Language Organization Structure

Asymmetrical communication is organized differently in different cultures. Mainstream English speakers use a sequential linear organization. Spanish speakers use frequent topic–associated digressions. A Navajo educator has suggested that Navajo thought is like frybread—"An idea bubbles up here, and another idea bubbles up over there."

Conversational discourse is symmetrical. Anyone can talk at any time and participants can assist one another in carrying on the conversation by helping each other find necessary words and clarify ideas. Testing involves asymmetrical communicative interaction; one person asks and the other answers. Asymmetrical communications require more language organizational skills because speakers are responsible for organizing the entire discourse in a manner that will be understandable to the listeners, and because they cannot rely on assistance from the listeners. Speakers must constantly remember the topic and make certain that each statement is related to the topic and to preceding and following statements. Speakers from both mainstream and culturally/linguistically varied communities may exhibit similar appearing difficulties in producing cohesive and coherent asymmetrical discourse, but for different reasons. Mainstream speakers with intrinsic, neurologically based language problems may have difficulty with asymmetrical discourse because they cannot simultaneously keep the topic and the individual statements in mind. Nonmainstream clients may experience problems because they have never been assisted in producing this type of discourse. Consequently, tasks such as telling a story may be overwhelming. The performance of the nonmainstream client may appear disorganized like that of the client with language-learning disabilities.

Formal testing generally cannot be used to determine if culturally/ linguistically different clients are language-learning disabled. Testing shows only if they are familiar with the culture of testing. Poor performance on testing may predict a client's performance in a school or work setting that requires skills similar to those on the tests, but it does not tell us if a client has an intrinsic language disability. We can make adequate evaluations of the speech and language of culturally different clients only over time by identifying their language learning needs in different situations, providing appropriate programming, and observing how quickly they learn what is taught.

EVALUATION OF NONMAINSTREAM AND POTENTIALLY ENGLISH-PROFICIENT CLIENTS

Dialect Variations

We must understand dialect variations and the process of second language learning if we are to provide appropriate assessment of individuals who do not speak the mainstream or standard variant of English and those whose first language is not English.

Some clients speak only English, but the English they speak is not the type that is heard on the 6:00 P.M. news. Not all English speakers use the same phonological, morphological, syntactic, semantic, and pragmatic rules. The variations in a language used by a racial, ethnic, geographical, or socioeconomic group are called *dialects*. Every dialect represents the phonological and grammatical rules used by persons in a speech community. Dialect variations may be at the word level (a can of Coke is a "pop" in western Pennsylvania and a "soda" in New York), at the phoneme level (in Australia the word "weight" sounds like the American word "white"), or grammar/syntactic level (the nonstandard English, "he don't got none" for the standard English, "he doesn't have any"). A dialect should not be considered deviant or deficient because it differs from the dialect of Standard American English. Consequently, persons with dialect differences should not be treated as though they have a speech disorder. Assessment of a client who speaks a nonmainstream dialect of English requires that we know the characteristics of the client's dialect. Some clients' language patterns may be influenced by multiple dialects. For example, a person's first language

> Some dialects have more social prestige than others. What dialects are considered prestigious in the United States and what dialects are not considered prestigious?

may be Cambodian. She may have first immigrated to France, then later immigrated to the United States where she learned English. Her speech and language patterns (dialect) in English may reflect characteristics of both Cambodian and French.

Our task, then, is to differentiate the elements of clients' language production that are characteristic of their dialect and those that may indicate a speech and language delay or disorder. In American English a glottal stop (/ʔ/) is not part of the phonological system, yet in Navajo and several Southwest Pueblo languages, it is the most common consonant. If an English speaking child frequently substitutes a glottal stop for other stops (p, b, t, d, k, g), it may be an indication of velopharyngeal incompetence. If a Navajo child frequently substitutes glottal stops for other consonants, it is possible that she has velopharygeal incompentence, but is it more likely that she is using it because in her language many of the other stop consonants cannot appear in word final position. Two major racial/ethnic dialects in the United States are Black English and Spanish-influenced English. Table 2–2 shows some common characteristics of Black English and Spanish-influenced English. Saying "baf" for "bath" in Black English may represent a dialect difference; while saying "ba" for "bath" may represent a speech disorder because Black English dialect would not omit the final sound in "bath."

Language Dominance/Language Proficiency

We sometimes refer to individuals who are learning English as a second language as limited–English proficient or as potentially English proficient. It has been suggested that we should consider these individuals as *language-enhanced persons* because they are capable of speaking more than one language. When we evaluate them, we must assess their *language proficiency* and their *language dominance*. Language proficiency refers to a client's ability to comprehend and produce language. Language dominance refers to the language in which a person is most fluent and proficient.

Commercial, standardized tests are available that reportedly assess language dominance. Such tests generally evaluate a person's vocabulary and syntactic knowledge in two languages by having the person select a picture that best represents a word or sentence. Language dominance is not, however, a stable phenomena. It is dependent on the situation and the people being spoken to. A client may be Spanish dominant at home, but English dominant at school or work. Clients may not have English words for items and events talked about at home; and they may not have Spanish words for items and events talked about at school or work. Hence, we cannot determine a client's language dominance by administering a test alone. We must also interview clients regarding the language they use in different situations and with different people. We need to be aware that a client may be dominant in a language, but not proficient. This is frequently true of students who are English dominant at school, but

A balanced bilingual is equally proficient in both languages. Being a balanced bilingual, however, is not necessarily indicative of a high level of language proficiency.

Contexts for language use are different for clients of different ages. What language contexts might you consider for a preschool child, a school-age child, and an adult?

Table 2–2. Common phonological and syntactic dialect variations.

Black English	Spanish-Influenced English
Phonological	
Consonant cluster reduction: *hol/hold; tes/test*	Substitutions because many Spanish dialects have no: /ɪ/, /ʃ/, /dʒ/, /z/ *confuse sheep/ship;* *choose/shoes;* *yellow/jello;* *sue/zoo*
Substitutions: *f/θ (baf/bath);* *v/ð (brover/brother);* *skr/str (skreet/street)*	
Consonant omissions: *r (cɑ/car; sto'y/story; potect/pro- tect);* *l (too/tool)*	Devoicing final consonants *k/g, f/v, t/d, p/b, s/z* One sound for /b/ and /v/
Devoicing final consonants *p/b, t/d, k/g*	Addition of /e/ for /s/ initial words *estudy/study*
Syntactic	
Nonobligatory plural markers on count nouns *(two dog)*	Adjectives follow nouns *house white/white house* *ball of tennis/tennis ball*
Nonobligatory possessive markers *(John cousin)*	No set word order for questions and no auxiliaries *When Mary came?*
Omission of copula and auxiliary be *(He a big dog. That your dog?)*	No auxiliaries in negative sentences *I no understand*
Multiple negation *(I don't got none/I don't have any).*	Double negatives *I not saw nobody*
Regularize third person *(he swim/he swims)*	Simple present used to refer to future *I see her next week*
Regularize plural copula/auxiliary *(I was, you was, he was, we was, they was)*	Possessives expressed with prepositional phrases *the book of Rosa*

speak another language at home. We must determine not only the client's language dominance, but also the client's degree of proficiency in the dominant language.

Language Loss

Evaluating speech and language skills in bilingual clients is complicated by the fact that clients, especially children, may be losing their first language while acquiring their second language. In such cir-

Children may also experience language loss because they elect not to speak their first language because they want to fit in. Expressive language loss is generally greater than receptive language loss.

cumstances, many children do not have age-level proficiency in any language. Figure 2–1 displays this situation. If children are monolingual, they generally exhibit a steady increase in language skills from the time of their birth. If a child is introduced to a second language at some point in time, the degree of exposure to the first language may be reduced. In such a case, the rate of language learning in the first language is slowed; and in some cases, first language learning stops and the child loses some or all of that language. At the time this is occurring, the child is not yet proficient in the second language. Consequently, such children are likely to appear delayed in both languages.

Adults who have been bilingual or multilingual and who have suffered strokes or traumatic brain injury show a variety of patterns of language preservation and recovery. Many first recover the language they have used the most recently, whereas others may begin to use a language they have not actively used for a number of years.

Evaluating Language Proficiency for Academic Success

Children who have academic proficiency in a first language develop academic proficiency in a second language more easily than children who have only an interpersonal proficiency in a first language.

Some writers distinguish between the language used in familiar social interactions (interpersonal language proficiency) and language necessary in school settings (academic language proficiency). The language skills for interpersonal proficiency are sufficient for everyday purposes of following directions, making requests, and sharing

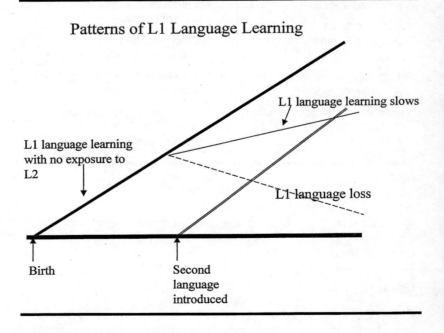

Figure 2–1. Patterns of L1 language learning.

and even paraphrasing familiar information. Academic language proficiency is required to use less familiar vocabulary and more syntactic complexity. Also, academic language proficiency involves the ability to use language to talk about language and to analyze, synthesize, and evaluate information. These language skills are particularly needed in social studies, science, and literature classes. Because students may sound fluent in basic interpersonal language skills, deficits in academic language skills often go unrecognized. Even in a supportive environment, it takes approximately 2–3 years to achieve proficiency in interpersonal language skills and 5–7 years to achieve academic language proficiency (Cummins, 1984).

Figure 2–2 carries this distinction further, identifying language activities that vary in terms of contextual support and cognitive demands.

Cognitively familiar, undemanding tasks or activities are ones the client has mastered and thus they require little active thinking. They require only interpersonal language proficiency. Unfamiliar, demanding tasks and activities require more active processing and do not rely on trained or rote responses. They require academic language proficiency. What might be a familiar task for one person may be an unfamiliar task for another person. For example, arroyos, cactus, and volcanos are familiar to persons living in Albuquerque, New Mexico, but not to persons living in Cedar Rapids, Iowa. We want to see how clients perform on activities that they have been specifically taught or should be familiar with and how they approach unfamiliar activities that should be manageable for their developmental level. Frequently we learn about those from the client, family members, or the client's teachers.

The context-embedded versus context-reduced dimension relates to the range of contextual support available for understanding and performing the activity. In a context-embedded activity, persons can rely on the people and objects in the environment to give them clues about meaning and feelings about how they are doing. Contextually reduced activities require reliance primarily on verbal instructions alone. Understanding these two continua will help us understand why a child's performance on formal assessments may differ from parental reports of children's abilities at home or a teacher's estimate of children's proficiency based on the language they use on the playground and in the cafeteria. Home, playground, and cafeteria activities are familiar and context embedded; many classroom activities and assessment tasks are unfamiliar and context reduced. Some adult clients may not have had formal educational experiences and are likely to have difficulty with unfamiliar, decontextualized language tasks, such as some of the tasks on formal, standardized tests.

Students who are learning English as a second language and students with language learning disabilities frequently experience academic difficulties as the literacy demands of the curriculum increase (that is, as more academic language skill is required). Assessment of

Review some tests that are commonly used. What items may be unfamiliar to a client? For example, have children ever seen a squirrel or a taxi?

Cognitively Undemanding

Exchanges greetings
Uses language to request & command
Carries on conversation
Follows spoken directions with
  contextual supports
Describes classroom objects & persons
Gives directions to peers

Relates personal experiences
Talks about familiar topics
  without contextual support
Reads notes, signs, directions
Writes from dictation
Answers questions about stories/text
  with familiar content

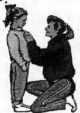

Context-Embedded   **Context-Reduced**

Follows directions for academic
  tasks
Understands contextualized
  academic content
Talks about less familiar topics with
  contextual support

Understands lectures on academic
  content
Uses language to predict, reason,
  analyze, synthesize, evaluate
Tells/ writes imaginary stories
Tells/writes explanations, persuasions
Engages in deductive thought
  experiments

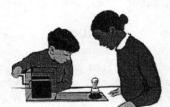

Cognitively Demanding

Figure 2–2. Framework for language assessment.

these students has traditionally employed an inside-out approach. In this approach, we look at what the student brings to the activity—cognitive and linguistic knowledge and skills and values and beliefs about subject content and school. If the student is experiencing difficulty with school tasks, it is often assumed that changes must be made in the student. Increasingly, it is recognized that adequate assessment must also consider an outside-in approach—an approach that considers the academic and participant structures of the lessons (Nelson, 1992; Westby, 1997). An outside-in approach considers both the academic demands of the lesson and the participant demands of the lesson (how students are expected to participate or interact in the lesson). Educators and speech-language pathologists have had considerable training in conducting inside-out assessments; they are just beginning to conduct outside-in assessments.

Such assessments are important for all students, but are critical for students from culturally/linguistically diverse backgrounds. When there is a discrepancy between the cognitive/linguistic knowledge and skills of the students and the cognitive/linguistic demands of the curriculum, we must determine what underlying skills and knowledge the students must have or must develop if they are to be successful with the curriculum. The obvious objective is to find out whether the differences between what students bring to school and what the curriculum requires is due to cultural/linguistic language differences or to neurological deficits. This is frequently difficult to determine, particularly if you have given only standardized testing. Whatever the reason for the discrepancy, however, students will need help if they are to succeed in school.

Now to the question of why students from nonmainstream backgrounds may be having difficulty even though they do not have intrinsic language learning disabilities. One suggestion is that there is a cultural conflict or incompatibility between socialization patterns in the students' homes and in schools (Tharp & Gallimore, 1988). Researchers who hypothesize that cultural differences between home and school contribute to students' academic difficulties have suggested that schools could facilitate the learning of nonmainstream students by employing culturally congruent teaching which involves teaching meaningful content using social participation structures that are familiar and comfortable to the students.

Other researchers have suggested that nonmainstream students have not been given access to the "culture of power"—the academic discourse patterns of the mainstream culture (Delpit, 1988; Ladson-Billings, 1994; de la luz Reyes, 1991). The emphasis is not only on the vocabulary and content, but also on discourse styles required for classroom success and how to participate in lessons. Ideally, education for these students should teach the "code of power" (academic discourse) in ways that are congruent both with the students' cultural background (what they know and how they best learn) and with the nature of the academic material they must learn (Lee & Fradd, 1998). Speech–language pathologists and teachers must develop a bridge between where the students are and where they need to be by providing them with the language and social skills necessary to succeed in schools (Figure 2–3).

We see a variety of clinical histories of children who are potentially English proficient. They mainly are affected by family education and the child's inherent abilities (Peña & Valles, 1995). Here are four possibilities:

In classrooms of mainstream students taught by mainstream teachers, teachers frequently call on students by name. Students bid for turns by raising their hands and only one student talks at a time. In classrooms of Hispanic students taught by Hispanic teachers, teachers pose questions to the entire class and students call out answers, with several students talking simultaneously.

Hawaiian children markedly improved in reading when teachers engaged them in "talk story" about the reading material. In the children's community, "talk story" is interactive narration, verbal play, and conversation that is enjoyed by several people as they build a story together.

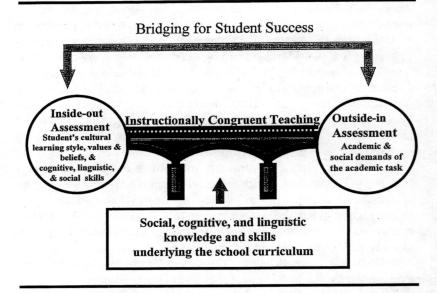

Figure 2–3. Bridging for student success.

Asian children are the most underrepresented "minority" group in special education and are identified later than children from other cultural/linguistic groups.

■ The child's family has a formal educational background; the child learns the second language (L2) quickly and does not have a language learning disability. Such a child may be thought to have a communication disorder only if he or she is transitioned too quickly into English only, or if academic language requirements of the curriculum are not recognized.

■ The child's family lacks formal educational background; the child learns oral language quickly, but has difficulty acquiring academic language because the family cannot support literate language learning. The child does not have a language learning disability, but may be so judged because of academic difficulties.

■ The child's family may or may not have formal educational experiences; the child learns oral language adequately, but experiences difficulty with academic language. The child does indeed have a language learning disability, but may not be referred because his or her oral language skills are appropriate.

■ The child's family lacks formal educational experiences; the child is slow to learn oral language and has difficulty with academic language. The child is language learning disabled, but may not be referred for several years because the child's delays are assumed to be due to background and to learning a second language.

Problems With Common Suggestions for Evaluating Potentially English-Proficient Clients

Schools, clients, and hospitals often require that we use standardized test procedures to document a client's disability and to justify treatment. Formal tests can be useful if you want to determine if an individual has the speech and language skills expected of mainstream individuals in a particular situation. The reasons for the poor performance of a nonmainstream person on such testing, however, are not easily interpretable. Without additional information, we cannot know if the person has done poorly because of an intrinsic, neurologically based language learning disability, or if the poor performance stems from unfamiliarity with the test items and the testing interaction patterns. Several methods have been suggested for ways to modify tests to make them more useful, but none seem wholly satisfactory (Damico, 1991; Vaughn-Cooke, 1983). As speech-language pathologists or audiologists we must be able to discuss effectively and convincingly the problems associated with these test modifications when administrators or supervisors suggest that we use these methods to evaluate culturally/linguistically different clients. That is, we must be able to explain why these methods do not successfully deal with the problem of validity. The following are some suggestions about how to do that.

1. *Translate the test.* Some concepts don't have a direct translation. For example, there is not a single word in Navajo that can be translated for the word *construction.* The concept is translated as "there is a man hitting a board with a hammer." Clearly, this sentence is not as complex as the word *construction.* Many aspects of English morphology and syntax do not have counterparts in other languages. For example, many Native American languages do not have gender pronouns. Vietnamese does not have plural and possessive markers. Even if test items can be translated from one language to another, the order in which concepts are learned may differ among cultures. When testing hearing of English speakers, audiologists use single syllable words and spondee words such as *baseball* and *hotdog* to assess speech reception. An equivalent Spanish test is not possible because the Spanish language has very few single syllable words and no spondee words.

2. *Standardize existing tests on minority populations.* Ethnic norms are potentially dangerous because they provide a basis for invidious comparisons between racial/ethnic groups. But the primary problem here is that there likely are differences among nonmainstream cultures in dealing with the concepts on the tests. As a consequence, the test results may well reflect cultural differences rather than innate potential.

3. *Use tests that include a small percentage of minorities in the standardization sample when developing tests.* This is a common

When asked to explain the term "learning disability" to Navajo parents so they would sign permission for special education, a Navajo interpreter reported that she told the family, "Your child can't do White people things in school. Sign the paper and they'll teach him to do White people things."

practice with commercial standardized tests. The problem with this approach is that the norms represent no one. The mean scores are below the mean for mainstream students and still above the mean for students from nondominant cultural groups.

4. *Modify existing tests in ways that will make them appropriate for clients from other cultures.* This is easier said than done. It is difficult to maintain similar complexity of content. We must have sufficient knowledge of the culture and be able to modify the tests in such a way so that the revisions provide the possibility of equal credit.

You can have a role in providing better services to culturally/linguistically diverse students by explaining to decision makers the difficulties in using standardized tests with nondominant clients.

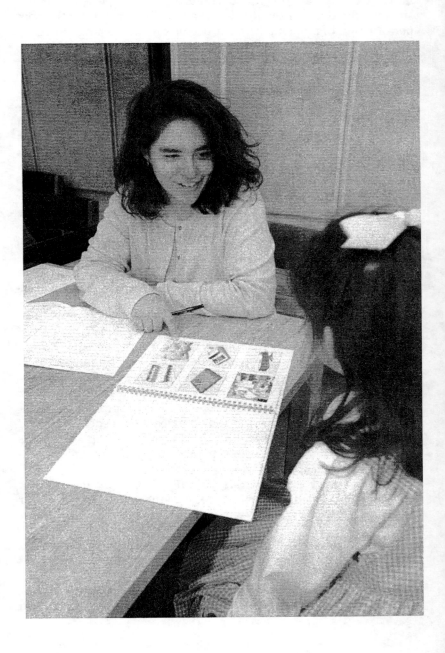

5. *Use a language sample and other observations.* Presently, we do not have adequate developmental information on nondominant cultural groups and non–English speakers. Without normative data we cannot evaluate the quality of a language sample or make a diagnosis regarding the normalcy of a client's language.

6. *Use criterion-referenced measures.* What should the criterion be and who establishes it? How do we know what the order of progression should be in the criterion? More data are needed about developmental sequences in children from nondominant cultural groups if we are to develop criterion reference measures.

Alternative Assessment Approaches

If formal tests are generally inadequate for assessing culturally/linguistically different populations, what is appropriate? There are three general approaches to consider.

Ethnographic Interviews

Ethnographic interviews enable us to attempt to see the world through the eyes of the clients and their families. In traditional interviews, professionals predetermine the questions that are to be asked and in some cases they predetermine the range of responses that can be given. In ethnographic interviewing, both questions and answers must be discovered from the people being interviewed. Different information is collected from different clients because the values, beliefs, strengths, and needs of each client vary as he or she functions within his or her culture.

We can gain a great deal of information by asking clients or family members to describe their typical day. As they discuss their typical day, you will note what is important to them—their concerns, what they like and do not like, what they do and how they do it, etc. Depending upon the reason for the referral, you can ask about specific activities or events. Types of information that are important for making speech and language assessment decisions may include normal language developmental patterns and beliefs about how children learn to talk; who talks to children and whom children talk with; topics of conversation for boys, girls, men, and women; reasons for talking (giving directions, asking questions, telling stories, joking); roles of boys, girls, men, and women in the culture; and how the culture defines and views a "handicap."

We want to know if other members of the client's culture view the child or adult as having speech and language differences or disorder. If they believe that a little girl, for example, has a speech and language disorder, it is likely that she does indeed have an intrinsic speech or language disorder. If they do not regard her as having a speech or language disorder, then, according to the standards of her culture, she does not have a disorder in situations that are common to her cultural community. She may, however, have an intrinsic disorder that is not recognized by members of her culture. This is par-

> You should approach the ethnographic interview with the attitude, "I don't know much about this person's point of view so I've got to encourage him or her to set the agenda for this interview," rather than with the attitude, "I know what I want to find out, so I am setting the agenda for this interview."

ticularly possible for language disorders that affect academic performance, because schools require structures and functions of language not required in other settings. If family members have not had much experience with the formal educational system, they may not recognize the reasons a child may be having difficulty.

Inventories and Work Sample Analysis

Inventories and analysis of collections of students' work samples, sometimes called *portfolios*, involve observing clients in naturalistic environments and evaluating their performance on authentic tasks. The observer considers the demands of the situation and the behavior and use of speech and language by others in the setting. We may observe the purposes for which the client uses language in a setting, such as a greeting; making a request; describing objects, events, and past experiences; reasoning and predicting what will happen; and projecting the thoughts and feelings of others. Also important is how he or she participates in conversation, such as initiating topics, taking turns, keeping to the topic (or not), elaborating topics, and repairing breakdowns.

> You may choose to be a passive observer or an active observer. Passive observers watch but do not interact with the client in the situation. Active observers participate in the activities with the client being observed.

For school-age students, we also need to evaluate the student's ability to comprehend the content of the school curriculum and to complete necessary written work. We can observe the student and ask the teacher to describe her concerns, with specific interest in the student's ability to deal with stories, comprehend complex sentence patterns and text material, and his or her ability to write in a variety of genres (narratives, descriptions, explanations, persuasions).

Dynamic Assessment

Dynamic approaches to assessment activities can be especially helpful in determining if a child may have a language disability rather than a language difference (Peña, 1996). Our interest is in how a child learns, or the child's potential for learning. Our major questions are: How easy is it for the student to learn a language task, to what extent does the student require instructional strategies that differ from those that have been used effectively with peers, and to what extent does the student exhibit off-task behaviors or inappropriate responses during instruction (Mattes & Omark, 1991)?

Evaluation of clients from culturally/linguistically diverse cultures should determine how easily their learning can be modified (Lidz, 1991; Peña, 1996). We design an evaluation to assess the child's ability to learn skills related to the area of concern. We assess the child using the tasks we have designed, and then we conduct a therapeutic program in which we mediate the child's learning by explaining expectations and by modeling and prompting how to do the task. Finally, we reassess the child. Children who respond well to the mediation by becoming involved with the activity and learning the tasks are unlikely to have a learning disability.

Coung and Tueyen were two fifth-grade Vietnamese boys in an Albuquerque school who were experiencing difficulty in language arts. They were no longer eligible for ESL (English as Second Language) classes because they had passed an oral language proficiency test. Their teacher, however, was concerned because Cuong and Tueyen could not tell or write a coherent story and could not comprehend the stories they read. The speech-language pathologist conducted a dynamic assessment to determine how modifiable the boys were for narrative skills. For the pretest she had the boys tell stories about two poster pictures. She then planned a series of lessons over a 2-week period in which she and the boys read short stories and identified the parts of the stories. Together she and the boys constructed a story with all the parts. After these activities were completed, she asked the boys to tell stories about two more poster pictures. Modifiability was determined from the students' responsiveness to mediation, the effort required by the speech-language pathologist to induce changes in the students, and evidence of the students transferring the narrative skills to their language arts class. Table 2–3 shows the results of mediation for Cuong and Tueyen. Cuong exhibited greater modifiability than Tueyen. He was more attentive to the tasks, retained the information better, and was better at self-monitoring.

A variety of creative approaches are being developed that have the potential to generate normative data regarding language learnability rates. These approaches use videos, puppet shows, or computer games to teach children unfamiliar vocabulary, morphological word

Table 2–3. Dynamic assessment results.

Strategy	Cuong	Tueyen
Attention	Attentive to all activities; rarely required reminders to pay attention	Lost interest part-way through lessons; required frequent reminders from the examiner to look at what they were doing
Style	Reflective; waited for instructions before beginning tasks	Impulsive; tried doing activities before examiner gave all the instructions; examiner had to keep materials out of his reach until they were ready to begin
Memory	Could tell the examiner what was done in a previous lesson	Examiner needed to give clues for student to remember previous lesson
Monitoring	Self-corrected omissions in his stories	Examiner had to remind him of the parts to include
Transfer	Recognized character goals in story read in language arts	Could relate beginning and ends of stories, but could not answer questions about the goals in stories

endings, or artificial languages and then present children with activities in which they must use what they have learned (Dollaghan, 1987; Jacobs, 1998; Oetting, Rice, & Swank, 1995; Roseberry-Kibbon & Connell, 1991). Persons who require more trials or variations in the rate of presentation of the trials on such tasks may have language learning disabilities.

INTERPRETING ASSESSMENT INFORMATION

As indicated in Chapter 4 (Morris), interpreting evaluation data to clients and their families is as important as conducting the evaluation. Several factors are particularly important to consider when interpreting assessment data with culturally/linguistically different clients and their families.

Using Interpreters

The gender, age, life experiences, race/ethnicity, language lls, and education of the person conducting the interpretive session can make a difference in what clients hear and how they hear it. If you work on a team, consider who would be the best person to conduct the interpretive session.

Under optimal circumstances, you should have a translator/interpreter assist in the session even if the client and family are able to communicate to some degree in English. You will be talking about unfamiliar concepts and using words that are not common in everyday English. Without a good interpreter there is likely to be significant misunderstanding. Ideally you want someone who is familiar with the concepts you are discussing; maybe you can even train them for the task. Certainly an interpreter should be acceptable to the client or family. Generally, you do not want someone who lives in the family's neighborhood. In this situation, the family may be hesitant to talk because they may be concerned that the interpreter will tell other people in the community about "their problems." If you are working with refugee families from countries where there has been armed conflict, you want to make sure that the interpreter is from the "same side" as the client. Several years ago I was working with a Vietnamese family who had three children with disabilities. I called Catholic Charities, the agency in town responsible for arranging for interpreters. They sent a person trained in interpreting in medical and educational settings, yet it was clear during the session that things were not going well. I later learned that the interpreter was an ethnic Chinese from Vietnam and because of the history of ethnic Chinese in Vietnam, neither the interpreter nor the family trusted one another. In the current world situation, you will need to be careful in selecting interpreters for refugees from Yugoslavia (Croatia, Bosnia, Herzegovina) and some of the Middle Eastern countries.

Avoid having children interpret for their parents. That can disrupt the culturally based parent/child roles and interaction patterns.

Include the Extended Family

Always include family members when assessing a child. Inform the parents that they can bring any other family members or friends they would like to have with them. In some cultures the parents do not make the decisions for the child's care. Grandparents, godparents, aunts, uncles, or tribal elders may determine if, when, and how medical, therapeutic, or educational services are sought and accepted, so they should be included.

Cultural Interplay

Be aware that miscommunication may arise because of differences in values, beliefs, and communication patterns. In some traditional cultures, men are reluctant to accept information given by a woman. A mother may not accept suggestions given by a clinician who does not have a child of her own. Different cultures use different rates of speaking and different patterns in taking turns in a conversation. These differing speaking rates and turn-taking patterns may affect the client's or family's ability to participate in a discussion with you.

In many cultures, particularly Asian cultures, it is important to maintain *face*, which is a negotiated public image that people want to portray in interpersonal interactions. Talking with a family about problems or difficulties their child has can put them in a situation of losing face. If you attempt to push your points, the family is not likely to openly disagree with you (they do not want to put you in a position of losing face), but they are likely to avoid you in the future by not being available for meetings or not following through on recommendations.

Persons from the Northeast United States have much shorter pauses between speaking turns than persons in the South and Midwest. When persons from the Northeast and the Midwest speak together, Midwesterners may think the Northeasterners are rude because they do not give the Midwesterners a turn; and the Northeasterners may think the Midwesterners are dull because they don't have anything to say.

Rudeness Bias

Mainstream professionals like to ask questions. These questions may appear rude and overly personal to some clients and families. Some topics may not be permissible topics for strangers to raise. When you must ask questions, explain why the questions are important. (For example, "The answer to this next question will help me know how to work with your child.")

Courtesy Bias

Most clients and families do not wish to cause problems or create friction. They wish to be polite or to "save face." They may not believe what you are saying and they may disagree with your recommendations, but often they will not tell you so. Instead, during the meeting they may agree to anything, although they have no intention of following your suggestions.

Racial Difference Bias

If families have had a history of negative experiences with individuals from your ethnic/racial group, they may not trust you or may not feel comfortable with you. If families have negative self–esteem for their own ethnic/racial group, they may not trust a professional from their own group. They may think that the professional is no longer part of the group, or they may think that the person is a token professional and does not really have the skills necessary to do the job.

CONCLUSION

Speech, language, and hearing evaluation of culturally/linguistically diverse clients is a complex task. It requires not only knowledge about development and disorders in mainstream populations, but also knowledge about cultural variations in the development and use of language, causes and manifestations of speech and language disorders, and values and beliefs associated with disabilities and intervention. Valid evaluations for all clients require sensitivity to their cultures.

REFERENCES

Battle, D. E. (1998). *Communication disorders in a multicultural populations* (2nd ed., pp. 3–29). Boston: Butterworth–Heineman.

Crago, M. B. (1988). *Cultural context in communicative interaction of young Inuit children.* Unpublished doctoral thesis, McGill University, Montreal.

Cummins, J. (1984). *Bilingualism and special education.* San Diego, CA: College-Hill Press.

Damico, J. S. (1991). Descriptive assessment of communicative ability in limited English proficient students. In E. V. Hamayan & J. S. Damico (Eds.), *Limiting bias in the assessment of bilingual students* (pp. 157–217). Austin, TX: Pro-Ed.

Delpit, L. (1988). The silenced dialogue: Power and pedagogy in educating other people's children. *Harvard Educational Review, 58,* 280–298.

Dollaghan, C. A. (1987). Fast mapping in normal and language-impaired children. *Journal of Speech and Hearing Disorders, 52,* 218–222.

Downs, M. (1985). Language disorders from hearing losses in multicultural populations. In L. Cole & V. Deal (Eds.), *Communication disorders in multicultural populations.* Washington, DC: American Speech-Language-Hearing Association.

Heath, S. B. (1982). Questions at home and school. In G. Spindler (Ed.), *Doing the ethnography of schooling.* New York: Holt, Rinehart, and Winston.

Jacobs, E. L. (1998). KIDTALK: A computerized language screening test. *Journal of Computing in Childhood Education, 9,* 113–131.

Ladson-Billings, G. (1994). *The dreamkeepers: Successful teachers of African American children.* San Francisco, CA: Jossey-Bass.

Lee, O., & Fradd, S. H. (1998). Science for all: Including students from non–English language backgrounds. *Educational Researcher, 27,* 12–21.

Lidz, C. S. (1991). *Practitioner's guide to dynamic assessment.* New York: Guilford.

Mattes, L., & Omark, D. (1991). *Speech and language assessment for the bilingual handicapped* (2nd ed.). Oceanside, CA: Academic Communication Associates.

Mayfield, S. A. (1985). Excess lead absorption and language disorders in Black children. In L. Cole & V. Deal (Eds.), *Communication disorders in multicultural populations.* Washington, DC: American Speech-Language-Hearing Association.

McWilliams, B. J., Morris, H. L., Shelton, R. L. (1990). *Cleft palate speech.* Philadelphia, PA: B. C. Decker.

Nelson, N. (1992). Targets of curriculum based language assessment. In W. Secord & J. S. Damico (Eds.), *Best practices in school speech-language pathology.* San Antonio, TX: The Psychological Corporation.

Oetting, J. B., Rice, M. L., & Swank, L. K. (1995). Quick incidental learning (QUIL) of words by school-age children with and without SLI. *Journal of Speech and Hearing Research, 38,* 434–445.

Peña, E. (1996). Dynamic assessment: The model and its language applications. In K. N. Cole, P. S. Dale, & D. J. Thal (Eds.), *Assess-ment of communication and language.* Baltimore, MD: Paul H. Brookes.

Peña, E., & Valles, L. (1995). Language assessment and instructional programming for linguistically different learners: Proactive classroom processes. In H. Kayser (Ed.), *Bilingual speech-language pathology.* San Diego, CA: Singular Publishing Group.

Post, R. H. (1964). Hearing acuity among Negroes and whites. *Eugen Quarterly, 11,* 65–81.

Reyes, M. de la luz (1991). A process approach to literacy instruction for Spanish–speaking students: In search of a best fit. In E. H. Hiebert (Ed.), *Literacy for a diverse society.* New York: Teachers College Press.

Roseberry-Kibbon, C., & Connell, P. J. (1991). The use of an invented language rule in the differentiation of normal and language impaired Spanish-speaking children. *Journal of Speech and Hearing Research, 34,* 596–603.

Scott, D. (1985). Hearing loss and sickle cell anemia. In L. Cole & V. Deal (Eds.), *Communication disorders in multicultural populations.* Washington, DC: American Speech-Language-Hearing Association.

Spector, R. E. (1985). *Cultural diversity in health and illness.* Norwalk, CT: Appleton-Century-Crofts.

Sue, D. W. & Sue, D. (1990). *Counseling the culturally different: Theory and practice.* New York: John Wiley.

Tharp, R. G., & Gallimore, R. (1988). *Rousing minds to life.* Cambridge, UK: Cambridge University Press.

Vanderas, A. O. (1987). Incidence of cleft lip, cleft palate, and cleft lip and palate among races: A review. *Cleft Palate Journal, 24,* 216–225.

Vaughn-Cooke, F. B. (1983). Improving language assessment in minority children. *Asha, 25,* 29–34.

Westby, C. E. (1997). There's more to passing than knowing the answers. *Language, Speech, and Hearing Services in Schools, 28,* 274–287.

RECOMMENDED READINGS

Battle, D. E. (1998). *Communication disorders in multicultural populations* (2nd ed.). Boston, MA: Butterworth-Heinemann.

Farr, B. P., & Trumbull, E. (1997). *Assessment alternatives for diverse classrooms.* Norwood, MA: Christopher Gordon.

Fradd, S. H., & McGee, P. L. (1994). *Instructional assessment: An integrative approach to evaluating student performance.* Reading, MA: Addison-Wesley.

Hamayan, E. V., & Damico, J. S. (Eds.). (1991). *Limiting bias in the assessment of bilingual students* (pp. 157–217). Austin, TX: Pro-Ed.

SECTION II

The Building Blocks

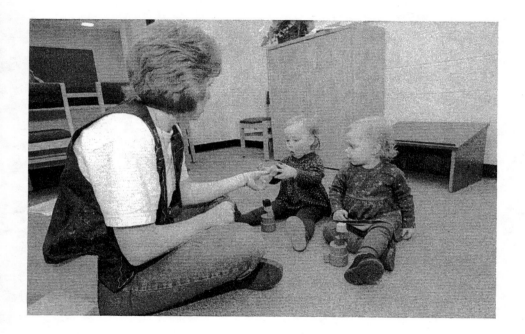

The next seven chapters deal with the central focus of this book. The first two are about aspects of diagnosis that involve both the clinician and the client and his or her family. In one, the emphasis is on obtaining information and in the other, the emphasis is on giving information. These two missions are alike in some respects and different in others. In the next chapter, Hall describes the step in which we examine the oral mechanism, the part of the human body that has to do with the mechanics of talking.

   The final four chapters in this section are about the parameters of speech and language: language, speech sounds, fluency, and voice. In each, the authors set forth their conceptual model of the parameter, some information about the disorder, and their approach to diagnosis of the disorder. This is the heart of the book.

CHAPTER

3

The Clinical History

Penelope K. Hall, M.A.
Hughlett L. Morris, Ph.D.

Our purpose in this chapter is to provide guidance in acquiring the skill of taking a clinical history. The term *clinical history* is used to refer to background information about the communication disorder so that we can better understand its nature and can assist in its treatment. In other words, we need to know what has come before, before we can proceed!

Common sense tells us that the "history" of a speech and language disorder varies with its nature and so the process of history taking must certainly be tailored to the disorder and the patient at hand. For example, the questions asked an adult with a recent onset voice problem will obviously be different from those asked a parent of a child who shows evidence of problems in language acquisition. In the first case, the informant is the woman or man with the problem, and information about childhood development is probably not relevant (although vocal use patterns during adolescence may be!). In the second case, the informant is the parent or the responsible adult and detailed information about development will probably be crucial to the clinical purpose. Health status, family, school/work status, and personal reaction to the problem will be important in both. However, it is important to keep in mind that every patient/client is

Sometimes it is difficult to determine when the problem "began."

an individual. Some will require the professional to obtain an extensive exploration of the individual's background, although many patients will not. Therefore the extensiveness of the history required in order to obtain an understanding of the person's background will vary. Even so, it seems reasonable that the beginning speech language pathologist is well advised to focus on several aspects of the clinical history interview that are common to all or the majority of patients with speech and language complaints.

Finally, as have other contributors to this text, we have taken some short cuts in our language use in this discussion for ease of reading. Sometimes we use the feminine gender and sometimes the masculine gender pronoun. We use *patient* throughout, but in some settings *client* would be preferred. In the context of history taking, we describe discussions with the *patient* but obviously, if the patient is a child, these discussions will be held with a parent or responsible adult. With these thoughts in mind, we proceed.

> As you read subsequent chapters be sure to extract information to help you develop questions about these specific disorders.

Why Do We Need to Know the Clinical History?

The clinical history tells us a lot about the problem under consideration, and the patient with the problem. It gives us ideas about what we can do to help. And, it saves time. Without the clinical history, we approach the clinical problem blindly, and in a vacuum. A good history taker is the hallmark of a good clinician.

When Do We Take the Information?

The clinical history begins usually even before meeting the patient. That an examination has been arranged tells us that there is a concern about some aspect of communication. It tells us further that the concern is important enough to seek our professional advice as a speech-language pathologist.

The setting in which we work may give some automatic clues to the nature of the disorder. The SLP who practices in a school setting quite naturally expects prospective patients to be children; the SLP who practices in a rehabilitation center expects patients who have chronic disorders that are frequently debilitating; the SLP who conducts a wide-range private practice can expect almost anything!

> Many professionals use the acronym "SLP" for "speech-language pathologist."

Age of patient provides some clues as well. The referral of a young child is likely to indicate a problem in development, a congenital disorder, or a pediatric disease. An older adult more likely has chronic disease, a neurologic disorder or disease, or deterioration of earlier functional abilities.

Information available from the request for appointment or from the referral may be useful in identifying the problem, depending on the level of sophistication with which the request or referral is made.

While the public and our colleagues from other disciplines are generally on target about whether there *is* a problem (after all, the public is the final authority about the matter), they frequently are poorly equipped to describe with any precision the *nature* of the "speech" problem. Frequently, the report is that the child or adult "can't talk plainly," "has trouble saying certain words," "repeats," "can't get the words out," "can't think of the right words," "doesn't talk much," "can't talk," "talks too slowly," "talks through her nose," "nobody can understand him," "her teacher can't hear her," "I don't sound like I used to," "I lose my voice a lot," "on the phone, people mistake me for a man (woman)," "I can't swallow right," and so forth. The experienced SLP can probably identify the general nature of the disorder from information like this.

On the other hand, all or most of this information can be misleading about the "real" problem, so the SLP must be on her toes to avoid a bias in expectation that interferes with her ability to make observations.

What we typically regard as the taking of clinical history takes place when we begin our interview with the patient and family. We use this occasion to get acquainted with the patient and to learn as much as possible, or as much as needed, or both, about the problem and the patient to add to our previous knowledge. Actually, we continue this process of learning throughout all our encounters with the patient, but this initial interview is the starting place.

From What Sources Does the Clinical History Come?

Usually we begin the clinical interview with background information in hand, noting particularly what we know thus far about why and how this initial appointment was made. We also are familiar with any available reports from colleagues, including those from other disciplines that have been requested—after the patient or responsible adult has given the proper written authorization for release of the information to us of course! These forms are always properly dated and kept on record. Sometimes clinics develop their own questionnaires which the patient is asked to complete prior to the appointment with you. These reports and forms will be in the clinical file along with information about previous examinations or treatment the patient has received in this clinic. Sometimes the patient will bring reports from other facilities to the interview.

In most cases, the heart of the clinical history is taken during the initial portion of the examination period. The main strategy is that of asking questions of the patient and family to gain information about the problem and to form an impression about the needs, restrictions, and motivations that seem relevant to the clinical problem.

Spouses, children, and other relatives may be helpful in providing such information when the medical problems of some adults limit their participation in gathering the clinical history.

Be sure to have clients sign appropriate forms so that you can request relevant information from other facilities.

How Shall We Interview the Patient and the Family?

Certainly we want to conduct the interview so that, when finished, we will have the information we need. That calls for considerable attention to *what* you want to ask. Before we consider the *what*, let's think about the *how*, the manner with which we talk to the patient and family about the problem.

Let's begin by agreeing that there's no one right way to do this. The patient has come for help and is anxious, if not always able, to tell you what she knows or suspects about the problem and how it affects her life. The patient also may not be aware of the extent of the problem. In the same way, by virtue of our interest in speech-language pathology, we proclaim a strong interest in people and an uncommon skill in talking with them. So the objective is to bring these two motivations together as well as possible for the benefit of the patient. Following are a number of questions that we must think about as we strive to accomplish that objective.

1. Can our manner during an interview be both friendly and professional? It may be difficult to describe in writing what constitutes a friendly manner, but most of us know one when we see one! Certainly, as described in Chapter 2, there may be variations among cultures in what constitutes "a friendly manner." In general, in North American culture, it includes smiles and handshakes. A professional manner is even more difficult to describe but, again, we know it when we see it. It includes discussion focused on the problem, in clear and direct language. It reflects a nonjudgmental attitude that makes it possible for the patient and family to answer questions, to confide, to relate feelings, and to ask questions without undue embarrassment. It assures the patient that all clinical information will be confidential within the appropriate clinical setting. It demonstrates interest and concern about the problem and the patient. It conveys the ability to discuss good news and bad news with equal clarity and compassion.

2. What can we do to foster a professional manner? We can seek to work in a physical environment that is adequate in size, comfortable, attractive but not distracting, and easily accessible to all. We can present a physical appearance that is pleasing, consistent with the standards of the community and work setting. That includes clothing and personal grooming. We can make arrangements about payment for our services (if there is an exchange of money) that are convenient, comfortable, and easily understood.

3. Can we use both technical and everyday language? Yes. Not only can we, but we must. Everyday language is needed to put the patient at ease and to help him feel confident of his ability to talk with you about the problem. Questions put in everyday lan-

Body language is important

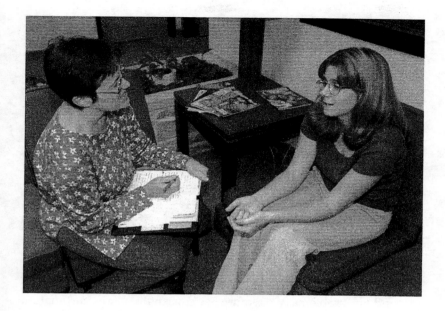

guage will lead to dependable, honest answers that will be useful to your purpose. At the same time, we also use technical language in our discussions. Frequently, technical language is more precise and more descriptive than everyday language: *phonological disorder* tells us more than *doesn't talk clearly* although for many purposes the two terms may be used interchangeably. When we use technical language, we must be certain that the patient knows what the words mean, how to say them, and how they are written (parents are sometimes embarrassed when they learn that *pharyngeal* does not begin with an *f*!). Acquainting the patient and the family with technical language gives them more confidence in their ability to understand the problem and, certainly, to ask better questions in the future.

Don't lose your patients by using professional "jargon."

4. Can we structure the interview for the sake of efficiency and yet make it possible, even easy, for the informant to volunteer information that may be useful? The question indicates the two competing objectives in this regard. In most circumstances, the time available for history taking is limited and so the discussion must be focused carefully to obtain the desired information. Yet it is crucial to pace the interview so that the patient has the easy opportunity to volunteer comments that, from her perspective, are relevant. If they are relevant, we must be prepared with follow up. If they are not, we must be able, in a friendly manner, to move on with the interview.

5. How can we be sensitive to cultural differences that are important to observe in interviewing? Obviously, there is no easy answer here, since North American peoples reflect such a large number of cultures that it would be impossible here to consider

number of cultures that it would be impossible here to consider them all in this regard. The key word, of course, is *sensitive*. That includes clear acknowledgment of the possibility and probability of important cultural differences among us, genuine efforts to learn about them and how they influence our professional practices as a speech-language pathologist, and our best attempts to incorporate these understandings in our daily dealings with patients and families. While sensitivity to these "ethnographic issues" is important during all our clinical activities, it is especially crucial in our first interviews since initial relationships set the stage for all that follows. Useful discussions of these ethnographic issues are provided in Chapter 2 and by Westby (1990), Battle (1998), and Kamhi, Pollock, and Harris (1996).

6. What about confidentiality? The SLP, like all professional workers who deal with human problems, is pledged to keep all information about the patient and her problem in confidence. That means that we maintain privacy of what we know about her and her problems. We require her consent to obtain information about her and her problem gathered as a result of professional services from another clinician, of any kind. One way to do this is to simply ask her to request that the information be sent to us. Another is to make the request ourselves, including her written release of information for this purpose in our request. Confidentiality also means that the results of her evaluation are discussed or shared only with her and with whomever else she gives written consent for that specific release of information. Otherwise we are ethically obliged to restrict our discussions of her problem to those of our colleagues within the institutional setting where we work who might provide additional helpful insights to our overall management of the patient.

7. How can we continue to improve our interviewing skills? We can improve by practice, by reflection, by observing others, by increasing our sensitivity, and by learning more about disorders we treat.

Some additional discussions of interviewing techniques are provided by Evans, Hearn, Uhlemann, and Ivey (1989) and Shipley (1997).

How Do We Ask Questions During a Case History?

Sometimes the clinical history is also called a case history.

We all recognize that the way in which questions are asked can influence the amount, quality, and specificity of the answers. Some types of questions give us factual information, while others clarify information, or give a sense of the informant's feelings about the problem. As we collect background information, we must be aware of the different types of questions and use them appropriately.

Some questions are requests for general information and can be regarded as "open" questions. Some examples are: "What are your concerns about your daughter?" "What do you do when you can't understand your son?" "Tell me about your husband's job" or "Describe your daughter's academic program." While we control the general background areas that are being explored, we do not control the range of responses we receive. Nor do we control how extensively an informant responds. However, open questions often allow us to help the informant expand on issues that need further exploration. These types of questions can even help an informant clarify her own thinking about an issue. Open questions allow the informant to be an active participant in the information-gathering process.

Other questions are ones that the informant can answer with very few words, and can be regarded as "closed" questions. Closed questions have a legitimate place in obtaining background information. For instance, closed questions help us get correct factual information about the patient, such as "What is your son's birthdate?" "Who was the speech-language pathologist who evaluated your wife after her stroke?" and "How old was your daughter when she began receiving remediation?"

Another example of closed questions are those that can be answered "yes" or "no." Yes/no questions can be useful, particularly when very specific information is needed to clarify what areas may need to be discussed further. Examples are: "Does your husband wear a hearing aid?" or "Is your son receiving physical therapy now?" On the other hand, yes/no questions are not likely to stimulate further discussion, and so should be used sparingly in most interview situations.

Another example of closed questions is one in which we provide several possible answers. This type of question can be helpful to the informant in recalling specific information, such as "Did your daughter take her first steps around the time she celebrated her first birthday, or did she do this at a later age?" or "Did a speech-language pathologist talk with your husband before he had his laryngectomy, or was it after the surgery?" After the specific information is recalled, use of other types of questions will help the informant give further expanded information about the situation.

Finally, we need to consider the limitations of an interview that consists solely of question-answer discourse. For many purposes and with many patients and families, the question-answer format needs seasoning with strategies that include "supportive" comments by the interviewer, such as "This is helpful information for me to know" or "I know it's hard to remember some of this information I'm asking for," that encourage the patient to spontaneously continue the discussion of the topic at hand or to change the topic to one not previously included in the interview. The ability to keep the interview on track, yet permit or even encourage such excursions from the routine questions, is the prime example of interviewing skill.

Try to do the question/answer discourse in a natural manner.

What Do We Want to Know?

We begin by carefully reviewing information that has been released to us prior to the appointment. Our interview then begins by asking what the problem is and we listen carefully to the answer. Most often the answer is consistent with our expectations but sometimes it is not. In either case, we continue to discuss the problem until we have a satisfactory understanding. Sometimes we need also to ask to whom this is a problem. Sometimes the answer is surprising. The patient may not consider the "problem" to be a problem; it is a problem to someone around her—parents, teachers, work supervisors. And, sometimes, after the total examination is completed, the "problem" is not considered a "problem" to us either! The information tells us about social, educational, and occupational perspectives of the problem and the patient and will impact how we manage or treat the problem, and the patient.

Next we ask when the problem began and how it has developed. Information about onset provides valuable clues about causes of a number of speech and language disorders and hence appropriate treatments. We ask also how the disorder has developed, seeking to understand whether the severity of the disorder is stable, improving, or worsening. We want to ask also about how troublesome the disorder is and in what ways it interferes with patterns of living (school, work, social interactions, health, etc.).

For many communication disorders, asking about variability of the problem has special significance for planning treatment, and so these questions merit careful consideration. If the answers indicate that the disorder varies, we need to ask specifically about when is it better, and when worse. Of equal importance is the question of whether, today, the disorder is "typical" (or better than usual, or worse than usual). If not typical, and especially if better than usual, we need to find ways to find out the usual severity of the disorder.

Information about previous treatment, or previous efforts to seek treatment, is vitally important. That sets the stage for our examination and treatment planning. We learn what the patient has done previously about the problem and whether she thinks it helped. Did she understand the examination and the recommendations? Did she follow the recommendations? If not, why? Did the problem get better? Sometimes we ask why she came to us rather than continuing with the previous clinical program.

Sometimes we ask the patient and family what they think has caused the problem. The answer provides insight into what the patient understands about the disorder in general and specifically in her case. It will reflect whether his understanding is a reasonable explanation or whether it is based on misconception. Frequently we refer back to this discussion at the end of the examination when we are reporting our findings and our recommendations.

Give careful attention to reports about variability. The information is useful in the later examination.

Another important group of questions are asked for the purpose of understanding family–social–school–work history and the interactions between the communication disorder and that history. For example, whether the patient is an adult or child, we want to estimate family and social relationships and the extent to which they are influenced by the disorder. For some disorders, especially those that have genetic implications, we ask whether other members of the family have this or other disorders of communication. If so, what are the disorders and what is the relationship? Also, has the problem been resolved?

We need information about daily life. We ask the child and his family about school activities. At what grade level is he placed? How is he doing academically? What kind of academic problems does he have? How are they being dealt with? If the child is in preschool, we want to know about child care or preschool arrangements. To what extent are the communication problems causing him problems? We ask the adult about daily life and activities. Again, how is his life influenced by the disorder?

In the school setting, the child's teachers are also valuable informants.

For some speech and language disorders, information is needed about general and specific aspects of health. We ask about a child's developmental patterns, illnesses, disorders, treatment, and medication. We ask the adult about general health, whether there have been diseases, and about their treatment including surgery. Does the informant see any connection between any health problem and this disorder? From whom is health care sought, and is there progress in treatment?

Our major focus in these questions about health is on matters directly relevant to the communication disorder. However, sometimes we need to know about health problems that have indirect relevance. Does she have visual problems or reading problems that interfere with our examination? How might his treatment program for dialysis influence a language therapy program for aphasia? Sometimes these factors become clearly apparent during the interview; other times we find out about them later.

What If the Informant Doesn't Have the Information You Need or Seems Reluctant to Give It?

In many instances, the informant does not have the information needed. Neither she nor her family can tell you much about her medical status or what medical or surgical treatment is planned. She is unclear when she became hoarse and whether the medical doctor who examined her was in general practice or was an otolaryngologist, and what the findings were. Another client is an adopted child, placed at age 4, and not much is known about his early development or his biologic parents. Yet another patient can't remember much about recommendations or treatment provided by a previous speech-language pathologist. If the information is crucial to the diagnosis, every attempt should be made to get it. Usually that requires action by the patient: "Please ask (the local speech pathologist, the special education resource teacher, the school psychologist, the pediatrician, the neurologist, the otolaryngologist, etc.) to send me a report about her findings and plans for treatment." Sometimes we offer to make the request, especially if we want to ask for specific information.

What if the informant seems hesitant to respond to questions or appears hostile? On occasion the patient or family have mixed feelings about the clinical appointment, and show their uncertainty by seeming uncooperative or even antagonistic during the interview. Or their demeanor indicates such feelings even if that is not their intention. The interviewer must be prepared to carry on in the face of such apparent reluctance to cooperate, taking care to explain why certain information is needed. If the perception of noncooperation continues, we must offer to terminate the interview and the clinical examination. In our experience, some offers are refused, with disclaimers that the perception is true, and the interview is continued with more success. Some are accepted, with obvious relief. When that happens, if the patient is inclined, we must offer another appointment or other assistance in a way that the offer can be accepted without loss of face.

How Can We Tell If the Information Given Is Dependable?

Remember to specify in the written report of the interview who provided the information, such as "Mr. Hernandez *stated* that his daughter walked at 24 months of age."

Our expectation is that the information we are provided prior to and/or during the examination is dependable. After all, the patient came, or was brought, to us for assistance and presumably wants to cooperate. Sometimes, however, during the course of the interview we notice sufficient inconsistency among various details that we must repeat questions or ask for further clarification. Usually that clears up the confusion. If not, we proceed as best we can, including in our written report of the interview our concerns about reliability.

When and How Do We Conclude the History?

As indicated earlier, we strive for a balance between a conservative use of time and a need to be complete. We make a judgment call about when we have the necessary information to proceed with the examination. Sometimes the transition between history and examination is indicated verbally. Sometimes we ask: "Is there anything else that you think we should talk about before we proceed?" In other circumstances the transition is hardly apparent. Certainly we all agree that the history taking process continues throughout this and subsequent interviews with the patient, as we learn more and more about the disorder and the patient.

Shall We Use a Previously Prepared Outline as We Ask Our Questions and When We Write Our Report?

Many SLPs prefer to use an outline to assist them in remembering to ask the relevant questions and to use time efficiently. An example of such an outline is presented in Appendix 3A. Other formats include those by Darley and Spriestersbach (1978), Meitus and Weinberg (1983), Haynes and Pindzola (1998), Shipley (1997), and Shipley and McAfee (1998). Other practitioners find it effective to have several leading questions in mind when the interview begins but to allow the informant considerable freedom in determining the direction of the discussion and the interrelationships among the various aspects of the problem. Probably, most of us seek a moderate path between the two extremes.

An outline is very helpful in writing the report, particularly if there is considerable similarity between one patient and another. In such cases, a checklist may even be sufficient. When there are differences among patients in the kind of information needed, each report must be tailor made, or nearly so. Differences in work settings also affect whether reports are written in accord to an outline. Again, it seems probable that most practitioners choose a moderate path between the extremes.

What Else Do We Learn About the Patient and the Problem in Addition to the "Facts"?

The history taking interview gives us, usually, our first impression of the patient as a speaker. We can judge for ourselves her conversational skills, what disorders are apparent, and their severity. We also can make observations about how easy or how difficult it is for her to discuss the problem and any influences it has on her life. We also get an impression of her personal and social interactions. These observations and impressions, so much a part of our clinical science and art, help us connect what we learn about the communication problem to those who live with the problem and who deal with it as best they can.

What Do I Need to Be Aware of When I Am Working With Persons From a Culture Different Than Mine?

As was noted earlier, ours is a multicultural society. As persons and as professionals we all need to be culturally sensitive and strive to be culturally appropriate. To be otherwise will likely negatively impact the patient's trust in you as a professional and your effectiveness in dealing with her and with the communication problem.

Wyatt (1998) addresses many relevant areas of which we need to be aware when dealing with individuals from varied cultures. As part of our preparation for appointments we need to become familiar with the specific cultures of our clients so that we can interact appropriately and conduct an examination which will be helpful to the patient. Factors that Wyatt suggests you need to understand and explore while preparing for an examination include the patient's likely familiarity with the health care system in which you work; beliefs that may impact the procedures you will conduct and how you will conduct them; beliefs about health, illnesses, and disabilities; and knowledge about specific illnesses with communication ramifications that may be prevalent in a particular racial or ethnic group. Issues specific to the case history process include how greetings are made; the "status" you have in the new relationship with the patient; understanding how verbal interactions are started and ended, and how conversational turns are taken; and use of such nonverbals as head-nodding and eye contact.

> Some religions do not permit the videotaping often used as a standard procedure in assessing communication disorders.

What Do We Do When the Patient Does Not Speak English?

When preparing for an examination of a patient who has no knowledge, or limited knowledge, of English, you will need, obviously, to engage a translator. You should schedule a planning conference with the translator so that he has knowledge of the procedures you plan to complete during the examination, including the case history. Reviewing the general areas you plan to explore in the history and previewing the actual evaluation procedures may allow the translator to help you by identifying areas which are culturally biased. Be sure too to give the translator enough time to prepare for the case history and examination since he may not be familiar with all of the vocabulary you will be using! Also be sure that the translator knows that he should translate precisely and should feel free to ask you and the patient for clarification when necessary.

> It takes considerable practice to work with a translator.

If your institution sees many patients with limited-English proficiency, you might consider having all paperwork such as authorizations forms to request information, release of information forms, and fee schedules, as well as history questionnaires, translated into the first language(s) of the patients. Of course, this will depend on the laws of your state regarding the legal status of second languages.

How Can We Use the History Taking Process to Make the Entire Clinical Relationship Effective and Efficient?

By many standards, this initial history taking interview sets the stage for all that follows. We want to show our genuine concern about the patient and her problem so that we can be effective. We want to create an atmosphere in which she has easy opportunity to express her concerns, impressions, and questions. We want to identify as quickly as possible aspects of the disorder for further examination so that time will be well spent. And we want to achieve all these goals as well as possible.

SUMMARY

The clinical history is our personal introduction to the patient. During the history interview, we hear the patient tell us about the problem and how it influences her life. We ask about onset, variability, and previous treatment. We identify her purposes in asking for our assistance. We structure the interview so that our discussion will yield useful information. We also set the pace so that she can ask questions or volunteer comments. During the interview we make our own judgments about the disorder and its severity. We observe the patient during the discussion for indications about attitudes and feelings that are relevant to our purpose. At the conclusion of the history taking interview, we expect to have considerable information to use as our basis for the clinical examination. Further, we expect to have formed a comfortable relationship with the patient so that we can proceed effectively with the evaluation. Later, the information gained during the interview process will become part of a written document, the evaluation report, describing the communication status and the potential impact that the patient's history may have had on the problem.

REFERENCES

Ethnographic Issues

Battle, D. E. (Ed.). (1998). *Communication disorders in multicultural populations* (2nd ed.). Boston, MA: Butterworth-Heinemann.

Kamhi, A. G., Pollock, K. E., & Harris, J. L. (1996). *Communication development and disorders in African American children: Research, assessment and intervention.* Baltimore, MD: Paul H. Brookes.

Westby, C. E. (1990). Ethnographic interviewing: Asking the right questions to the right people in the right ways. *Journal of Childhood Communication Disorders, 13,* 101–111.

Wyatt, T. (1998). Assessment issues with multicultural populations. In D. E. Battle (Ed.), *Communication disorders in multicultural populations* (2nd ed.). Boston, MA: Butterworth-Heinemann.

Interviewing Techniques

Evans, D. R., Hearn, M. T., Uhlemann, M. A., & Ivey, A. E. (1989). *Essential interviewing: A programmed approach to effective communication* (3rd ed.). Pacific Grove, CA.: Brooks/Cole.

Shipley, K. G. (1997). *Interviewing and counseling in communication disorders: Principles and procedures* (2nd ed.). Boston, MA: Allyn and Bacon.

Case History Forms

Darley, F. L., & Spriestersbach, D. C. (1978). *Diagnostic methods in speech pathology* (2nd ed., pp. 58–59, 61–95). New York: Harper and Row.

Haynes, W. O., & Pindzola, R. H. (1998). *Diagnosis and evaluation in speech pathology* (5th ed., pp. 415–417). Boston, MA: Allyn and Bacon.

Meitus, I. J., & Weinberg, B. (1983). *Diagnosis in speech-language pathology* (pp. 60–70). Austin, TX: Pro-Ed.

Shipley, K. G. (1997). *Interviewing and counseling in communication disorders: Principles and procedures* (2nd ed., pp. 233-242). Boston, MA: Allyn and Bacon.

Shipley, K. G., & McAfee, J. G. (1998). *Assessment in speech-language pathology: A resource manual* (2nd ed., pp. 14–16). San Diego, CA: Singular Publishing Group.

RECOMMENDED READINGS

Emrick, L. L., & Haynes, W. O. (1986). *Diagnosis and evaluation in speech pathology* (2nd ed., Chapter 2). Englewood Cliffs, NJ: Prentice-Hall.

Haynes, W. O. & Pindzola, R. H. (1998). *Diagnosis and evaluation in speech pathology* (5th ed., Chapter 2). Boston, MA: Allyn and Bacon.

Meitus, I. J., & Weinberg, B. (1983). *Diagnosis in speech-language pathology*, (Chapters 2, 9, & 10). Austin, TX: Pro–Ed.

Nation, J. E., & Aram, D. M. (1984). *Diagnosis of speech and language disorders* (2nd ed., Chapter 4). San Diego, CA: College-Hill Press.

Peterson, H. A., & Marquardt, T. P. (1994). *Appraisal and diagnosis of speech and language disorders* (3rd ed., Chapter 2). Englewood Cliffs, NJ: Prentice-Hall.

Shipley, K. G., & McAfee, J. G. (1998). *Assessment in speech-language pathology: A resource manual* (2nd. ed., Chapters 1, 2, & 3). San Diego, CA: Singular Publishing Group.

Appendix 3A

Basic Case History Outline*

Name: _____   Date history taken: _____

Birthdate: _____   Interviewer: _____

Address: _____   Informant(s) (Full name and relationship

_____   to speaker): _____

Adapt this outline for appropriateness for child or adult patients

Complaint:

- What do they think the problem is? (State in informant's own words, if possible.)
- Is this the only problem? Are there other concerns as well?

Referral:

- Name of individual or agency making referral.
- Indicate relationship to patient.

History of Speech Problem:

- When did the communication problem begin?
- Age of patient when first regarded as having a communication problem.
- Who first became concerned about the communication problem? Under what circumstances?
- How did the communication problem begin?
- Are there any factors that may have caused the problem?
- Is the problem variable? If so, when does it get better? Worse?
- Have treatment programs been attempted? If so, what type?
- What is the name of the clinician(s) and their agencies with whom the patient has worked?
- Has progress been made with treatment programs? If so, describe the progress.
- Has the patient been seen by any other specialists because of the communication problem? If so, who? When?
- Have family members made any effort to correct problem at home? If so, what has been done?
- Have changes occurred in the communication status as a result of family assistance? If so, describe the changes.
- Has the patient made any effort to improve his or her speech? If so, what has been done?
- Have patient efforts resulted in changes in communication? If so, describe.
- Overall, has the problem changed over time? Has it become better or worse?
- Parents'/family members' estimate of present severity.
- Patient's own estimate of present severity.
- What things have seemed to affect the severity of the problem?
- What is the patient's first language?

(continued)

- Does anyone else in the immediate and extended family have similar, or other types, of communication or educational problems? If so, describe familial relationship to the patient and the communication problems.
- Does the communication problem cause adverse comments or teasing?
- Have adverse comments been made in the patient's presence?
- What is the patient's attitude toward the communication problem? Are there variations in the attitude depending on the situation? Has he or she withdrawn from speaking or other situations because of it?
- What is the attitude(s) of family members toward the communication problem?

Birth and Developmental History

- How was the health of the mother during the pregnancy with the patient? Any illnesses, accidents, injuries, operations? Any medications taken? Any alcohol or substance abuse?
- How long was the pregnancy?
- How long was the labor? How difficult was the labor? What was the type of delivery? Were there any unusual circumstances about the labor and delivery?
- What were the Apgar ratings?
- What was the color of the newborn?
- Did/does the patient have any problems sucking? Swallowing? Chewing? Eating? Choking? Drooling?
- What were the ages for achieving the listed communication milestones?
    Babbling
    Cooing
    First word of any kind
    First word with meaning
    Two-word combinations
    Three-word combinations
    Asking questions with "wh-" words (why, what, when, who, where, how)
- What were the ages for achieving the listed developmental milestones?
    Crawling
    Sitting
    Standing
    Walking
    Riding tricycle/bicycle
    Feeding self finger foods
    Using eating utensils
    Using crayons, pencils, scissors
    Dressing self
    Bladder control
    Bowel control
- What hand does the client prefer to use? How would you estimate the patient's manual dexterity and general coordination?

Medical History

- What is the status of the patient's general health at this time?
- What illnesses has the patient had? Include the age when illness occurred, severity, length, and any complications. Indicate if the patient is currently immunized for any of the illnesses.

Asthma
Bronchitis
Chicken pox
Cytomegalovirus (CMV)
Ear infections
Encephalitis
Hepatitis
Influenza
Measles
Meningitis
Mumps
Pneumonia
Rubella (German Measles)
Sickle cell disease
Whopping cough
Other

- What other medical problems has the patient had? Include age, severity, length, and complications.
Allergies
Colds
Convulsions/Seizures
Croup
Dizziness
Headaches
Noise exposure
Sinusitis
Tinnitus
Other

- What injuries has the patient sustained? Include age, extent of injury, and management.
Broken bones
Lacerations
Other

- What surgeries has the patient undergone? Include age, where operation took place, severity of problem.
- Has the patient been hospitalized? If so, for what problem?
- Is the patient currently taking any prescription drugs? If so, what? For what medical problem? What is the length of time the medication(s) has been taken?
- Does the patient abuse alcohol? Abuse drugs and/or substances?
- What is the present condition of the tonsils and adenoids?
- Is there a history of mouth breathing?
- Does the patient wear glasses or corrective lenses?
- What is the estimated status of hearing and vision?

Educational History

- Did the patient attend preschool? Where? For how long?
- What was the age when the patient entered school?
- Has the patient ever failed or skipped a grade?
- What is the present grade placement, school setting, and school attending?

(continued)

- What kind of grades/evaluations does the patient receive?
- Are there any subjects/classes that are especially difficult for the client?
- Are there any subjects/classes in which the client does especially well?
- Does the patient receive any special academic support services? If so, when were these initiated? How many minutes per day/week is the patient involved with them? Is there a current IEP (Individual Educational Plan)? What are the main objectives of the IEP?
- Has the patient received evaluations because of educational problems? If so, by whom? When? How old was the patient? In what grade was the patient?
- How does the patient get along with teachers and schoolmates?
- If in high school, what are plans following graduation?
- If the patient is an adult, what was the highest grade/degree that was completed? Where was it completed?

Work History

- Is the patient currently employed? If so, where? For how long? What is the work schedule? Who is the employer?
- Has the patient previously been employed? If so, where? For how long?
- What type of educational or vocational training was necessary to prepare for the current job? Where was this completed?

Family an ' Social History

- With whom does the patient live?
- What are the ages of the patient's family members?
- What is the health status of family members?
- Are there other immediate and extended family members who have communication and/or educational problems? If so, describe the problems.
- What are the leisure-time activities of the family and of the patient?
- Does the patient and/or family participate in community activities? If so, what are they?
- Describe family relationships.
- Describe relationships with peers. What are the ages of peers? In what activities do the patient and friends engage?
- How does the patient play when by himself? When he is with friends?
- Describe the discipline practices.
- Describe the personality characteristics of the patient.
- Are there any behavior abnormalities of the patient, e.g., thumb sucking, tempter tantrums, destructiveness, hyperactivity.
- What languages are spoken in the home?

Comments on Interview

- Comment on the subjective aspects of the interview, such as ease of the development of rapport, nature of informant's language behavior, expressive movements, emotional reactions, insight, interest and knowledge about the problem, your perceptions of accuracy of the information given to you.
- Any other important observations.

CHAPTER

4

The Exit Conference

Hughlett L. Morris, Ph.D.

Certainly there is the expectation on the part of the patient/client and family that, after the diagnostic interviews and tests are done, the results will be discussed with them in an exit conference. This expectation is reasonable and must be considered carefully by the clinician. The emphasis is on explaining what has been done; what has been learned; what, if any, new questions have been uncovered; and what to do next.

The word *counseling* has been used by some writers in discussing this clinical transaction. I'm going to avoid that word because, to me, that notion goes beyond the objectives I want to focus on, those just named in the previous paragraph. Counseling implies helping the patient deal with the problem or situation. That intent is frequently part of an exit conference in diagnosis. But, in my view, counseling calls for technical skills beyond the scope of this text. And so I leave that for others to discuss (Crowe, 1997; Dunst, Trivette, & Deal, 1988; Luterman, 1984).

What follows here is a series of questions to be asked by the examining clinician of her or himself as she or he concludes the diagnostic process and prepares to wrap up the session with the patient/client and the family. The beginning clinician most likely will need to be systematic in considering these and other questions before the exit conference. With experience, they come to mind along the way during the examination. Either way, the answers to the questions are the basis for the discussion in the conference. Mind you, I said

> Tell them early on that there will be a wrap-up conference after the examination.

discussion, implying a two-way street. Some of the questions call for information given by the clinician; others, two in particular, call for participation in the discussion by the client/patient and the family.

All of these questions and others that may come to your mind as you think about the matter will, I hope, seem like common sense. That's good, because if they do, it will be easy to remember them and their importance.

One last comment. The productive clinician in a busy clinic is always pressed for time. Diagnosis in speech-language pathology is time consuming, and time is money, regardless of the economic basis for the clinic. But we must always allow sufficient time in the busy schedule for the exit conference. Not to do so will defeat the entire purpose at hand. So try to plan ahead!

In practice, it's really easy to forget this!

THE QUESTIONS

1. Have I got the information, to the best of my ability and the resources available to me, to answer the questions asked by the patient and family when they come for a diagnosis?

Be sure you know the questions!

First, when the appointment is made, there must be some way to determine that the problem is essentially communication, not personal adjustment or medical. Or, stated another way, that the diagnostic appointment is suitable to the purposes of the clinic. If not, everyone involved will be frustrated by the mismatch and the time poorly spent.

At another level, the clinician must examine his information to determine whether he has enough information, or the right kind, to deal with the diagnostic questions with professional confidence. If the answer to either is no, then he must be straightforward in talking about that in the exit conference. That may be unsatisfying to the patient and family, but it's better to be up-front and truthful than to try to conceal the matter.

The issue of "resources available to me" is frequently a problem. If you had more time with the client for interviewing and testing, if you had more precise equipment, if you had more time to research available information about the disorder, if, if, if . . . . But in almost every clinical situation, we deal with limitations. And usually they are not so constraining that we can't proceed in a satisfactory, and ethical, manner. Certainly this matter of needing to do more is related to decisions about referrals, considered in discussions below.

Finally, if over time, the clinician is impressed repeatedly with inadequacies of diagnostic procedures for disorders more and more often encountered, better to do something about that. Pronto. Maybe more training is needed, or additional resources, or a change in the focus of the clinic.

2. Are there other aspects of the communication disorder that the patient and family have not considered or identified in their recognition of the "disorder" and questions they have about it?

This can be tricky. The family asks about a stuttering problem and you do language testing also. And then, in the exit conference, you spend more time talking about language than stuttering. The aphasic woman turns out to be having problems of aspiration during eating. There are other examples of patients for whom the nature of the clinical problem changes character or emphasis during examination. Clearly you want to indicate these shifts in focus as the examination proceeds. Explaining why you are doing what you're doing as you go will minimize the probability of surprises on the part of the patient and family during the conference.

This issue of "other" aspects of the communication disorder, besides the one specifically asked about, brings to mind a warning to us as clinicians. It is that, like the patient and the family, we can focus too easily on one aspect to the exclusion of others. The child with cleft palate may, in addition to indications of velopharyngeal dysfunction, also demonstrate slow development of language skills. The adult with a speech sound disorder may also be disfluent in stressful social situations. Careful history taking and observation throughout the diagnostic session is needed to find out about these "other" problems.

At the same time, we need to guard against being too "long-eared." A child with delayed speech and language may also sound hoarse to your trained ear. The family may be dealing well with the speech and language delay but have not recognized the hoarseness as a problem. Depending on the case, it may be unwise to make such an issue of the hoarseness that they worry about voice also. In this example, of course, as discussed in Chapter 9 (Verdolini), hoarseness in children is frequently observed as a maturation process. So be careful what you stir up!

> Of course, if the patient who is hoarse is an older man, attention must be paid. The symptom might indicate laryngeal cancer!

3. How can I organize my information so as to help the patient and family to understand my understanding of the "problem"?

The rule of thumb here is to begin at the beginning ("As I understand it, your main concern is . . ."). Then tell what you've done ("I did some general testing about . . . and some specific tests about . . ."). Tell what you found ("As you suspected, she clearly has difficulty . . . but she is also doing pretty well in . . ."). Tell them any normed findings if they ask or, depending on the circumstances, even if they don't ask ("On the test of . . . she compared with normal children of age X."). Tell them other observations ("Based on my short time here with him, and in my conversation with him, he's pretty worried about . . . I take that to mean that he would welcome some help.").

Obviously, the above scenario is written toward the family about a child. The language will be different if the patient is an adult, although the approach may well be the same.

There is the issue of whether you encourage or discourage questions along the way. That, of course, is related to the next question to be considered (how to present findings). But it also has to do with organization. I've done it both ways. Sometimes I want very much to present my clinical findings in an orderly way, and to be sure that I don't leave anything to chance or leave some key point out completely. In that case, I might request that no questions be asked until I'm done with my information. The risk here is that you seem to be discouraging questions or even condescending to the patient and family. Other times, I sense that getting the information to them is going to be difficult to accomplish if I'm too assertive. In that case, I encourage them to ask questions along the way and try to keep track of various points to be made as the conversation continues. The risks here are that I may get sidetracked from the main issues and forget something that I intended to include. Getting sidetracked is a particular danger if the person you're dealing with is talkative and intent on telling you about topics that seem irrelevant to the task at hand.

The emphasis on organization is important for communicating your findings, impressions, and recommendations in an efficient, careful way. But organization is also important with regard to time. The more limited is the time for this exit conference, the more important is organization of presentation.

4. How can I best present this information to them so that they regard this diagnostic examination as satisfactory?

We're still talking about the manner in which the information is presented. The last question was about organization. This one is about other aspects.

As we indicated in Chapter 3 (Clinical History), we need here to be both friendly and professional. In taking history, we want to gain cooperation in order to get information we need. In the exit conference, we want to give information in a way that it can and will be received, accepted, and remembered. Use terminology that they are likely to know. Don't talk down to them. Repeat key ideas, using different language. Watch carefully for indications that they are or are not understanding what you are saying. If the news is bad, try to include some good ("She's having problems with this but doing well with that."). Qualify when you need to ("As far as I can tell . . . ," "Our findings today indicate . . ."), but don't go so far as to cast doubt in their minds about what you're telling them; that is, if you are certain of what you are telling them!

In Chapter 2, Westby reminded us of the importance of sensitivity to cultural differences in almost every aspect of diagnosis. Certainly

Especially accepted and remembered.

that is crucial in history taking and equally so in the exit conference when we want to give our information, again, so that it will be well-received, accepted, and remembered. Not only is the verbal language used very important for that purpose but also our demeanor, our attitude (as they perceive it), our body language, our directness, even our manner of eye contact; all may influence the degree to which we communicate with them during this exit conference.

All these hazards are multiplied when the news is bad. The family may have suspected their child was slow to develop language but your comparison of her skills on the normed test really brings it home to them. The man who stutters may have been kidding himself about severity until he had to face up to some of the "difficult" tasks you presented to him. So, in these cases and others like them, we must be especially careful with what we say and how we say it in the wrap-up conference. How you do that may well influence whether they act on your advice about treatment. But resist any urge you have to sugar-coat the findings. You owe it to them to be honest, candid, and straightforward.

Sometimes you will find yourself in the uncomfortable position of reporting findings, impressions, and diagnoses that are contrary to what the patient and family have been told previously, and told by clinicians or others whom they trust. The family doctor says their 8-year-old boy will outgrow the stuttering. A grandmother insists that all the children in her family were slow to talk and they got better on their own. The classroom teacher says the problem is that the child is not trying hard enough. The plastic surgeon who surgically repaired the cleft palate is certain the oral structure is okay and that speech therapy will cure the persistent nasal speech. And on it goes. In cases

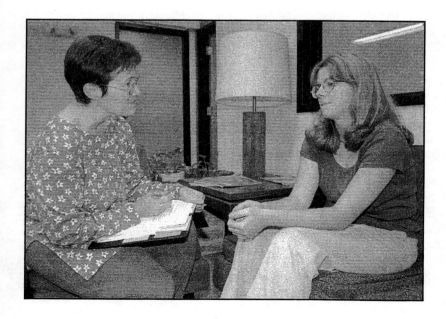

To the degree possible, in circumstances like these, be friendly but firm in your professional opinion.

like this, if you are certain of your findings, stick to them. Explain that though there may be differences of opinion, you are trained to understand and deal with speech and language disorders and that you are confident of your findings and what they mean. And that if they want to get a second opinion, you can suggest sources to locate your colleagues who do the same kind of work as you do. If they continue to be skeptical, do not try to persuade. Restate your position and then terminate the conference, trying to ensure that they feel comfortable in contacting you again should they decide to do so.

5. Do I know enough about the "problem" to recommend treatment (or not)?

There's no way to answer this question in a general fashion. It is a proper question, one that must be answered each and every time at the end of a diagnostic procedure. Understandably, the beginning clinician may have doubts about the findings, more likely the clinical impression, that experienced clinicians may not have. With experience comes perspective. But even the experienced clinician may wonder whether she "knows enough" to make a decision about management. If the decision is for treatment, in this case therapy, the rationale must be clearly identifiable, not only for the patient and family but for the clinician also. The clinician must be able to state clearly on paper, for the world to see, what the goals of therapy are and the time frame within which improvement is expected. Without that specification, the recommendation is open-ended and may well lead to confusion and misunderstanding on the part of everyone. That is especially important when therapy is planned for one aspect of the problem but not another.

Lots of opportunity for confusion here.

An excellent example is the case of therapy planned for delayed language shown by a child with physiological velopharyngeal incompetence, for which speech therapy is not the effective treatment (Chapter 14, Peterson-Falzone). The parents and the surgeon may be misled by the decision to provide therapy, confusing language delay with physiological velopharyngeal incompetence.

Every speech-language pathologist I know sometimes recommends trial therapy. I've done that, many times. It is a good thing to do, for the very objective the label indicates ("I'm not sure this will work but let's try it for awhile, and see"). As before, the clinician needs to specify clearly the objective of the therapy and, in particular, what seems to be a reasonable "trial" period. And certainly an end point, at which time we take stock to see where we are.

Finally we must be aware of the same pitfall that other clinicians face who do both diagnosis and treatment. The danger, of course, is the perception of drumming up business for ourselves. For that reason, we need to be sure that the client and family know about any other speech-language pathologists in the area who provide treatment for this problem.

6. What other diagnostic procedures or examinations might be useful to them?

Obviously this is another version of Question 1: Have I got the needed information? There are many variations. One is that we are pretty sure of the nature of the problem but some fine tuning is needed to be more specific about the underlying mechanisms. Another is that, frankly, we haven't got the expertise and resources to do a proper job of this, and we need help. When this is the case, referral to a colleague in speech-language pathology who specializes in this problem is needed. To discuss that idea, of course, we need to be familiar with our colleagues in the area, and what they do, and how to refer to them.

Get to know your colleagues. This is an important reason, along with continuing education, for membership in and attendance to local and regional professional meetings.

Sometimes we sense or are told outright that the patient and family are skeptical about our diagnosis. In that event, we need to indicate to them, freely, that they may well want a second opinion. And suggest to them how that might be obtained.

Then there is the circumstance in which, in your opinion, the need for assistance is from another professional, technical area: psychology, medicine, dentistry, and so forth. That's good thinking. After all, we are members of the larger healthcare team and we must be aware of the larger picture. Again, referral to a specific physician (or dentist or psychologist) is to be avoided, but rather the referral should be generic, with suggestions about ways to locate an appropriate provider. Usually I try to give the patient and family a written "referral" that they, in turn, give to the other examiner, specifying the status of my examination and why I think additional information of a different kind is needed, and a request for a report about her or his impressions. That takes the burden off the patient and family of having to remember the details of the story.

In this regard, we need to be careful in that referral to avoid asking any question that seems to ask the opinion of another profession whether speech-language therapy might be useful. That determination is ours to make, not theirs. We seek further information of the kind we are not technically qualified to obtain or interpret in order to make the best plan for *our* further treatment of the disorder. On the face of it, this sometimes seems like a matter of semantics, but it is not. The issue is our professional autonomy to diagnose and treat speech and language disorders.

Be careful here.

7. Have I given them sufficient opportunity to ask questions, to express their feelings, and to sort out decisions about what to do next (if anything)?

To the degree that the word *counseling* fits in this sort of exit conference, it fits here. Up until now we've thought mostly about the conference for the purpose of information giving. But clearly this is a two-way street. Whether our information is received effectively will depend on the extent to which we give the client and the family a voice in this discussion. What else do they want to know? What needs to be repeated? Can the message be restated in simpler terms? Are they surprised by my findings, my impressions, and my predictions? Do they want to talk about what's next, or do they need more time to think about it?

Sometimes it is really difficult to allocate enough time to deal with this question. We are inclined to be quick and to the point about what we found and what we make of what we found, tell

Personally, I have to work hard to do this.

them what we think is next, and thank them and say goodbye. And sometimes that's all we need to do. But we must not be so routine in our attitude and our conduct that we miss indications, overt or not, that more is needed. Certainly that is the case when the news is "bad" or unexpected. But it may also be true otherwise. We must be always sensitive to the need to spend that extra bit of time!

SUMMARY

The mission of diagnosis in speech–language pathology is not completed until the findings and clinical impressions are discussed with the patient and family in ways which they can easily understand. Usually, that takes place in the exit conference. Here we have considered the process mainly as one in which the clinician makes her best attempt to share what she has learned and what she makes of it. The last question posed emphasized the fact that in many instances the process is also a dialogue between the clinician and the client and her family. Taken farther, the word *counseling* has been used to describe this dialogue. We consider that important but beyond the scope of this text to be described in any further detail.

Rather our focus is on technical competence of the examining clinician and his ability to apply the models described in Chapter 1 (Tomblin) to arrive at a clinical impression of the speech-language disorder based on his best efforts at history and examination.

Now follow discussions of specific disorders in which some of these technical aspects are described, remembering always the necessity to consider characteristics of the patient and the family, and the cultural context in which they live.

REFERENCES

Crowe, T. A. (Ed.). (1997). *Applications of counseling in speech-language pathology and audiology.* Baltimore, MD: Williams and Wilkins.

Dunst, C., Trivette, C., & Deal, A. (1988). *Enabling and empowering families.* Cambridge, MA: Brookline Books.

Luterman, D. M. (1984). *Counseling the communicatively disordered and their families.* Austin, TX: Pro–Ed.

CHAPTER

5

The Oral Mechanism

Penelope K. Hall, M.A.

As you know by now, the clinical process is one of asking questions with the goal of solving problems. Questions that must be asked for each and every client or patient include: "Are there any problems with the mouth that might be the cause of, or contribute to, the communication disorder?" and "If there are problems with the mouth, what specific communication disorders might we suspect?" The purpose of this chapter is to help you determine what observations need to be made, and then explain how to interpret these observations in order to answer the question of possible relationships between the structures and the functioning of the speech-producing mechanisms and the presenting communication problems.

Mouths and oral structures come in a variety of shapes and sizes and with different degrees of mobility. Some of the observations discussed in this chapter will give you only gross, general information. Some are of uncertain reliability, especially for the beginning clinician. Some yield only approximations of the information you are seeking, with more precise information requiring instrumentation that is not readily available in most clinic settings. But despite these limitations, a diagnostic examination for a speech and/or language problem needs to include a careful evaluation of the peripheral oral mechanism. Thus, clinical judgment, gained from your clinical experiences, will form the basis for many of the interpretations you will need to make when evaluating structural and functional adequacy of a patient's oral mechanism.

Even general information about the oral mechanism can be helpful.

This chapter presents fairly extensive and detailed descriptions of tasks and observations to be made when evaluating the function of the speech mechanism. It is hoped that these will be helpful in your learning about the procedures themselves and how to interpret them. However, it is stressed that during a single diagnostic evaluation you will seldom complete all the tasks presented in the chapter. Instead, you will be selective and complete tasks which will help answer the specific questions asked of you or that you have developed for each of your individual clients.

WHY DO WE WANT TO ASSESS THE SPEECH MECHANISM?

In the minds of many people, "speech" is the most readily apparent part of the communication process. And, if there are problems with "speech," the problem must be related to how the mouth works, because "speech" is produced by the mouth. Further, the "speech" problem might be solved by "fixing" the part of the mouth that is "broken" or "not working well." Even though this is not the case for most speech and language problems, it is true for some communication disorders. As a result, the speech-language pathologist must be skillful in estimating the degree to which the oral structures and functioning are normal. When conducting an examination of the speech mechanism we evaluate the face, lips, tongue, teeth, hard palate, soft palate, and pharynx.

WHAT DO WE WANT TO LEARN ABOUT THE SPEECH MECHANISM?

We examine the oral mechanism to answer our questions about how adequate each structure of the mechanism is for the production of speech, and how well each structure functions for the production of speech. To determine adequacy for speech production, each physical structure within the mechanism and the function of each structure needs to be evaluated individually and then, again, as part of the entire mechanism. From these observations, we can make estimates about the speech mechanism's structural and functional adequacy, each of which must be considered separately, as they are very different aspects.

Structural adequacy deals with the normalcy of the structures and their normalcy in relationship to each other. Some questions to ask about structural adequacy include: Is the tongue normal in size and appearance? Is there an unrepaired cleft palate? Are any front teeth missing? Also, assessment of the structural adequacy of the speech mechanism includes whether any problems of the physical structures might interfere with speech production. *Functional adequacy* is concerned with how well these structures, regardless of intactness and relationships to each other, move and perform during speech production. For example, the following questions may give you information about the functional adequacy of the speech mechanism: Does the tongue move normally? Is there the ability to open and close the velopharyngeal port rapidly?

Attempting to understand the difference between structural adequacy and functional adequacy is fundamental to the evaluation of the peripheral speech mechanism. Also, it is important to understand that problems with structures of the mechanism may or may not be related to the functional use of the mechanism for speech. For example, your client's mechanism may exhibit many structural "problems," but function adequately for speech. In contrast, another patient's mechanism may be structurally "perfect," but may not have adequate function during speech.

Some structural abnormalities are present from birth and are known as congenital problems. An example is cleft lip and/or palate. Structural abnormalities may also be acquired through accidents or diseases, such as traumatic injuries to the mouth or surgical removal of parts of the oral structures because of cancer.

> See Chapter 14 for more information on cleft lip and palate and Chapter 13 for additional information on head and neck cancer.

Frequently, assessment of the functional adequacy of the oral mechanism is more difficult than assessing the structural adequacy. In arriving at judgments, the speech-language pathologist looks at the *rate* at which speech productions, or movements, are performed, as well as the *accuracy* of the productions. As with structural abnormalities, difficulties with the functional adequacy of the speech mechanism may be the result of developmental problems, problems acquired as a result of trauma or disease, or may simply be for reasons unknown. We may find problems with the functional adequacy of the speech mechanism in patients exhibiting cerebral palsy and those who have had neurological insults as the result of strokes, traumatic accidents, and neurological system cancers. These functional problems sometimes may be more narrowly specified, such as dysarthria or apraxia. For other clients, problems in functional adequacy may be apparent even though the basis for the problem is not clear. With still other clients and patients you will find problems in the function of the speech mechanism during speech, but will be unable to describe it as a specific type of disorder; in these cases the mouth just doesn't seem to "work" very well during speech.

> Discussions about dysarthria and apraxia are continued in Chapters 7 and 12.

HOW MAY WE LEARN ABOUT THE SPEECH MECHANISM?

With the majority of your clients, the evaluation of the speech mechanism will be a clinical procedure that relies heavily on observations, estimates, and clinical judgments. There are a few direct measurements that can be made, such as the dimensions of a cleft palate and the measurements of dental occlusion and dental relationships.

> Clinical judgments are often required when conducting a speech mechanism examination.

However, the relationships between these measurements and the production of speech are unclear. Further, the equipment to perform these and other measurements is often not readily available to most speech-language pathologists, nor have most speech-language pathologists been trained to make the measurements.

There are some tasks that have been standardized through "norm-referenced" information that will help you in interpreting a patient's performance on a task. These norms compare a given client's performance of a specific task to the performance of a group of persons with "normal" speech doing the same task. "Norm-referenced" information is available for some tasks used to assess the speech mechanism, such as some diadochokinetic rates. Such norm-referenced information may be helpful in understanding the functional adequacy of a client's mechanism. The norms can also be used to obtain "client-referenced" information, as when we compare a particular patient's performance on assessment tasks conducted across time. Client-referenced information can be particularly helpful in determining if there has been a change in the client's performance over a period of time. These changes may indicate that such aspects as remediation, maturation, or spontaneous recovery have or have not helped the patient use the speech mechanism with improved rate and accuracy during specific tasks.

WHAT EQUIPMENT DO WE NEED?

There are a few pieces of equipment that you will need when conducting an examination of the peripheral oral mechanism. A flashlight is essential for observation of the structures and movements at the back of the mouth. Other equipment you will need includes sterile, individually wrapped tongue depressors; a stopwatch; and a small mirror that will fit comfortably under a patient's nostril, sometimes known as a "nasal mirror." The use of examination gloves also is required when doing a physical examination of the oral cavity.

HOW DO WE ASSESS THE SPEECH MECHANISM AND WHAT MIGHT OUR FINDINGS MEAN?

Test Forms

The physical examination of the speech producing mechanism goes by various names, including the "speech mechanism examination," "oral mechanism examination," "peripheral speech mechanism examination," "oral peripheral examination," and "orofacial examination."

There are a number of formats that can be used as the basis of your assessment. Some of these forms providing an outline for recording results are commercially available, with others having been developed by clinicians working to solve their own professional assessment needs. Some forms are very general, while others are developed for very specific populations of clients with communication disorders. A list of forms is included at the end of the chapter under Recommended Readings.

Speech mechanism examination forms should be thought of as "guides" to help you organize your assessment and observations, ensuring that your evaluation is comprehensive. Although the actual organization of the assessment forms will vary and the suggested tasks may differ, most address the structural and functional adequacy of the various parts of the face, mouth, and oral cavity.

Diadochokinetic Tasks

A special type of task is often used in examination of the oral mechanism. Patients are asked to attempt "diadochokinetic" tasks to evaluate the functional adequacy of the oral mechanism. These tasks call for the rapid repetition of either a speech or nonspeech task. The purpose is to assess how *consistently, accurately,* and *rapidly* the patient is able to make the repeated movements. Diadochokinetic tasks place "stress" on the speech mechanism, because we rarely (if ever) use our most rapid possible rate of speech. But when the maximal movement or speech rate is attempted, you have the opportunity both to observe how well the mechanism works as a whole and to assess how well the individual articulators function in the task.

There are two ways in which diadochokinetic tasks are performed. In the first method, the client produces the speech or nonspeech task for a specified period, often 5 seconds, which is then repeated for a total of three or more trials. The average number of productions *per second* is then calculated. The second method involves having the patient produce a specified number of productions or movements, with the speech-language pathologist timing the trial to determine how much time the client needs to complete the entire task.

Norms are available for some of these diadochokinetic tasks, although there are two reasons why the norms should be used with caution. First, much of the research that includes diadochokinetic information was conducted with small subject groups. Second, the age groups for which the norms were developed are sometimes very narrow or, in other cases, are not precisely specified. Available research findings also indicate that diadochokinetic rates increase with age, starting at age 2 years, 6 months. However, when norms are available for a task, an "average" performance range, summarized from the research literature, will be reported in the margin notes in this chapter. It is hoped this placement will help you quickly find the information when needed. However, you may find it helpful to memorize these average rates, which can assist you in evaluating the function of the mechanism. At the end of the chapter is a reference list that contains the sources of these diadochokinetic norms.

Diadochokinetic tasks involve repetitive movements or speech sounds, such as repeating the syllable "tuh" or opening and closing the lips as fast as possible.

Speech Versus Nonspeech Tasks

The function of many of the oral structures is assessed using several different types of tasks: tasks that involve nonspeech movements and tasks that involve speech movements. Comparing the performance of the various parts of the mechanism for these varying tasks will help you to determine if there are problems with the mechanism and, if so, of what type. However, there is disagreement about the degree to which information about nonspeech movements is predictive of speech movements. Even if they are not predictive, the use of nonspeech tasks in your speech mechanism examination will give you some idea of how well the structure can function in various ways. This includes the range of movement, the duration of movement, and the strength of movement. The *range* of movement indicates how far a structure, such as the tongue, is able to move. The *duration* of movement indicates how long a single or repeated movement can be maintained or sustained. The *strength* of movement indicates how well a structure can achieve and maintain a position when an external force is applied.

There is additional discussion of speech and nonspeech tasks used diagnostically in Chapter 12 (Clark, Stierwalt, & Robin).

Getting Started

It is best to establish a degree of rapport with the patient before conducting the oral peripheral examination because some clients are hesitant to have you look into their mouths. Before you begin the actual examination, briefly explain what you will be doing and why it is an important part of the total diagnostic evaluation. Remember that for some clients the things we are asking them to do may be new to them or they may feel uncomfortable in performing them. Some young children may even refuse to do the tasks or will do so only after you go to considerable efforts to make a series of "games" or "challenges" out of the tasks. Explanations and encouragement help assure patients that you respect them and their dignity.

WHAT KINDS OF OBSERVATIONS AND EVALUATIONS DO WE MAKE?

The Face

The face is a part of the speech mechanism evaluation because of the important role facial expression plays in nonverbal communication. The examination will give you clues about muscle weakness and possible problems with the innervation of the face and mouth, which can be associated with problems of speech production as well as facial expression. Such problems need to be documented and may also give us hints that other parts of the speech mechanism, such as the tongue, might also demonstrate similar problems.

Part of the assessment of the face can be done by observing the client during conversation, perhaps as part of rapport-building or as you obtain background information. Look at the external features of the face: the forehead, nose, lips, and jaw. Look at the general symmetry of the face when it is at rest. Is there a drooping of the corner of the mouth? Is an eyelid partially or completely closed? Is the mandible, or jaw, drooping on one side?

The symmetry of the face can also be assessed by asking the patient to make specific movements. Ask him to open his mouth as far as possible. Does the jaw move, or deviate, to one side or the other? Can he raise both of the eyebrows? Can he close both eyes tightly?

Please see Figure 5–1 to review the structures associated with the nose and lips.

Summary of Procedures

To assess the structural adequacy of the face you can ask the client to do the following after having observed the general symmetry with the face at rest:

1. Open the mouth as far as possible.

2. Raise both eyebrows.

3. Close both eyes tightly.

Lip Structure

The lips are very important in the production of speech; they are used to impound the air for the plosives /p/ and /b/, to restrict air flow for the fricatives /f/ and /v/, and to help shape the oral cavity in the production of vowels. The ability to seal the lips so that they remain closed is important in the swallowing process by holding food or liquids within the mouth. Deviations in the structure of the lips may interfere with these roles. We must also recognize that the entire oral mechanism has a great capacity to compensate for and overcome structural problems.

There are several observations you need to make of the lips when they are at rest. Look for symmetry, general contour, or shape of the mucocutaneous ridge, and the condition of the lips. A lack of symmetry may indicate the presence of a neuromotor problem and may be apparent as you look at general facial symmetry. Does there seem to be an adequate amount of vermilion tissue in the lips? Can the lips be closed? Do you observe drooling? Does the lip tissue appear healthy or are there indications of inflammation, infection, or growths that might need medical attention?

You also may see a cleft lip, which may be a unilateral (on one side only) cleft or a bilateral cleft. The cleft may not have yet been repaired, particularly in infants and very young children. For most

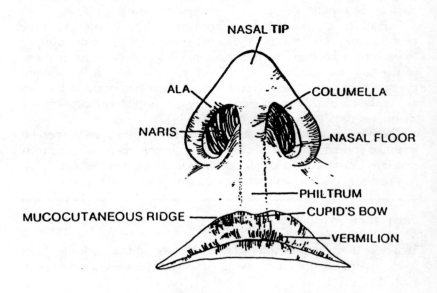

Figure 5–1. Physical structures of the lip and nose. (From Meitus, I. J., & Weinberg, B., *Diagnosis in Speech Language Pathology.* Boston: Allyn & Bacon, 1983. Reprinted with permission.)

patients, however, look for a scar line in the nose and lip areas that may indicate a cleft lip repair. Remember that not all scars in the lipline are the result of a cleft lip repair. If present, note the shape of the scar(s) and how tight the tissue appears to be.

Lips are usually very mobile and, as stated previously, are used to compensate for many structural deviations. Thus, the explosion of air needed to produce the /p/ or /b/ sounds can usually be achieved even if either the upper or lower lip is very short or thin. Clinical and research findings tell us that, except in extreme cases, even an unrepaired cleft lip does not cause significant problems with speech sound production. However, you must look at the "total client" and question the possible negative impact of a scarred and uneven upper lip on the person's self-concept and personal adjustment.

Summary of Procedures

To assess the structural adequacy of the lips, you can make a number of observations.

1. Observe the lips at rest for symmetry, contour, condition, and an adequate amount of tissue.

2. Observe any presence of scar tissue.

Lip Function

Nonspeech Movements

There are a number of nonspeech tasks that you may use to assess lip function. You may begin by asking the client to make "static" movements, movements that are made and then "held in place." Examples are the unilateral retraction of the lips to each side of the face and the bilateral retraction of the lips. Remember, this is not a "smile," so requesting a smile for this movement is an inappropriate "prompt," (things that clinicians can do to help their client's attempts to achieve success with the requested movement or speech act).

The adequacy of lip function also needs to be assessed with nonspeech diadochokinetic tasks that require the lips to move, as opposed to remaining in static positions. An often-used task is to have the patient alternatively protrude and retract the lips by giving her the directions to "pucker, then smile, pucker, then smile," and so on. This is an example of a "reciprocal" movement task where the lips alternately make a series of backward and forward movements. Another task is to ask the patient to approximate, or open and close, the upper and lower lips without making any speech sounds. While the client is performing these series of movements, be sure to look for the symmetry of the movement, how easily the movement seems to be made, how rapidly the movements are made, and how long the client is able to continue making the movement series.

> The normal adult is able to open and close the lips without sound 5–6 times per second.

Clients who have problems accomplishing these nonspeech movements with their lips may have neuromotor deficits, which, in turn, require further evaluation and may result in referrals for medical examination. Or, the client may have a history that indicates neurological problems, so the problems the client has in making nonspeech movements may not be a surprise to you. However, when you observe patients having problems with nonspeech movements, you should not automatically assume that these are caused by underlying neurological problems. Perhaps the requests seemed "silly" and unnecessary to the client. Perhaps they are movements that the patient has seldom made and are, therefore, "unpracticed." Should you suspect the latter, the client's performance may improve in subsequent trials with the tasks.

You may find that prompts using the patient's auditory, visual, and tactile-kinesthetic sensory modalities are necessary to help achieve the best performance the person is capable of giving on nonspeech tasks. These sensory prompts are often used in a hierarchy, so that at first only verbal requests are made by the speech-language pathologist. If the client has problems performing the task after receiving only auditory cues, you can provide visual cues by modeling the movements yourself and/or using a mirror for the patient to visually self-monitor after watching you. If the visual clues do not result in successfully made movements, you can provide tactile cues by lightly touching the part of the face that is to make the movement.

Summary of Procedures

Nonspeech tasks that may help you assess the functional adequacy of the lips are:

1. Unilateral retraction of the lips to each side of the face.

2. Bilateral retraction of the lips.

3. Series of "pucker, smile."

4. Series of upper and lower lip approximations.

Speech Movements

A reciprocal speech movement task that can be used to help assess the functional adequacy of the lips, and that is diadochokinetic in nature, involves asking the client to make a series of the vowels /u/ and /ɪ/ (e.g. /uiuiuiui/ etc.). Remember that this task is different than the nonspeech task of completing a "pucker, smile" series. There are no known norms for this task, so you need to observe accuracy, smoothness, and rate during the task. Another diadochokinetic speech task used to assess the functional adequacy of the lips is the diadochokinetic repetition of the monosyllable /pʌ/ ("puh").

The normal diadochokinetic rate for /pʌ/ is 3–6 per second for c   dren, and 6–7 per secondfor adults.

Summary of Procedures

The functional adequacy of the lips during speech can be assessed by:

1. Repetitions of /uiuiui/.

2. Repetitions of /pʌ/.

Lip Strength

The strength of the labial seal can be assessed by asking the patient to puff out each, and then both, cheeks, sealing the air by tightly closing the lips. Then, you gently press on each cheek, and both cheeks, with the flat of your hand to see if the labial seal is broken with the air escaping out the mouth.

Summary of Procedures

The strength of the lip seal can be evaluated by:

Requesting that the patient puff out the cheeks, then pushing against each cheek, and both cheeks.

Teeth

Teeth are involved in the production of a number of consonant sounds by channeling the airstream. These phonemes are the labiodental (/f/, /v/), the linguidentals (/θ/, /ð/), and the fricatives (/s/, /z/, /ʃ/, /ʒ/). As the teeth are easily observable, dental deviations are often blamed as the cause of a speech sound disorder. In fact, this may or may not be correct. We need to be very aware that most speakers are able to make major compensations for dental deviations, such as children who continue to produce correct /s/ and /z/ sounds despite the loss of primary ("baby") central incisors and the gradual growth of new, larger, permanent teeth. But it is important to be able to identify clients whose dentition actually may be a factor in their communication problems.

You need to learn the names of teeth and the typical ages when the permanent teeth emerge. This information is important because you may be dealing with children who are in the process of losing their deciduous teeth and gaining their permanent ones, as shown in Table 5–1.

You must also assess the dental "occlusion," which is the relationship of the upper and lower dental arches and the alignment of the teeth when the jaw is closed. This is done by telling the client to "bite down" on the back teeth and then to spread the lips or to "show the gums," which prevents the client from thrusting the jaw forward. This allows you to see the first upper and lower molars easily, which is crucial to the determination of occlusion.

Many dentists use the Angle classification system to describe occlusion and malocclusion, and you also will find our adaptations of it helpful.

The four occlusions with which you need to be familiar are:

1. *Normal occlusion*
   The cusps, or points, of the first upper molar should fit into the "groove" between the two anterior and posterior cusps of the lower molar. A handy way to think of normal occlusion is that the mandibular (lower) first molar is "half a tooth ahead" or in front of the maxillary (upper) first molar, as shown in Figure 5–2. It is important to keep in mind that a normal occlusion is not the "average" occlusion. Very few individuals have an occlusion that is "normal" in every way.

   You will need to modify this evaluation for young children who do not have permanent first molars. For these youngsters, you can examine the most posterior teeth that are in place. Then, line them up the same way you would when viewing the first permanent molars.

2. *Neutroclusion (or Angle's Class I)*
   When a person presents with a neutroclusion, the upper and lower dental arches are in correct occlusion, but individual teeth are misaligned. For instance, a tooth, or teeth, may be rotated or teeth may be jumbled.

Table 5–1. Eruption of dentition.

Teeth	Age of Eruption
PRIMARY DENTITION	
Maxillary	
Central incisor	7.5 months
Lateral incisor	9 months
Cuspid	18 months
First molar	14 months
Second molar	24 months
Mandibular	
Central incisor	6 months
Lateral incisor	7 months
Cuspid	16 months
First molar	12 months
Second molar	20 months
PERMANENT DENTITION	
Maxillary	
Central incisor	7–8 years
Lateral incisor	8–9 years
Cuspid	11–12 years
First bicuspid	10–11 years
Second bicuspid	10–12 years
First molar	6–7 years
Second molar	12–13 years
Third molar	17–21 years
Mandibular	
Central incisor	6–7 years
Lateral incisor	7–8 years
Cuspid	9–10 years
First bicuspid	10–12 years
Second bicuspid	11–12 years
First molar	6–7 years
Second molar	11–13 years
Third molar	17–21 years

Source: Adapted from *Pediatric Dentistry: Infancy Through Adolescence* by Pinkham, J. R., Casamassimo, P. S., Fields, H. W., McTigue, D. J., and Nowak, A. J., 1988. Philadelphia: W. B. Saunders Company. Adapted with permission.

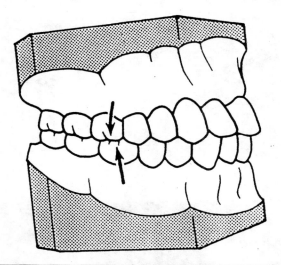

Figure 5–2. Normal occlusion. The arrows indicate the normal occlusion relationship of the first molars. From "Speech Defects Associated with Dental Malocclusions and Related Abnormalities" by H. H. Bloomer, 1971, (p. 727). In *Handbook of Speech Pathology and Audiology*, L. E. Travis (Ed.) Englewood Cliffs, NJ: Prentice-Hall. Reprinted with permission.

3. *Distoclusion (or Angle's Class II)*

A distoclusion occurs when the lower dental arch, or mandible, is "too far back" in relation to the upper dental arch or maxilla. This is apparent when you align the upper and lower first molars, as illustrated in Figure 5–3. It often also is apparent when the individual's mouth is closed, because the chin looks as if it is receding.

4. *Mesioclusion (or Angle's Class III)*

Mesioclusion exists when the mandible is "too far forward" in relation to the maxilla. Thus, the lower dental arch overlaps the upper dental arch, which can be observed when you align the first molars, and as seen in Figure 5–3.

You also will need to be familiar with several other aspects of dentition as you conduct your speech mechanism examination. One involves the relative positions of the front (anterior) parts of the upper and lower arches. These terms and explanations are:

Openbite is the lack of contact between the upper and lower anterior teeth (incisors, cuspids, and bicuspids) when the first molars are in normal occlusion. (See Figure 5–4.)

Overbite, or *closebite,* is the excessive vertical overlapping of the lower anterior teeth by the upper anterior teeth, as shown in Figure 5–4. The upper central incisors normally cover one-half to one-third of the lower central incisors.

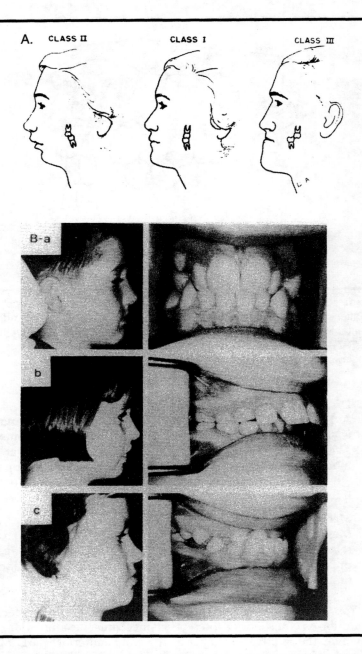

Figure 5–3. **A.** Three types of malocclusions showing Angle's classification, facial profile and relationship of the first molars. Left to right are: distoclusion (Class II), neutroclusion (Class I) and mesioclusion (Class III). **B.** Photographs of dental occlusions and affects on profiles. B-a shows a balanced profile of a child with a neutroclusion; B-b illustrates a profile with a receding chin and a distoclusion with an overjet (note how the lips reflect the overjet); and B-c reveals a lip posture in profile which reflects the mesioclusion. (From *Cleft Palate Speech* [2nd ed.], by B. J. McWilliams, H. L. Morris, & R. L. Shelton, 1990, p. 91. Philadelphia: Mosby-Year Book, Inc. Reprinted with permission.)

OVERJET   **OVERBITE**   **OPENBITE**

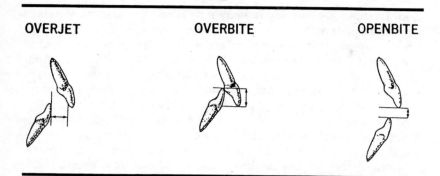

Figure 5–4. Illustrations of overjet, overbite, and openbite. *Overjet* is horizontal projection of the upper incisors in front of the lower incisors. *Overbite* is the overlapping of the upper anterior teeth over the lower anterior teeth vertically. *Openbite* is the vertical distance between the upper and lower incisors that are not overlapping. (From "Orthodontic problems in children" by D. J. Hall & D. W. Warren, 1983, p. 966. in *Pediatric Otolaryngology, Volume II*, C.D. Bluestone, & S. E. Stool, Eds. Philadelphia: W. B. Saunders. Reprinted with permission.)

Crossbite is a lateral, rather than a parallel, overlapping of the upper and lower dental arches. When a crossbite occurs, it appears as if the lower jaw is located either to the right or left of a normal, central position relative to the upper jaw.

Overjet is the excessive horizontal distance between the surfaces of the incisors, as illustrated in Figure 5–4. The upper central incisors are normally 1–3 mm ahead of the lower central incisors. An overjet is sometimes seen in children who have a history of thumb sucking.

Underjet is a lack of normal horizontal distances.

In addition, there are terms that describe the relative positions of individual teeth in the dental arch. These are:

Labioversion (a tooth tilting toward the lip)

Buccoversion (a tooth tilting toward the cheek)

Linguaversion (a tooth tilting toward the tongue)

Edentulous space(s) (a missing tooth or teeth)

Supernumerary/extraneous teeth (extra teeth)

While you are conducting this portion of the speech mechanism examination, be sure to note the general, overall condition of the teeth. How clean do the teeth appear to be? Are there any spots or areas that could be caries, or cavities?

You also can encounter several different types of dental appliances or prostheses while conducting a speech mechanism examination. *Dentures* are commonly known as false teeth, and may consist of all the upper and/or lower teeth, or only selected groups of teeth. There may be *orthodontic appliances* (braces). Do not be surprised to see orthodontic appliances on adults as well as children, as orthodontia is helpful to persons of all ages. *Obturators* and *palatal lift appliances* are similar in appearance to the more familiar dental retainers used in orthodontia, except that they are longer and have bulb-like structures at the end. These are very special prosthetic appliances constructed to help the speech become easier to produce and to understand when there are problems with the function of the soft palate and velopharyngeal mechanism. These situations are addressed later in this chapter and in Chapter 14.

You need to evaluate dentition because of the possibility that dental abnormalities *may* have adverse effects on speech production. Sometimes you may conclude that there is a relationship between missing or misaligned incisors and errored productions of the fricative phonemes, such as the client who distorts sibilants (/s/, /z/, /ʃ/, /ʒ/, etc.) and who also has incisor dentition problems. Occasionally misaligned teeth may also intrude into the shape or the size of the mouth and result in speech errors. An example of this may be with a child who is unable to make the bilabials /p/ or /b/ because of an overjet of the upper incisors. Instead, the child may make a labiodental stop that closely resembles an /f/. The presence of dental appliances may cause some potential problems in how the tongue moves and where it is placed during speech attempts. However, the oral mechanism is able to compensate for many dental deviations.

Summary of Procedures

The dentition should be structurally assessed by:

1. Noting dental development and condition of teeth.

2. Observing the occlusion.

3. Observing any deviations in the positions of the anterior teeth.

4. Observing any deviations in the position of other individual teeth.

5. Noting dental appliances or prostheses.

Tongue Structure

The tongue is used in speech to channel and obstruct the air stream in the production of consonants. It also influences vowel productions and voice resonance by contributing to the shape of the oral cavity. Further, it is crucial in the process of swallowing.

Tongues vary in size and shape, as do overall mouth sizes (Figure 5–5). The size and shape of the tongue and mouth must be appropriately related to one another and they usually are. The determination of this relationship is a subjective judgment about which you will develop confidence with clinical experience.

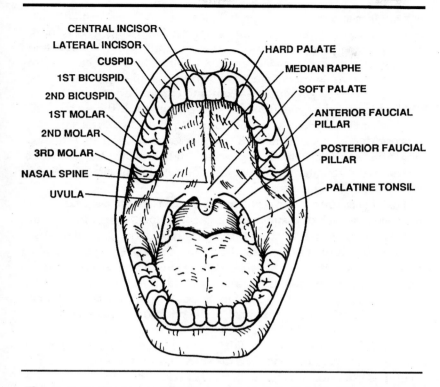

Figure 5–5. The physical structures of the mouth. (Adapted from *Diagnosis in Speech-Language Pathology* by I. J. Meitus, & B. Weinberg, Eds., 1983, p. 43. Austin, TX: Pro-Ed. Adapted by permission.)

You begin your assessment of the tongue's structure by observing it at rest. Note the size of the tongue. Does it appear to be atrophied (shrunken) or furrowed on one side? Are there any fasciculations (involuntary movements) seen with the tongue at rest? Are there any other involuntary contractions or twitches along the edges of the tongue? Next, ask the patient to protrude the tongue as far as possible. Does the tongue deviate to one side? If so, this may indicate a weakness in the musculature or innervation on one side. Should this be the case, the tongue deviates *toward* the side on which there is a problem. This is because the muscles on the affected side are unable to exert enough force to "balance" the force produced on the unaffected side—thus, the tongue moves toward the weaker side. Does the tongue protrude very little or not at all? This may be an indication that there is a bilateral weakness in the musculature or innervation. Any of these problems may indicate that there is peripheral nerve damage, which can result in a neuromotor speech problem known as dysarthria, or in swallowing problems, known as dysphagia.

You also will need to determine if there is tissue missing from the tongue. This information can be obtained during the case history or during the oral mechanism examination. Missing tongue tissue will have most likely resulted from injury or surgical removal,

Dysphagia will be more completely discussed in Chapter 15. Assessment procedures of this disorder exceed the scope of this chapter.

called glossectomy. Total or partial glossectomy is performed when there is a disease process, notably cancer. Following glossectomy, the remaining part of the tongue is frequently very adaptable and capable of compensatory movements. The resulting speech may not be evaluated as "normal," but may be understandable, although the extent of the excision must be taken into consideration.

Next, look at the general condition of the tongue. Is there a coating? If so, what is the color? A coating on the tongue may reflect a disease process, the client's general health, or medication the person is taking. Also note whether there are any lesions on the surface, underside, or edges of the tongue. If so, medical consultation is needed, as the lesion(s) may be cancerous.

The *lingual frenum* or *frenulum* also needs to be assessed. The frenum is the web of tissue that connects the underside of the tongue to the floor of the mouth at the midline of the tongue. You can observe this structure as you investigate the underside of the tongue. You also need to observe the possible effects of the length of the frenum while the tongue is protruded. If the frenum is short, the anterior, or front, part of the tongue may be limited in the amount of protrusion it is able to make. The resulting appearance of the protruded tongue is that the anterior portion is "heart-shaped" because of the frenum's inability to allow for the extension of the midline of the tongue. The center of the tongue tip is thus unextended as the surrounding tissue of the tongue margin is extended, giving the heart-shaped appearance.

> When the lingual frenum is determined to be too short and restricts tongue movement, a "tongue tie" may be said to be present.

Summary of Procedures

The structure of the tongue can be assessed by the following tasks:

1. Observing the tongue at rest for shape, completeness, and condition.

2. Asking the patient to protrude the tongue.

3. Observing the length of the lingual frenum.

Tongue Function

The normal tongue is highly mobile and is able to move rapidly and precisely. The next step in the evaluation of the speech mechanism is to assess these functions of the tongue. This is done to determine if there are limitations in tongue function and, if so, what these are and how the limitations might affect speech production. Some limitations in the function of the mechanism may be from underlying neuromotor problems. However, problems in performing tasks assessing tongue function do not always indicate a neuromotor etiology.

Functional assessment of the tongue is done with both nonspeech and speech tasks.

Nonspeech Tasks

The first of several procedures you can use to evaluate nonspeech tongue function is to request that the patient open the mouth slightly, and make repeated elevations of the tongue tip to the alveolar ridge, while producing no sound. Observe how accurately and smoothly this task is performed. Because you will have no auditory cues, you will need to observe and count the number the times the elevation is completed within a selected time period. Thus, you will need to place your stopwatch near the mouth so you can monitor timing as well.

During this, as well as other diadochokinetic-type tasks, some clients may employ "mandibular assist." Assist is said to occur when the jaw, rather than the tongue, makes the required movements. Use of mandibular assist needs to be noted, although the assist may be normal in clients below the age of 7 to 8 years. You should try to determine if the tongue movement can be made without the accompanying jaw movement. Have the patient attempt to stabilize the jaw by holding his chin to reduce or eliminate the movement of the mandible during the speech task. If this does not work, you should stabilize the jaw by holding it during additional trials of the task. By doing this, you can acquire information about whether the tongue is capable of making the movements or whether the assistance provided by the jaw movement is a necessary compensation for the patient to complete that particular movement.

The "tongue wiggle" is the second nonspeech procedure you can use. The "wiggle" consists of alternate lateral touching of the corners of the mouth during several trials. Again, because there are no sounds being produced, you will need to watch the mouth to count excursions, so you also will need to place your stopwatch near the mouth. When counting, use only the full excursions from one side of the mouth and back again to signify a single unit. You also may find that the rate at which this task is performed is similar to the norms for the previously described elevation of the tongue tip to the alveolar ridge and for the diadochokinetic production of the syllable /tʌ/, which will be discussed later in this chapter. In addition to the rate at which the tongue can make these lateral moves, you will also want to evaluate how accurately and smoothly the trials are performed and to note if the performance deteriorates or remains consistent across trials.

The "tongue circle" is another nonspeech task that taxes the function of the tongue. The "circle" is completed by having the patient open the mouth slightly, and then attempt to move the tongue around the resulting circular–appearing mouth opening. Many patients find this a very difficult task because it involves a constant change in the direction of the tongue movement. There are no norms for the task. However, the procedure is an excellent way to gain subjective judgments about the smoothness, accurateness, and coordination of the tongue. When repeated over several trials you also can check the consistency with which the client is able to do the task.

> The average diadochokinetic rate for elevating the tongue to the alveolar ridge with no sound is 4.5 to 5.0 per second.

> The rate at which children and adolescents between 4½ and 14½ years of age can produce alternate lateral tongue movements is 10 repetitions in 3–5 seconds. Another norm is an average of 4.5–5.0 excursions per second.

Summary of Procedures

Nonspeech tasks that may assist in the evaluation of the functional adequacy of the tongue are:

1. Repeated elevation of the tongue tip to the alveolar ridge without sound.

2. The tongue "wiggle."

3. The tongue "circle."

Speech Tasks

A speech task that can assess function of the tongue tip is the diadochokinetic production of /tʌ/. Typically, the syllable is repeated for several trials. Should you observe mandibular assist, attempt to stabilize the jaw in order to separate the tongue and jaw movements.

Several additional diadochokinetic tasks will help you assess tongue function. Diadochokinetic production of /kʌ/ assesses the function of the posterior part of the tongue in a speech task. Another diadochokinetic task that evaluates the patient's control of the tongue, as well as the lips, is production of the multisyllabic nonsense word /pʌtʌkʌ/. Some young clients may not be able to produce this nonsense string of sounds. They may be able to perform a similar task that has meaning to them, however. The words "patticake" and/or "buttercup" accomplish much the same purpose as /pʌtʌkʌ/ in your assessment procedures.

In addition to the rate of production, the *accuracy* of the sequences of sounds in the multisyllabic words is also very important. For instance, observe if the correct order of the syllables is maintained over the repetitions, as well as being maintained over multiple trials. Problems with consistency in maintaining correct productions and syllable order is a characteristic of clients with apraxia of speech, a motor speech disorder.

With some patients it also may be necessary to assess the impact of what appears to be a restricted lingual frenum, or possible tongue tie. The tongue tip needs to move the furthest to produce the /l/, /n/, /t/, and /d/ sounds. During assessment you need to incorporate these sounds into speech tasks. Some clients with a frenum that appears restrictive may be able to produce these sounds accurately and with good rate. Other clients may have developed compensatory ways of producing the sounds to accommodate for the restrictive frenum. Still other clients may be unable to reach the alveolar areas or to compensate adequately to produce the sounds. In such a case, it is necessary to refer the patient for medical management by a surgeon. However, it has been our experience that, although some clients show short frenums, these rarely impact negatively enough on speech skills to justify the surgery.

Typical diadochokinetic rates for /tʌ/ are 3.5–5.5 per second for children between the ages of 2½ and 5 years, and 5.5–6.5 per second for adults.

Average diadochokinetic rates for /kʌ/ e 3.5–5.5 per second for children and adolescents 2½ to 15 years of age, and 4–6 per second for adults.

Eight-year-old boys can typically produce /pʌtʌkʌ/ at a rate of 1.0–1.5 per second.

Chapter 12 will discuss the speech characteristics of apraxia and dysarthria, both of which are motor speech disorders.

Summary of Procedures

The functional adequacy of the tongue can be assessed via use of:

1. Diadochokinetic productions of /tʌ/.

2. Diadochokinetic production of /kʌ/.

3. Diadochokinetic production of /pʌtʌkʌ/ or real words with a similar structure of their syllables.

4. In the case of a suspected restrictive frenum, production of the /l/, /n/, /t/, and /d/ in various speech tasks.

Tongue Strength

To assess tongue strength you will need to use a sterile, individually wrapped tongue depressor. First, ask the client to protrude his tongue and then to resist your efforts to force the tongue to the right, left, and back into the mouth with the tongue depressor. A second task to assess tongue strength is done by asking the patient to place the tongue tip against the inside of the cheek, and then to resist your efforts to move the tongue toward the midline of the mouth with the flat of your fingers placed on the outside of the cheek. When a weakness is present, it is easier to force the tongue inward on the side which is opposite the weakness than it is to force the tongue on the side of actual weakness. Thus, if a weakness is on the right side, it will be easier to force the tongue inward from the left side of the mouth. This is because the force you apply on the left side meets little or no resistance from the weakened right side. If, during your assessment of tongue strength, you detect weakness, the speech and/or swallowing disorder that brought the patient to you may have a neuromotor basis or component.

Summary of Procedures

Tongue strength can be assessed by:

1. Asking the client to protrude the tongue and provide resistance when you apply force with a tongue depressor on the left, right, and center of the tongue.

3. Asking the patient to place his tongue against the inside of the cheek and provide resistance as you apply force.

Hard Palate Structure

The role of the hard and soft palates during speech and swallowing is to provide a barrier between the nasal and oral cavities. The hard palate, or roof of the mouth, is a bony structure that must be assessed for structural intactness or adequacy. If a hard palate is not intact, air may inappropriately escape from the mouth into the nasal cavity and out through the nose, resulting in nasalization of speech.

The structure and color of the center or midline of the palate need to be assessed. The normal midline structures may consist of a midline *raphe*, or indentation, or a bony line and bump, called a *torus*. The normal colors at the midline of the hard palate are pink and white. The posterior (back) edges of the hard palate usually are located near the last molar. Its shape should be scalloped and be continuous across the palatal vault.

Be sure to note the presence of an unrepaired, or a partially repaired, cleft in the hard palate. If the palate has been surgically repaired, be alert for the possible presence of small openings, or holes, along the repair line. These are called *fistulas*, which allow air to escape into the nasal cavity. You also will need to note the presence of lesions, or growths, on the hard palate, which require medical attention. Also note if there has been surgical removal of any of the hard palate because of disease or trauma. Finally, note the presence of any prostheses, such as dentures, obturators, or palatal lifts.

> Fistulas are small holes resulting from breakdown of surgically repaired tissues.

A variation of cleft palate is the *submucous cleft palate*. The term submucous is descriptive, because the cleft is not apparent during visual inspection. The bone defect that constitutes the submucous cleft of the hard palate is beneath the intact mucous membrane (literally, submucous). The bony defect is a notch in the posterior margin of the hard palate, where the posterior nasal spine normally is found. The notch cannot usually be seen, and must be palpated, or felt, with a finger. The notch of the submucous cleft palate has no ill effects on speech or voice production.

The overall size and contour, or shape, of the hard palate or palatal vault also needs to be examined. Note the height and width of the vault. Make special note of hard palates that appear to have flat, low vaults or high, narrow vaults. These two contours can potentially result in problems with voice resonance and make articulation difficult for the lingua-alveolar sounds of /l/, /n/, /t/, and /d/. The impact of the vault shape on speech can be determined by assessing the ease and accuracy with which the patient can make these four speech sounds.

Velopharyngeal Mechanism Structure

The velopharyngeal port is known by several names, including the "VP port" and "palatopharyngeal mechanism." This mechanism is comprised of the velum, or soft palate, and the pharynx, which includes the "back wall" as well as the side walls of the throat. Please refer to Figure 5–5 to help you identify these structures and their relationship to one another. The velopharyngeal port mechanism opens and closes the area at the back of the throat that separates the oral and the nasal passages to allow safe swallowing and normal speech production. Specifically, the port is closed during swallowing so that food and liquid (including saliva) are forced downward into the esophagus and not permitted into the nasal cavity. Generally, the velopharyngeal port is also closed during the speech production of plosives and fricatives, but is open during production of nasals. However, it is important to remember that, even in normal speakers, there is considerable variation in the opening and closing of the port, depending on the speech task.

As is true elsewhere in the oral mechanism, there frequently is disparity between the structures and function of the velopharyngeal port mechanism. The structures may appear normal, but demonstrate disordered function. We need to remember that it is the function, not structure, that should be our focus during this part of the examination. Sometimes the apparent disparity between structure and function is because we are able to see only part of the mechanism, as the nasal surface of the soft palate and pharyngeal walls—the components of the velopharyngeal mechanism that cause closure—are hidden from our view by the oral surface of the soft palate. So, our view is incomplete, and we must be very careful in interpreting our observations. Still, examination of the velopharyngeal structures available to our limited visual inspection is worth our time.

It is important that the structures are in a position similar to that used when the client is talking, rather than distorted, as when the patient's head is tilted back. A tilted head distorts the musculature of the structures, as well as the typical way in which the structures move. You need to make your examination with the client's mouth at your eye level. With children, this can perhaps best be done by asking them to sit on a table or to stand. In addition, the patient's mouth should be only three-quarters open, because full mouth opening also distorts the musculature that needs to be assessed.

A major observation is whether the soft palate, or velum, and uvula (the most posterior portion of the soft palate) are intact, or whether there is a physical cleft or opening of another kind. Note if there is an unrepaired, or a repaired, cleft of the soft palate. If there is a history of a surgically repaired cleft palate, look for the presence of fistulas. The color of the soft palate at midline may give you a clue to a submucous cleft that is not detectable by visual inspection. Normally the soft palate is the same color as the hard palate. If there is a bluish color running throughout or partway through the palate at midline, suspect the possibility of a submucous cleft, which needs to be palpated. A submucous cleft of the soft palate consists of a muscle defect and results in diminished bulk, length, or movement of this component of the velopharyngeal mechanism. The client's speech may be uncontrollably nasalized. Also be suspicious of a submucous cleft if you see a *bifid*, or split-looking, uvula. You may need to use a sterile tongue blade to determine the degree of intactness or bifidness of the uvula. This is done by stroking the uvula forward in an effort to separate the individual-appearing parts of the structure. Also note scars, holes, or tears in the palatal tissue which have resulted from trauma.

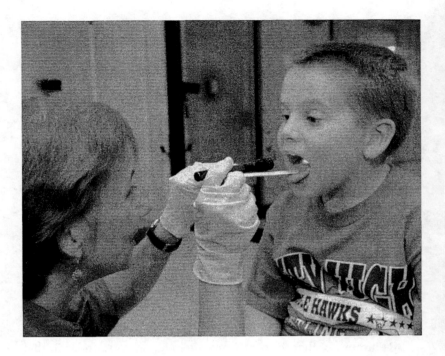

While looking at the palate at rest, observe the symmetry. Should the velum appear to be asymmetrical, with one side resting at a lower level than the other side, ask the patient to produce sustained or repeated /a/ sounds and observe if the palate continues to appear asymmetrical. If so, a unilateral muscular weakness or a problem with innervation may be present. In this situation, the uvula will move toward the unaffected side. With other clients you may think that the palate is generally too low when at rest, which could indicate a bilateral weakness. In this situation ask the patient to produce a sustained /a/ or series of /a/s to see if there is any change in position of the velum. If bilateral weakness is present, you will see very little, if any, movement.

Other structures that need to be noted are the faucial pillars and tonsils, which, when present, are located between the anterior and posterior pillars (see Figure 5–5). Tonsils, one on each side, are usually very easy to identify in children, because the masses are often enlarged. The size of tonsils is not usually of concern *unless* they are red and inflamed and/or have white matter on them, indicating that they may be infected. Problems with the size of the tonsils also can occur if they are so large that the airway is obstructed, and if the movement of the posterior part of the tongue is affected. These problems may be severe enough to warrant a referral to a physician, whose management may include a tonsillectomy, or surgical removal of the tonsils. You may have to look very carefully for tonsils in many of your adult clients; this tissue naturally atrophies, or shrinks, as an individual matures and reaches adulthood.

You will need to make subjective judgments about the depth and width of the oropharynx, which is the space at the back of the mouth. Clinical experience will help you make these subjective judgments. The oropharynx must be shallow enough in depth to allow the soft palate to extend back and elevate slightly for achievement of velopharyngeal closure with the back wall of the throat, or pharynx. As well, the velum must be long enough to reach the back wall of the pharynx. The width of the oropharynx is also important. The space must be narrow enough to allow the side walls at the back of the mouth to move inward, or mesially, a movement that helps to close off the nasal airway from the oral airway.

Not usually apparent during the speech mechanism examination, but important to the velopharyngeal structure and function, are the adenoids. Adenoids (and tonsils) are lymphoid tissues and are presumably a part of the immunologic system protecting an individual against disease. Like tonsils, the adenoids are most prominent in childhood, and least prominent, if present at all, after adolescence. When the tissue is at maximum size, the enlarged adenoidal pad can provide considerable help in reducing the size of the velopharynx. In fact, if the adenoids are too large they may block the nasal passageway, creating denasal voice quality. If a patient's soft palate is short, the enlarged adenoidal pad may help the child compensate in closing off the velopharyngeal port; the velum makes contact with the enlarged adenoids rather than the back pharyngeal wall. However, if the child had an adenoidectomy, this compensatory structure for closing the port is no longer present, so velopharyngeal dysfunction may result because the palate is unable to reach the pharyngeal back wall. Likewise, adolescent patients may be referred to you because of concerns about the gradual increase in nasally emitted air during speech. This could be velopharyngeal dysfunction resulting from the gradual atrophy of the adenoids, which also reduces and eventually eliminates a compensatory means for closing the velopharyngeal port.

> Hyponasality is another name for denasal voice quality.

Summary of Procedures

The structural adequacy of the VP mechanism may be assessed by:

1. Observing the soft palate for intactness and symmetry at rest and during productions of prolonged and repeated /a/.

2. Evaluating width and depth of the oropharynx.

Velopharyngeal Function

As indicated earlier, assessing the ability of the VP port to function in its task to separate the nasal and oral airways is difficult. There are a number of structures that are involved in the necessary movements,

Instrumental techniques for evaluation of velopharyngeal and swallowing functions are described in Chapter 14, dealing with cleft palate, and Chapter 15, dealing with swallowing disorders.

and these movements must be made in a coordinated manner. You also need to be aware that some important movements are hidden from view during clinical physical examination of the mechanism. In fact, it is not possible to evaluate velopharyngeal function by physical examination alone. However, observations of the mechanism performing both speech and nonspeech tasks may be helpful in assessing this function as well as with instrumental approaches. Instrumental assessment procedures are needed to objectively measure velopharyngeal function. These include various radiological and aerodynamic techniques, oral endoscopy, and nasal endoscopy. They are described in some detail in Chapter 14 (Peterson-Falzone).

Speech Tasks

Important initial clues about the function of the VP port mechanism come from listening to your patient's speech in conversation with you. Is there hypernasality? (Does it sound to you as if too much air is coming through the client's nose during speech?) Is air actually escaping out the nose when the patient is producing nonnasal phonemes? Do you see the nares (nostrils) flaring when the client is talking with you? Do you hear "funny" sounding phonemes that could be transcribed as glottal stops or pharyngeal fricatives—speech sounds that are being made too far back, perhaps as a way of trying to help close off the nasal airway?

A simple assessment technique that can be helpful in determining if air really is escaping during nonnasal sounds is through use of a "nasal mirror." Ask the client to produce sounds in isolation, syllables or words that target the specific phonemes you think might be produced with "nasal emissions" during your general observations of connected speech. Hold a mirror under the patient's nares, or nostrils, and watch for clouding during nonnasal sound production. This clouding would indicate that the VP port is not closing appropriately. This is, of course, not a precise measure of velopharyngeal function, but a very useful and inexpensive method to gain some information about the VP mechanism function during speech.

Have the client open his mouth (approximately three-quarters of the way) and observe the VP mechanism during two tasks—production of a prolonged /a/, and production of short, repeated /a/s. A sterile tongue depressor may be necessary for holding the tongue down so you can get a good view of the oropharynx during these tasks.

During production of the prolonged /a/ you should see two definite movements. The soft palate should move "up and back" so that the posterior pharyngeal wall is reached. You also should see the lateral pharyngeal walls and faucial pillars move mesially, or inward, toward the center of the throat. These two movements (posterior and mesial) should close the pharyngeal port, and the closure should be maintained as the /a/ continues to be produced. The movements occur simultaneously and quickly, so you need to be observant and know what you are looking for. As indicated earlier, it is possible to gain only part of the picture of the adequacy of velopharyngeal port movement during the oral examination; recall that many of the structural relationships and movement patterns within the velopharynx are not visible to you.

During the first /a/ produced in the series of short, repeated /a/s, you should see the posterior and mesial movements described for the prolonged /a/. However, these movements occur only on the first /a/; very minor movements occur during the remainder of the /a/ series.

Another speech task that can help assess the function of the VP mechanism is to determine if the diadochokinetic rates for /pʌtʌkʌ/ are better with the nares occluded or open. If the velopharyngeal mechanism is leaking air, the patient will find that having the nares occluded may help the overall efficiency of the speech system and the diadochokinetic rate will improve.

Summary of Procedures

Speech tasks which can assist in the evaluation of the functional adequacy of the velopharyngeal port are:

1. Observation of conversational speech.

2. Use of the nasal mirror during simplified speech tasks.

3. Observing prolonged /a/.

4. Observing repeated /a/s.

5. Measuring diadochokinetic rates for /pʌtʌkʌ/ with the nares (nostrils) open and closed.

Nonspeech Tasks

The functional adequacy of the velopharyngeal port can also be assessed by various tasks that do not involve speech. One such task is having the client blow out a birthday candle or a match in the usual oral way. Does air leak through the nose during the task? If it does, a comparison can be made with the nostrils open, requesting that the client make his best attempt to direct the air orally, and with the nostrils occluded (closed), as you are manually preventing air from escaping nasally. If you can detect a difference in performance between the nostrils being open and when they are occluded, the chances are good that the patient has a velopharyngeal closure problem. *A caution:* Be alert for the possibility of nasal congestion from upper respiratory infections or allergies when performing these or other tasks in assessing how well the VP port is functioning.

A final nonspeech task you can conduct to assess functional adequacy of the VP mechanism is to attempt to elicit a gag reflex. This is an unpleasant experience for the client, so do not make this a part of your typical examination of the speech mechanism. Rather, elicit the reflex only if you hear hypernasality, have documented the presence of nasal emission during speech, and see little or no movement during the prolonged /a/ and repeated /a/ tasks. With these conditions, you need to estimate the maximal movement of the velopharyngeal mechanism in an attempt to establish if there is innervation to the port area. The gag reflex can be elicited in numerous ways by use of a tongue blade, such as touching the palate, touching or stroking the pharyngeal wall, or placing pressure on the back of the tongue. If the reflex is present, you will see a great deal of posterior palatal and mesial wall movement. If you see asymmetrical or little movement during the gag reflex, suspect neuromotor weakness. Place this task at the very end of your speech mechanism examination; few patients will let you have "another look" into their mouths after having had the reflex elicited!

Summary of Procedures

Functional adequacy of the VP port mechanism can be assessed by the following nonspeech tasks:

1. Impounding air to blow out a candle or match.

2. Eliciting a gag reflex.

The speech mechanism examination requires much practice—and the sooner you can start this practice, the better. You will need to overcome feelings of invading another person's very personal space. You will need to gain an important base that will help you learn to make subjective clinical judgments. You will need to begin acquiring the observations necessary to gain a concept of how large the range of "normal" structures and "normal" function really is. You will need to learn how to work efficiently when doing this examination; know what you need to look for when you ask the client to open the mouth and then gain this information with a minimal number of mouth-opening requests to your patient. Practice doing the procedures involved in the speech mechanism examination to become a proficient professional when you do it "for real" with your first client.

ARE THERE CULTURAL FACTORS THAT I NEED TO BE AWARE OF WHILE CONDUCTING A SPEECH MECHANISM EXAMINATION?

In a word, yes! For instance, Salas-Provance (1996) discusses the often contradictory results in studies of the facial, physiological, and acoustic characteristics of African Americans and their speech productions. However, many studies appear to support craniofacial differences by race. For instance the columella portion of the nose tends to be shorter and the nasal base wider in African Americans than in Hispanics and Caucasians. Other studies have found greater soft-tissue thickness in the lower lips, and more anteriorly based upper jaws, with fewer distoclusions and mesioclusions with African American subjects when compared with White subjects. As well, you will find it helpful to know that with African American patients any scarring resulting from repair of a cleft lip may include depigmentation. And, when examining the oropharynx of African Americans, any inflamed mucous membranes will appear to have a purple hue rather than a red coloration found with clients of other racial groups.

Religious beliefs also can impact how we interact with our patients while examining the oral mechanism. Davis, Gentry, and Hubbard-Wiley (1998), discuss factors involving the beliefs of Confucianists, Buddhists, and Hindus of which we need to be aware. For instance, it is offensive to have the head touched and it is considered rude to show one's teeth in public. The prohibition for touching the head is held also by Muslims. The relationships between the genders are also factors that clinicians need to understand in the practice of their professions. Thus one must be aware of, and sensitive to, the many facets of cultural beliefs and practices when conducting an examination of the speech mechanism.

WHAT DO WE DO NEXT?

After we have made the observations and taken the measurements necessary to assess the structural and functional adequacy of the oral mechanism, we need to describe results. However, we must be *very* careful in relating these descriptions to the speech problems we have also observed and assessed. You must be very logical when thinking about cause-and-effect. The information you gain during the speech mechanism examination should be used to help you support or refute the hypotheses you have developed about the client's problems with communication. Some patients with structural problems of the speech mechanism also have articulation or resonance problems. However, the relationships among these are not always predictable. For instance, remember that some individuals can compensate for very large abnormalities in the structure and/or function of the mechanism, with other clients seemingly unable to compensate for what appear to be lesser problems with the mechanism. And, other patients may have problems with the mechanism that are so severe that the person's communication skills probably are not going to improve without assistance beyond what you will be able to provide. Finally, with some clients you will conclude that, even though there are structural and functional deviations in the speech mechanism, these do not have any relationship to the communication problem.

You also must develop recommendations for your client as a result of your diagnostic evaluation. Recommendations may be based on your examination of the speech mechanism. Perhaps you will want to recommend a period of trial remediation to see if the patient is able to improve speech skills despite the problems you may have observed in the structure or function of the mechanism. Or, you may want to determine if the client is able to learn some compensatory movements that will improve the speech skills. You may need to refer some patients to professionals in other fields, such as the family physician, dentist, orthodontist, or otolaryngologist. You also may refer some clients to other speech-language pathologists who have special expertise in dealing with specific kinds of communication or swallowing disorders. In some job settings these recommendations come from you alone, while in other job settings they are made by a team of professionals from different fields—each with input into the recommendation–making process on what needs to be done to best serve the client's present and future needs.

SUMMARY

An examination of the peripheral speech mechanism needs to be a part of the evaluation process, to a greater or lesser extent, for all clients. Through these results you will be better able to address the questions of whether or not there are problems with the structure and/or function of the mouth that might be the cause or might contribute to the patient's communication or swallowing problems, as well as obtain clues as to the specific nature of these disorders.

REFERENCES

Battle, D. E. (1998). *Communication disorders in multicultural populations* (2nd ed.). Boston: Butterworth-Heinemann.

Davis, P. N., Gentry, B., & Hubbard-Wiley, P. (1998). Clinical practice issue. In D. E. Battle (Ed.), *Communication disorders in multicultural populations* (2nd ed.). Boston: Butterworth-Heinemann.

Kamhi, A. G., Pollock, K. E., & Harris, J. L. (1996). *Communication development and disorders in African American children: Research, assessment and intervention*. Baltimore, MD: Paul H. Brookes.

Sales-Provance, M. (1996). Orofacial, physiological, and acoustic characteristics: Implications for the speech of African-American children. In A. G. Kamhi, K. E. Pollack, & J. L. Harris (Eds.), *Communication development and disorders in African-American children: Research, assessment, and intervention*. Baltimore: Paul H. Brookes.

RECOMMENDED READINGS

Examination Forms

Dworkin, J. P., & Culatta, R. A. (1996). *Dworkin-Culatta oral mechanism examination and treatment system*. Farmington Hills, MI: Edgewood Press.

Dworkin, J. P., & Culatta, R. A. (1980). *Dworkin-Culatta oral mechanism examination*. Nicholasville, KY: Edgewood Press.

Enderby, P. M. (1983). *Frenchay Dysarthria Assessment*. Austin, TX: Pro-Ed.

Mason, R. M., & Simon, C. (1977). An orofacial examination checklist. *Language, Speech and Hearing Services in Schools, 8*, 155–163.

Nation, J. E., & Aram, D. M. (1984). *Diagnosis of speech and language disorders* (2nd ed., pp. 354–360). San Diego, CA: College-Hill Press.

Peterson, H. A., & Marquardt, T. P. (1981). *Appraisal and diagnosis of speech and language disorders* (pp. 191–192). Englewood Cliffs, NJ: Prentice-Hall.

Robbins, J., & Klee, T. (1987). Clinical assessment of oropharyngeal motor development in young children. *Journal of Speech and Hearing Disorders, 52*, 277.

Shipley, K. G., & McAfee, J. G. (1998). *Assessment in speech-language pathology: A resource manual* (2nd ed., pp. 91–94). San Diego, CA: Singular Publishing Group.

Spriestersbach, D. C., Morris, H. L., & Darley, F. L. (1978). Speech mechanism examination. In F. L. Darley & D. C. Spriestersbach, *Diagnostic methods in speech pathology* (pp. 339–343). New York: Harper & Row.

St. Louis, K. O., & Ruscello, D. M. (1987). *Oral speech mechanism screening examination, revised*. Austin, TX: Pro-Ed.

Vitali, G. J. (1986). *Test of oral structures and functions*. East Aurora, NY: Slosson Educational Publications.

Diadochokinetic Rates

Blomquist, B. L. (1950). Diadochokinetic movements of nine-, ten-, and eleven-year-old children. *Journal of Speech and Hearing Disorders, 15*, 159–164.

Canning, B. A., & Rose, M. F. (1974). Clinical measurements of the speed of tongue and lip movements in British children with normal speech. *British Journal of Disorders of Communication, 9*, 45–50.

Ewanowski, S. J. (1964). *Selected motor speech behavior of patients with parkinsonism*. Unpublished doctoral dissertation, University of Wisconsin, Madison.

Fairbanks, G., & Spriestersbach, D. C. (1950). A study of minor organic deviations in "functional" disorders or articulation: 1. Rate of movement of oral structures. *Journal of Speech and Hearing Disorders, 15*, 60–69.

Fletcher, S. G. (1972). Time-by-count measurement of diadochokinetic syllable rate. *Journal of Speech and Hearing Research, 15*, 763–770.

Irwin, J. V., & Becklund, O. (1953). Norms for maximum repetitive rates for certain sounds established with the Sylrater. *Journal of Speech and Hearing Disorders, 18*, 149–160.

Kreul, J. E. (1972). Neuromuscular control examination (NMC) for parkinsonism: Vowel prolongation and diadochokinetic and reading rates. *Journal of Speech and Hearing Research, 15*, 72–83.

Lundeen, D. J. (1950). The relationship of diadochokinesis to various speech sounds. *Journal of Speech and Hearing Disorders, 15,* 54–59.

Robbins, J., & Klee, T. (1987). Clinical assessment of oropharyngeal motor development in young children. *Journal of Speech and Hearing Disorders, 52,* 271–277.

Sprague, A. L. (1961). *The relationship between selected measures of expressive language and motor skill in eight-year-old boys.* Ph.D. dissertation, University of Iowa, Iowa City.

Yoss, K. A., & Darley, F. L. (1974). Developmental apraxia of speech in children with defective articulation. *Journal of Speech and Hearing Research, 17,* 399–416.

Cultural Issues

Battle, D. E. (1998). *Communication disorders in multicultural populations* (2nd ed.). Boston: Butterworth-Heinemann.

Davis, P. N., Gentry, B., & Hubbard-Wiley, P. (1998). Clinical practice issue. In D. E. Battle (Ed.), *Communication disorders in multicultural populations* (2nd ed.). Boston: Butterworth-Heinemann.

Kamhi, A. G., Pollock, K. E., & Harris, J. L. (1996). *Communication development and disorders in African American children: Research, assessment and intervention.* Baltimore, MD: Paul H. Brookes.

Sales-Provance, M. (1996). Orofacial, physiological, and acoustic characteristics: Implications for the speech of African-American children. In A. G. Kamhi, K. E. Pollack, & J. L. Harris (Eds.), *Communication development and disorders in African-American children: Research, assessment, and intervention.* Baltimore: Paul H. Brookes.

Instrumental Assessment and Techniques

Karnell, M. P., (1994). *Videoendoscopy: From velopharynx to larynx.* San Diego, CA: Singular Publishing Group.

McWilliams, B. J., Morris, H. L., & Shelton, R. L. (1990). Instrumentation for assessing the velopharyngeal mechanism. In *Cleft palate speech* (2nd ed., pp. 163–196). Philadelphia: B.C. Decker.

Shprintzen, R. J. (1997). Nasopharyngoscopy. In K. E. Bzoch, *Communicative disorders related to cleft lip and palate (pp. 387–409).* Austin, TX: Pro-Ed.

General

Haynes, W. O., & Pindzola, R. H. (1998). *Diagnosis and evaluation in speech pathology* (5th ed., pp. 303–307). Boston: Allyn and Bacon.

Kent, R. D. (1997). *The speech sciences.* San Diego, CA: Singular Publishing Group.

Meitus, I. J., & Weinberg, B. (1983). *Diagnosis in speech-language pathology* (Chap. 2). Austin, TX: Pro-Ed.

Peterson, H. A., & Marquardt, T. P. (1994). *Appraisal and diagnosis of speech and language disorders* (3rd ed., Chap. 7). Englewood Cliffs, NJ: Prentice Hall.

Shipley, K. G., & McAfee, J. G. (1998). *Assessment in speech-language pathology: A resource manual* (2nd ed., pp. 88–96). San Diego, CA: Singular Publishing Group.

Appendix 5-A

EXAMINATION FORM:
Speech–Producing Mechanism

The Face

- At rest: Symmetrical_____ Asymmetrical_____
  - Drooping corner of mouth____
  - Drooping mandible_____
  - Eyelid closure_____
  - Other_____

- Requested movements:

	Symmetrical	Asymmetrical
Open mouth as far as possible	_____	_____
Raise both eyebrows	_____	_____
Close eyes tightly	_____	_____

- Observations / Comments:

Lips: Structure

- At rest:

	Adequate	Inadequate
Symmetry	_____	_____
Contour	_____	_____
Condition	_____	_____
Amount of tissue	_____	_____

	Yes	/	No
Presence of scar tissue	_____		_____

- Observations / Comments:

Lips: Function

- Nonspeech movements

	Adequate	Inadequate
Unilateral retraction to each side of face	_____	_____
Bilateral retraction of lips	_____	_____
Series of "pucker, smile"	_____	_____
Series of opening and closing lips	_____	_____

  - Trial 1:
  - Trial 2:
  - Trial 3:
- (Adult norm: 5–6 / second)

(continued)

- Speech movements

Adequate / Inadequate

Repetitions of /uiuiui/   _____   _____

Repetitions of /p8/   _____   _____

         Trial 1:

         Trial 2:

         Trial 3:

     (Adult norm: 6–7 / second)

     (Child norm: 3–6 / second)

- Observations / Comments:

Lips: Strength

- Patient puffs out cheeks and seals lips—assess strength of seal by gently pushing against:

Adequate / Inadequate

     Right cheek   _____   _____

     Left cheek   _____   _____

     Both cheeks   _____   _____

- Observations / Comments

Teeth

- Missing primary or permanent teeth
- Condition of teeth
- Description of occlusion, bite, and tooth position:

     Normal occlusion   _____

     Neutroclusion (Angle's Class I)   _____

     Distoclusion (Angle's Class II)   _____

     Mesioclusion (Angle's Class III)   _____

     Normal bite   _____

     Openbite   _____

     Overbite / closebite   _____

     Crossbit   _____

     Overjet   _____

     Underjet   _____

     Labioversion   _____

     Buccoversion   _____

     Linguaversion   _____

- Presence of any dental appliance or protheses
- Observations / Comments:

(continued)

Tongue: Structure

- Tongue at rest:

                                          Adequate / Inadequate

    Size   _____   _____
    Completeness   _____   _____
    General condition   _____   _____

                                          Yes   /   No

    Presence of lesions   _____   _____
    Presence of atrophy   _____   _____
    Presence of fasciculations   _____   _____
    Presence of twitches and   _____   _____
    involuntary movements

- Patient protrudes tongue

                                          Yes   /   No

    Deviations to right   _____   _____
    Deviations to left   _____   _____

                                          Adequate / Inadequate

    Extent of protrusion   _____   _____

- Patient elevates tongue

    Length of lingual frenum   _____   _____

- Observations / Comments:

Tongue Function:

    Nonspeech tasks

                                          Adequate / Inadequate

- Repeated elevation of tongue tip
  to alveolar ridge with no sound   _____   _____
            Trial 1:
            Trial 2:
            Trial 3:
    (Norm: 4.5–5.0 / second)

- Tongue "wiggle"   _____   _____
            Trial 1:
            Trial 2:
            Trial 3:
    (Norm: 4.5–5.0 / second)

- Tongue "circle"   _____   _____

(continued)

Speech Tasks

Adequate / Inadequate

- Repetitions of /tʌ/   _____   _____
  - Trial 1:
  - Trial 2:
  - Trial 3:
  - (Child norm: 3.5–5.5 / sec)
  - (Adult norm: 5.5–6.5 / sec)
- Repetitions of /kʌ/   _____   _____
  - Trial 1:
  - Trial 2:
  - Trial 3:
  - (Child norm: 3.5–5.5 / sec)
  - (Adult norm: 4–6 / sec)
- Repetitions of /pʌtʌkʌ/ OR word
  word with similar syllable structure   _____   _____
  - Trial 1:
  - Trial 2:
  - Trial 3:
  - (Child norm: 1–1.5 / sec)
- Observations / Comments

Tongue: Strength

Adequate / Inadequate

- Client protrudes tongue—
  assess resistance when tongue
  depressor is applied:
  - On the right side   _____   _____
  - On the left side   _____   _____
  - To the tongue tip   _____   _____
- Patient places tongue inside cheek—
  assess resistance when force is applied:
  - On the right side   _____   _____
  - On the left side   _____   _____
- Observations / Comments

Hard Palate: Structure

Adequate / Inadequate

- Description
  - Midline intactness   _____   _____
  - Midline structures   _____   _____
  - Midline color   _____   _____

(continued)

- Size   _____   _____
- Height   _____   _____
- Width   _____   _____

- Observations / Comments

Velopharyngeal Mechanism: Structure

Adequate / Inadequate

- Velum, Uvula
    Intactness   _____   _____
    Color   _____   _____
    Symmetry   _____   _____

- Faucial pillars   _____   _____
- Oropharynx
    Depth   _____   _____
    Width   _____   _____

- Observations / Comments

Velophary..geal Mechanism: Function
Speech tasks

Present / Absent

- Hypernasality / nasal emissions
  during conversational speech   _____   _____

Adequate / Inadequate

- Movement during prolonged /a/   _____   _____
- Movement during repeated /a/   _____   _____
- Rate comparison for /pʌ/tʌ/kʌ/, nares
  open and nares closed   _____   _____
Nonspeech tasks
- Blow out candle or match   _____   _____
- Movement during gag   _____   _____

SUMMARY

Structural adequacy of the mechanism:

Functional adequacy of the mechanism:

Overall adequacy of the mechanism for speech production:

CHAPTER

6

Language Disorders

Amy L. Weiss, Ph.D.,
J. Bruce Tomblin, Ph.D.,and
Donald A. Robin, Ph.D.

The purpose of this chapter is to introduce you to the process of language diagnosis. We have included information for evaluating language abilities regardless of the age of the client or whether concern about language is one of many reasons or the only reason for referral. Language problems are pervasive in the individuals we serve and because of the need for language competencies in our daily activities the diagnosis of a language disorder will be a common clinical challenge to you. Language diagnosis is particularly challenging because of the complexity of language and the varied nature of language disorders. Due to this complexity, it is essential that you have in mind a model or road map concerning the nature of language, a clear understanding of the diagnostic problem solving process, and a clear sense of the clinical standards used to make decisions in this area. This chapter will attempt to provide you with a general, usable framework to use in your diagnosis of language disorders. As discussed in the introductory chapter, this will be one of the "generic" chapters that can be used in conjunction with those chapters appearing later in the text that discuss individuals with more specific diagnoses, for example, cleft palate or neurological deficits. In later chapters covering more specific disordered populations where

Many clients referred to us for other reasons also may have a language disorder.

language disorders may represent a portion of the client's communication problem, you will be referred back to this chapter for appropriate language-related information.

AN OVERVIEW OF LANGUAGE AND LANGUAGE DISORDERS

A Model of Language for Diagnostic Purposes

Our perspective is that *language* is a socially shared code comprised of a set of arbitrary symbols, used primarily for communication, and that language can be conveyed verbally, manually, or in written form (Owens, 1996). This definition emphasizes the first aspect of our model of language diagnosis: the modalities of language usage. That is, we believe that no assessment of our clients' language can be considered complete without evaluating both *language comprehension* (understanding) and *language production* (expression). Further, with some clients—particularly those with acquired language disorders—we include both the spoken (if speech is the output mode used by the client) and written forms of language in our evaluation. Thus, our definition of language is not equivalent to, but instead is broader than, our definition of speech. *Speech* represents only one mode of language expression and, although it is probably the mode we will spend the most time evaluating, it will not tell us the whole story about a client's language abilities. Broader even than the term *language* is the concept of *communication*. Our goal in evaluating the language abilities of our clients is to determine how successfully they can convey as well as interpret information in their daily activities because that is the all-important function that *communication* serves. In fact, for our very young clients or those who are significantly delayed in language development who are not yet producing real words, we will observe their use of gesture and/or vocalizations (nonverbal vocal productions) in context to determine the presence of nonverbal precursors to verbal communication in their expressive repertoires. Our interest, then, is not just in cataloguing the words and sentences our clients may produce; our underlying goal is to investigate all their attempts at purposeful communication regardless of their form.

In keeping with current descriptions of the language system and to facilitate our discussions of assessment procedures, we have divided language into five different components: *phonology*, which represents the sound system of a language and includes the rules that organize that system and generate allowable sound combinations; *syntax*, which characterizes the allowable patterns of word combinations that form, for example, declarative or interrogative sentences; *morphology*, which describes the set of inflections that allows us to alter words to indicate, for example, number, tense, and possession (e.g., bus*es*, walk*ed*, and Mommy*'s*, respectively); *semantics*, which deals with vocabulary development as well as the roles that words can play when combined with one another (e.g., agent, action, object); and *pragmatics*, which concerns the use of language in context to express communicative intent, presupposition, and conversation rules (Roth & Spekman, 1984). Note that this division of language into these component parts is done for the sake of convenience only. The student of language development and language disorders should appreciate the interdependence and influence we know that these parts of language actually exert on one another in language development (Prutting, 1979), language disorders (Panagos et al., 1979) and in day-to-day language use (Crystal, 1987). For example, Campbell and Shriberg (1982) demonstrated that children with multiple speech sound errors were more likely to produce their error sounds correctly when the error sounds were embedded in a word that represented new information—information more critical to communication. So, in this instance, it appears that the children's ability to use what they know about phonology and pragmatics was interconnected.

> The various interactions among the components of language makes language evaluation even more challenging.

Those approaching language evaluation often differ in how they visualize the interactions and primacy of these different language components. Some believe that the components of language are equivalent and that, although these systems must interact in order for language to work properly, the status of these components can be evaluated separately and eventually treated separately. Others propose that pragmatics is the primary component of language, determining the choices of specific words and sentence types that are used based on context. Advocates of the latter orientation are wary of only collecting diagnostic information from structured language assessment techniques because these measures typically evaluate each com-ponent separately, often outside of the naturalistic contexts of pragmatics. Thus, you can see that your approach to the nature of language will influence the way you go about your language diagnosis. Figure 6–1 illustrates the relationships among the component parts of language.

The Relationship Between Language, Sensation, Perception, and Cognition

There is nearly universal agreement about the close relationship between language and other systems that are required for successful language development and use. Obviously, if spoken language is to be acquired and understood, it will be necessary for the person to be able to hear (*sense*) the auditory message and to *perceive* the complex frequency and temporal information contained in the signal. Further, higher level cognitive processes must be intact including the ability to represent experiences and ideas or *concepts*, store this information (*memory*), and focus *attention* on information to accomplish *problem solving*. For many years researchers tried to determine whether cognitive abilities were prerequisite for lan-

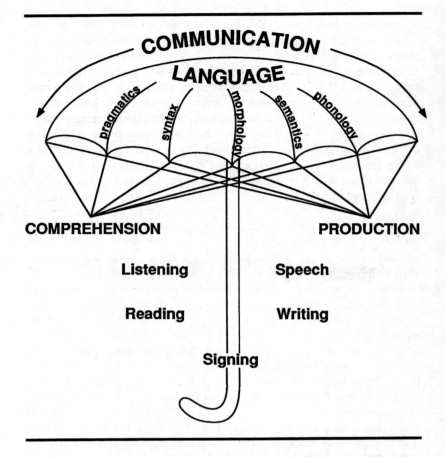

Figure 6–1. The relationships among communication and the component parts of language as they relate to the areas of assessment for language disorders.

guage learning and were impaired following acquired language problems. Researchers also tried to determine whether linguistic operations depended on cognition. Today it is generally believed that cognition and language develop interactively and that this interaction continues in adulthood, meaning that the two areas are interconnected and mutually dependent.

Later we will discuss the need to make a range of clinical decisions regarding the cause of a client's language disorder, as well as its prognosis and treatment options. Information concerning the sensory, perceptual, and cognitive abilities of the client will be essential in making these decisions, and so we need to know about those abilities in our efforts to diagnose language problems. Some of this information you may be able to obtain yourself during the examination; other information may come from colleagues in other professions. As part of your professional education, you will be trained to perform basic audiometric testing to screen for a hearing loss; however, in most instances you should refer clients who may be at risk for hearing loss (for example, those with language delay) to an audiologist for evaluation. Likewise, you may be able to obtain some information about general cognitive ability from your own tests, but most speech-language pathologists rely on psychologists for information about their clients' cognitive and intellectual functioning. Specifically, psychologists can be called on to answer questions about how an individual learns best and whether there are any cognitive or behavioral impediments to learning. This information may prove very useful when it is time for the speech-language pathologist to make recommendations concerning the type of special services needed by the client to facilitate changes in communication competencies. For older clients with acquired language disorders, the assistance of a psychologist may be needed in the differential diagnosis of an aphasia versus dementia or in evaluating and later treating the depression that may follow a cerebral vascular accident and hinder progress in treatment.

As you use information from cognitive testing, you need to keep in mind that many of the popular tests administered by clinical psychologists, such as the *Wechsler Intelligence Scale for Children— Revised* (Wechsler, 1974), require clients to have considerable prerequisite language ability. This requirement for language ability puts the client with a language disorder at a disadvantage, because language ability becomes confounded with intellectual ability. This is true both for clients with developmental language disorders as well as for those with acquired language disorders (individuals who suffer a loss of language ability following their acquisition of the language system). For these clients who have language problems, tests that emphasize nonverbal performance rather than verbal skills are preferable. See Sattler (1988) for a comprehensive discussion of this issue. A note of caution must be extended here because even performance scale tests are not always a perfect solution. Careful examination of the particular performance measure should also be made in that many "nonverbal" tests are performed with verbal strategies. For example, people often code nonverbal memory test items with names to assist in the task. This being the case, what may have been meant as a performance scale using nonverbal means to measure intelligence may actually invoke the use of verbal coding strategies.

An example of a performance scale task would be the matching of blocks with related patterns. The *Leiter International Performance Scale* is an example of a test that uses tasks of this type.

We have now laid out a general model of language and its relationship to information processing systems. This model will provide you with guidance as you work through the complex terrain of language.

A DEFINITION OF LANGUAGE DISORDERS

We just described language as a complex system of knowledge having to do with the function, meaning, and form of messages. Further, people must be able to use this system of knowledge with facility in the understanding and expression of ideas. When this complex system works well, people can engage in communication with few difficulties and with little effort. On the other hand, there are some children and adults for whom this system does not work well and in such cases we regard the person as having a language disorder. These people may have difficulty understanding things said to them, or they may have difficulties formulating messages, or both. Language disorders, therefore, occur when individuals do not possess the language skills required of them by their linguistic community and as a result find themselves confronted with frequent communication failure.

This way of defining a language disorder emphasizes the relationship between the expectations and demands of the person's community and the person's language abilities to meet these expectations. By emphasizing the community expectations, we admit that there is no fixed standard of what is considered "normal" or "good" language performance. Rather, the standard is whatever the person's community expects. Notice that in this statement we mentioned the person's linguistic community. If you are not very good at French and you go to Paris, you will face a good deal of communication difficulty. However, we would not say that you have a language disorder, unless you are a native French speaker and a part of the French society and you were still demonstrating significant communication difficulty. This issue also extends to instances of dialect. People are not considered to have a language disorder simply because they use a variant of a language that is different from the standard form so long as the variant is viewed as acceptable within their own community.

In our definition of language disorder, we have been using the concept of expectations. Even within an individual society, the expectations may vary for different members. In mainstream American culture, adjustments in expectations for language performance are made according to a person's age, and by the same token, we adjust our own speech and language when communicating with those we perceive as less linguistically competent than we are to increase the likelihood of communicative success. Thus, we do not expect 2-year-olds to be able to talk at length on a topic and, furthermore, we are not surprised when they do not use adult phonologic and grammatic forms. On the other hand, if an adult were to have the language skills of a 2-year-old, it is likely that the adult would face grave difficulties in maintaining interpersonal communication, obtaining an education, and living independently. Because of this, the speech-language pathologist also makes adjustments in assessment of the language skills of children. This is often done by incorporating norm-referencing in our interpretation of many of our language measures. In this case the child's performance is compared with that of other children of the same or a very similar age. Children who demonstrate language skills below one standard deviation (below the 16th percentile) for their age are usually regarded by both speech-language pathologists and classroom teachers as having unacceptably low language

We all speak a dialect or variant of some language; "nonstandard" dialects represent language differences, : disorders.

Interestingly, we can observe young, normally developing children—even those who are very limited in their own expressive repertoires—making similar adjustments in the speech and language they use to children they perceive as being younger than they are.

abilities and therefore these children are likely to be diagnosed as language impaired. There is evidence that not everyone uses the same criterion for the diagnosis of language impairment, however. Records and Tomblin (1994) suggested that children are more likely to be diagnosed as language impaired when their language scores fall below one standard deviation below the mean. More recently these researchers (Tomblin et al., 1996) reported that, when they used a criterion of 1.25 standard deviations below the mean on two of five composite language scores (representing comprehension, production, narration, vocabulary, and grammar) as their cutoff, their diagnoses of language impairments closely matched ratings made by clinicians.

Similar adjustment for age may also be made for older clients, thus recognizing that some language facility does decline with the normal process of aging. Many tests of adult language are normed on young adults ages 18–40 and thus comparison of the typical stroke victim age 60 or older is inappropriate. Note, however, that not all of the news about language use and advancing age is bad news. Older adults are often credited with larger vocabularies and greater skill at story telling!

Subtypes of Language Disorder

So far we have been talking about language disorder in its broadest form, and many of the questions you will be asking during language diagnosis, as well as the methods you will use to address these questions, will be applicable to all forms of language disorders. However, we need to consider at this point that there are two major subtypes of language disorder and at various points during this chapter we will be pointing out special diagnostic issues that pertain to these groups.

Developmental Language Disorders

As the term "developmental" implies, these are problems of language acquisition. Affected clients present a pattern of delays in language development from the early stages of language learning that often persists throughout childhood and that remains during adulthood in the form of a limited facility with language. Because a developmental language impairment can be viewed as a limitation in a growth or developmental process, we describe the language problem in terms of the level of development obtained by the client in the various domains of language function. Because of this, the assessment process for developmental language disorder often involves having the client perform language tasks along a continuum from early developing language skills to those that are acquired later in life. Notice that this approach to characterizing the language problem assumes that most clients with developmental language disorders are very similar to younger normally developing individuals—

an assumption of "language delay" that has received fairly strong support over the years.

Acquired Language Disorders

In contrast, an acquired language disorder is characterized by a clear reduction in language abilities and is therefore viewed as a disturbance of an already successfully developed system. In most instances, the client has developed language normally but, as the result of trauma to the brain or some disease process affecting the brain, has lost some degree of language ability.

Acquired language disorders may range in severity from subtle problems finding a word to a nearly complete inability to understand things said. In addition to variation in severity, acquired language disorders may differ in the areas of language affected. For example, some clients may have considerable difficulties understanding things said but have fairly good expressive language ability. In contrast, others may have considerable difficulty expressing themselves but have good comprehension abilities. Individuals with right hemisphere damage or traumatic brain injuries may perform normally on tests of basic linguistic abilities but fail on higher level material that involves such abilities as inferencing or sequencing. Some adults may have language impairments that are secondary to more general cognitive problems such as attentional and memory problems. Many of these differences are due to the side and areas of the brain damaged, as well as the particular cause of the brain injury.

Unlike developmental language disorders, persons with acquired language disorders may not present language skills that are like normal language users at a younger level. Instead you will observe that their difficulties with language often appear in the form of language usage errors that are very uncommon in most normal language users. These errors are often associated with increases in the information processing demands of the language task. Thus, long sentences may place a heavy burden on the client's memory and lead to frequent comprehension failure, whereas shorter sentences may place less demand on memory and as a result be easier to understand. Because of this, when speech-language pathologists assess the language problems in acquired language disorders, they will vary the information processing complexity of the language task and then note the type and frequency of language errors made. Moreover, as noted earlier, many of these individuals' problems may be related to more general cognitive problems. We will provide basic information on the diagnosis of acquired language disorders here, but more specific information can be found in Chapter 11.

The reader can see that, although we are going to be looking at many of the same dimensions of language regardless of whether the client presents a developmental or acquired language impairment, our view of the basic nature of two forms of language impairment will influence the way in which we characterize the language problem.

THE GOALS OF LANGUAGE DIAGNOSIS

The goals of language diagnosis are similar to the goals of diagnosis for any other disorder area: We are seeking to gain a clear understanding of the client's communication problem and to use this information to make decisions regarding the clinical management of the problem. In fact, our goals must fit into this broader diagnostic frame, since our language evaluation will usually be a part of a general consideration of the client's overall communication status. Often clients seeking our services do not already know that their problems involve the language systems concerned with communication. All they know is that they are having problems communicating. Also, many of the communication problems we see in the clinic are not isolated to language systems alone. For instance, many acquired language disorders are also associated with problems of speech production in the form of dysarthria, apraxia, or cognitive impairments. Therefore, our diagnosis of language is usually placed within the broader context of the diagnosis of communication disorder.

Chapter 1 pointed out that a number of issues are often addressed as a part of diagnosis. Although all the issues listed are important, in this chapter we will focus on the following diagnosis of language disorder issues:

1. Determination of the nature of the complaint.

2. Determination of the existence of a language disorder.

3. Determination of concomitant factors.

4. Prediction of the course of the language problem.

We will look at each of these now and consider what information we need to answer them and how we can go about obtaining this information.

DETERMINATION OF THE NATURE OF THE COMPLAINT

When a client with a language disorder comes to us with concerns about communication, our first step will usually be to guide whoever is the primary informant (the client, a parent or spouse, a teacher, a nurse, etc.) in describing the nature of the problems the client is having. It is during this initial conversation with the informant that you will begin to suspect that the problem may be one involving language. Complaints having to do with language will contain concerns over difficulties formulating ideas into wellformed utterances. If the client is a child, the parent may express concern that the child is using very limited word combinations or that the child's sentences have an immature quality. In addition, the parent may note that the child becomes quite frustrated when trying to communicate and may give up at the first sign of a misunderstanding or breakdown in communication. For some young children, the parents may note infrequent attempts to communicate even by means of gestures and/or vocalizations. If the client is older and has had normal language competencies, the complaint will contain comparative information about what the person cannot now do that he or she used to be able to do. Also in the case of an acquired language disorder, there will usually be strong evidence of a medical event such as a head injury or stroke associated with the onset of the language impairment. Although informants are less likely to initially provide you with concerns about language comprehension problems, once you ask—and it is wise to always specifically inquire about language comprehension—you will often be told that the client does have difficulty following directions, etc. It is also common to be told that the client has no problems understanding. Accept this as a possibility, but realize that sometimes clients can appear to be understanding more than they do. In fact, it is quite common for caregivers to overestimate young children's language comprehension skills due to children's reliance on nonlinguistic cues, including adults' frequent use of gesture when they are unable to understand all of the linguistic information given. This is something you will want to confirm later.

> Clients often guess the meaning of things being said by using nonverbal cues. This may lead us to believe that they have better language skills than they actually have.

You can see that, rather quickly, you are going to have information that may suggest that at least part of the communication problem may be based on problems with language. If this is the case, you will then move to the next question having to do with establishing the presence of a language impairment. See Figure 6–2 for several suggestions of questions that might lead to a discussion of the complaint with the family and other relevant persons.

---

1. What are your concerns about (client's) communication?

2. When he talks with you does he ask questions, ask you to get things, tell you about things that have happened?

3. Can you have a conversation with him?

4. When he talks with you, does he speak in full sentences, short phrases, or mainly words?

5. When you talk with him, do you believe he can understand the things you say to him?

6. What situations make it easier or more difficult for him to understand you?

Figure 6–2. Common questions you might ask while obtaining complaint information.

DETERMINING THE EXISTENCE OF A LANGUAGE DISORDER

If the complaint suggests that there may be a language disorder, we then begin posing questions having to do with the client's language status in the various areas of language according to the model of language we presented earlier. This model will guide us as we gather information about the client's language, and we will want to establish the client's status in each area of language provided by this model. This information can be obtained through the use of a variety of tasks ranging from standardized language tasks to very naturalistic conversations. Your job is to select tasks that will provide you with reliable and valid information and provide you with this information in an efficient manner. In so doing you will want to consider some of the issues raised in Chapter 1 regarding the reliability and validity of measures.

GENERAL COMPONENTS OF THE ASSESSMENT BATTERY

By now it should be clear that a comprehensive characterization of the language abilities of a client will require you to employ several different tasks within which you can observe the client's language performance. As a result, you will need to construct a battery of tasks to be used for your evaluation. There are some standardized tests that cover both language comprehension and production areas. For example, the *Test of Language Development* (TOLD-P:3), a language test for young children (Newcomer & Hammill, 1997), contains seven subtests, three of which address areas of language comprehension; the remaining four tests serve to evaluate language production competencies. Comprehensive tests of aphasia such as the *Boston Diagnostic Aphasia Examination* (BDAE; Goodglass & Kaplan, 1981) and the *Porch Index of Communicative Ability* (PICA; Porch, 1968) also examine both production and comprehension. Other standardized tests are more selective and focus either on language comprehension, for example, the *Peabody Picture Vocabulary Test-R* (PPVT-III; Dunn & Dunn, 1997) and *The Revised Token Test* (McNeil & Prescott, 1986) or on language production, for example, the *Carrow Elicited Language Inventory* (CELI; Carrow, 1974). So, it is important, when evaluating the usefulness of a test for inclusion in a particular client's test battery, that you identify which area or areas of language are being assessed and how these areas match up with both the presenting complaint and your own informal observations of the client's language competencies.

Within the general heading of language comprehension or language production, you need to know which subcomponent or subcomponents of language are evaluated. For example, the PPVT-III specifically addresses receptive, single-word vocabulary. Carrow-

Woolfolk's *Test of Auditory Comprehension for Language-R* (1985), on the other hand, is a language comprehension measure that evaluates three aspects of receptive language: single-word vocabulary, sentences, and the roles and relationships words have within a sentence. Therefore, a clinician could argue that using both of these tests as part of the same test battery would be redundant and a waste of time. Many speech-language pathologists, however, would consider the PPVT-III a more intensive clinical tool for evaluating receptive vocabulary and a well-respected test instrument due to its reliability and validity and might decide to find the time for both tests. One additional rationale for using both tests could be that one measure of receptive vocabulary would have the potential of substantiating the findings gleaned from the other one.

You will also be guided in your selection of testing materials by the presenting complaint. For example, if a child is perceived to have difficulty participating in classroom discussions, then a portion of the evaluation should focus on the child's classroom performance, as described in Chapter 10. Similarly, if a wife is concerned that her husband who has had a stroke appears to be most frustrated by his inability to respond to questions within a reasonable time frame, you will want to gather some data focusing on response latency to evaluate this ability.

Informal Observation

In our desire to derive supportive numbers through test administration as evidence for diagnosis, we sometimes overlook the importance of observing our clients. As mentioned, scores resulting from standardized tests can be easily criticized for not reflecting typical behaviors of language use or for the limited sample of language skills they reflect. As a consequence, we usually need to supplement the information we can gain through formal testing by observing our clients in activities of daily living. Ideally, this would involve several different "coconversationalists" in several different situations to provide a more comprehensive picture of how our clients' abilities correlate with their language needs and the flexibility with which they use the language in their repertoires. In addition, observation of clients with family members and other individuals even for 5 or 10 minutes enables us to form some opinion about the strategies used by these other individuals to interact with the client. For example, we may notice that a mother is very responsive to her child's conversation attempts, accepting both nonverbal and verbal bids from the child. At the same time we may observe that the child is much more likely to engage a sibling in conversation than either a parent or an unfamiliar adult. These two observations may help us down the road when we are planning intervention.

For school-age children, observation in the classroom setting is strongly recommended so that we can observe the child's ability to

Because language is a complex system, we need to observe it in natural settings to see how the system works as a whole.

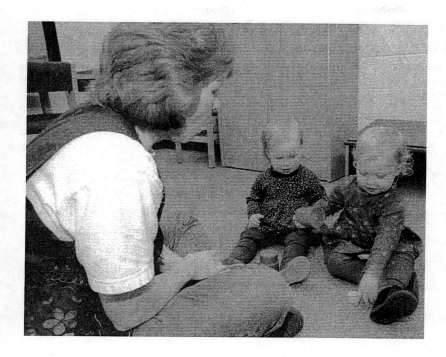

cope with the language demands of that classroom. Adults should also be observed in settings that more closely approximate their daily language use than do typical testing situations so that we can get an accurate and comprehensive picture of whether and to what degree their language abilities are compromised. When working with adults with acquired language problems it is also useful to observe the client in a variety of interactions between the client and other healthcare providers (e.g., nurses, physicians) because these different coconversationalists may also have an effect on the frequency and complexity of the client's language output.

THE TASKS USED TO COLLECT RECEPTIVE AND EXPRESSIVE LANGUAGE DATA

From what we have said, you can see that you are likely to be using several assessment methods in order to obtain information needed to determine the client's status in the various areas of language. Let's look at the most common methods used and see what information they provide. We will describe these methods in generic terms; however, as we do so, we will identify some of the common standardized tests that employ these methods (Leonard et al., 1978). Figure 6–3 illustrates all of the tasks that will be described for assessing receptive and expressive language abilities.

We cannot directly observe what clients understand when they hear an utterance. Therefore, we need tasks that allow the client to reveal what was understood.

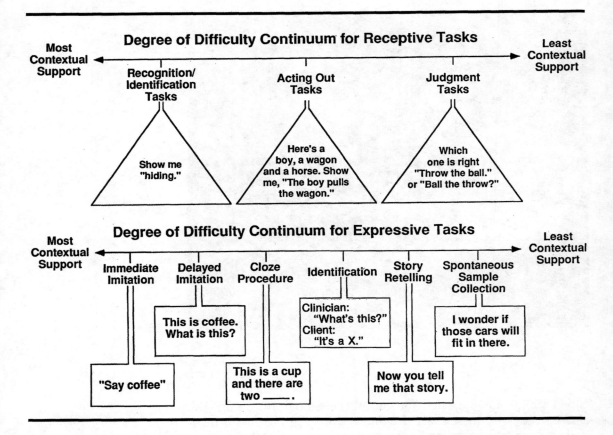

Figure 6–3. Tasks typically used to assess receptive and expressive language abilities depicted on a continuum representing most to least contextual support.

Receptive Language Testing

Three basic tasks can be used to evaluate receptive language: *recognition/identification*, *acting out*, and *judgment* tasks. Because these tasks are designed to reflect receptive language testing, they require no language production from the client. For that reason, they are often good tasks to begin with when working with a reluctant or reticent client. It is surprising how many young clients are already aware of their limited success with expressive language. If we do not tax their expressive abilities at the start of our testing, we may be more likely to gain the child's cooperation for the tougher tasks that lie ahead.

In *recognition/identification tasks*, the client is asked to listen to a language stimulus, which may be a single word, a phrase, or a sentence. After hearing the language stimulus, the client is expected to identify the object or event described in the word, phrase, or sentence from an array of nonverbal stimuli. These stimuli may be three-dimensional objects such as toys, but more often they are sets of pictures. Figure 6–4 shows the array of items used to test the client's understanding of "the girl pushes the boy." Notice that the other pictures serve as foils for alternate meanings that could come from the sentence. When using pictured material, it is very important to consider how well the meaning is depicted in the picture; otherwise, you may find that you are measuring the client's ability to interpret the picture, rather than to interpret the language stimulus.

Acting out tasks present clients with another venue for conveying information about language comprehension. Manipulable objects are made available to the client who is then asked to perform some task like, "Show me the boy pushes the wagon." Clients are then expected to maneuver the items in such a way that they "act out" the sentence or word combination (e.g., "hug baby") presented. It should be noted that acting out tasks have been criticized because they may underestimate language comprehension due to the number of different cognitive components that may contribute to performance on the task (Tyler, 1992). That is, other abilities in addition to language comprehension are required for these tasks to be accurately completed. This potential problem has been noted for testing adults with aphasia (Tyler, 1992) and children with language disorders (Crain, 1982). In some quarters, then, caution has been recommended when judgments of language comprehension ability have been made based largely on the results of acting out tasks.

In the third type of task, *judgment tasks*, the client is asked to make a judgment whether statements by the examiner are acceptable (according, presumably, to the client's internalized standards for

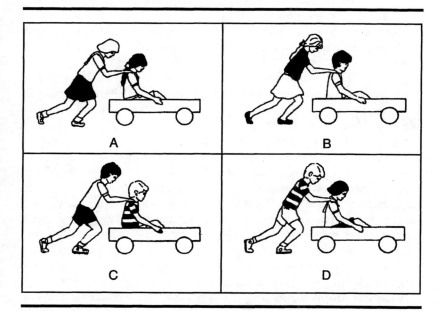

Figure 6–4. Picture material used to test comprehension of the sentence, "The boy pushes the girl."

language use). For example, the clinician says, "The sheeps are grazing" and asks the client for judgment of acceptability, such as, "Is that okay or not okay?" "silly or not silly," "right or wrong," and so on. The specific terms used should be selected based on the cognitive and language ability already demonstrated by the child or adult. In fact, the decision to use judgment tasks at all should be made carefully, since this is a task that involves a metalinguistic use of language. Metalinguistics refers to a conscious, formal, and non-communicative use of language. Metalinguistic tasks are cognitively demanding; therefore, as a general rule, judgment tasks may be too complex for children who have not achieved a mental age of at least 5 years, or with an adult who has known cognitive impairments. Using a judgment task with a child who is cognitively too immature to handle the task's demands or with an adult who has cognitive impairments could result in test scores that reflect poor understanding of the task, and not necessarily a lack of language comprehension for the targeted language items.

The responses we obtain on tasks involving identification, acting out, and metalinguistic judgment are usually scored on a right/wrong basis. Usually the client's overall performance on one of these tests takes the form of a total score (raw score) reflecting the number of correct or incorrect items. Sometimes, when time is limited, we use a shortcut in administration, called a basal-ceiling procedure. For example, the PPVT-III is designed to measure receptive vocabulary in individuals from 2:6 to 90+ years of age and does this by using a maximum of 204 items. Because the items on this test are scaled from early learned to later learned, we can avoid giving all the items by using the basal-ceiling method.

The basic idea with this method is that many of the items on a test such as the PPVT-III will be either very easy for the client or very hard. That is, they will be well below the client's developmental level or well above it. There will also be a set of items that represent a transition from well-known words to words that are not known. If we can identify this region and give only test items slightly below the transition region on up to items that are slightly above it, we can then determine the client's level of development without having to give all items. This is accomplished by establishing a basal level for the client. This is a set of test items in which we observe very high levels of accuracy. Therefore, we will credit the client with correct performance below this basal level because we assume that, if we had administered these items, the client would have gotten them correct. Once we establish the basal level, we then progress through the test administering items above it that are increasingly difficult and we expect that the client will be making an increasing number of errors. Finally, we should reach a point at which the client's performance is simply a guessing game, because the items are unknown and therefore too difficult. This is the point of ceiling performance. Giving more items beyond the ceiling will not be useful because all we would be doing is measuring the client's guessing performance.

Therefore, we can stop and assume that the client will get no more items correct except by luck. The client's raw score using this basal-ceiling approach will be the number of items the client got correct up to the ceiling level plus the number of items below basal, since we are giving the client credit for these. You will find the basal-ceiling procedure used in many tests designed for developmental assessment of language and in particular those measuring receptive language skills. You will need to look at the test manual in each case to determine specifically how the basal and ceiling levels are to be determined, since this will vary from test to test.

Expressive Language Testing

There are a number of different tasks that can be used to assess a client's expressive language. Among these are: *confrontation naming; imitation,* both direct and delayed; the *cloze technique; retelling;* and *spontaneous language sampling.* Each task can be viewed as a method of eliciting or increasing the likelihood that the client will produce language targets of interest.

Confrontation Naming

In this task the client is presented with a picture or an object and has to name that picture or item. *The Expressive One-Word Vocabulary Test* (EOWPVT; Gardner, 1979) and the *Boston Naming Test* (Kaplan et al., 1983) are examples of tests that utilize this task. Most tests designed to assess the speech sound system also employ picture identification. Of course, in that case the fact that the client can or cannot identify the picture is secondary to whether or not he or she can produce the target sound(s) embedded in the name of the picture. Sets of pictured stimuli or three-dimensional objects are presented and the clinician asks the client, "What's this?" or "Tell me what that is." Error responses from the client may come in the form of "not knowing," and therefore not giving a word, or they may be in the form of some type of response that is not correct. Clients with developmental language disorders will usually either give "I don't know" responses or an incorrect word. Clients with acquired language problems will also give these types of error responses, but they also may provide responses that are not real words. This latter type of error is called "neologistic paraphasia." Responses to confrontation naming can also be measured with respect to the speed of the client's response, which reflects the client's facility with word retrieval.

> Expressive language skills are usually impaired in individuals with language impairment.

Performance on these tasks may be used to establish the level of vocabulary development attained by the client. This is what is provided by the EOWPVT. Alternatively, you may use this type of task to determine if the client has difficulties retrieving and using words that he or she knows; that is, you are interested in determining if there is a *word-finding problem.* When we are using confrontation naming to evaluate for word-finding problems, we must have some way of demonstrating that the client knows the word for the pictures being presented. Therefore, when the client cannot name the picture, we can assume that it is due to a failure in retrieving the word rather than the word not being in the client's vocabulary. There are two common ways of determining that the client knows the word. The first approach is to demonstrate that the client can recognize the word in a receptive vocabulary task. The other approach is to show that the client can use the word in other naming activities. Evidence for word-finding problems is usually based both on frequent problems using words that are known, and on slow response rates during confrontation naming.

Imitation

These tasks represent a quick way to elicit information from a client. The client is told to repeat what the clinician says; younger children are sometimes told that they are playing a "copycat" game with the clinician. In a *direct imitation* task, the expectation is for the client to repeat back the clinician's production without any delay or intervening language. When some delay factor is imposed, either a brief time interval or additional language, the task becomes a *delayed imitation* task. Of the two imitation types, we assume that the delayed imitation task presents a greater challenge than the direct imitation task because it requires the client to hold information in memory longer before answering. The *Carrow Elicited Language Inventory* (CELI) is an example of a language test that employs a direct imitation task. The client is asked to repeat a set of 51 utterances one at a time after they are spoken by a clinician, starting with very brief, simple sentence structures and ending with much longer, more complex sentence structures. Most comprehensive tests of aphasia include imitation (repetition of speech) subtests. Some speech-language pathologists assert that performance on imitation of words and high- and low-frequency sentences assists in classification of aphasic patients into various subtypes of aphasia or syndromes such as Broca's aphasia versus transcortical motor aphasia.

Some have criticized imitation tasks because they have concluded that they may underestimate a client's language performance in more natural language usage tasks. This seems counterintuitive since imitation seems to be a simple task. However, imitation has some of the qualities of a metalinguistic task since imitation is not a communicative use of language and, as we noted earlier, metalinguistic tasks tend to be demanding. Therefore, clients may fail to imitate sentences with certain grammatical structures correctly, yet show clear evidence of being able to use the grammatical form in spontaneous speech. Imitation tasks have been criticized occasionally as more indicative of short-term memory than language ability. However, there are data to the contrary. There is considerable evidence that the sentence imitation performance of children and adults correlates well with their level of grammatical use in spontaneous speech. Thus, clients who are more advanced grammatically or who have better language production skill following a brain injury tend to imitate sentences better than clients who have poorer grammatical skills. This means that we can use sentence imitation tasks to provide us with an index of the child's growth status or as an estimate of the adult's expressive language capability, but we do need to be cautious about looking at specific grammatical errors made during imitation and assuming that they indicate that the client cannot use the form in spontaneous speech.

Sometimes imitation tasks are employed because they can elicit a language sample very quickly. When pressed for time, this can be a helpful strategy for clinicians so long as they remember that there is a potential "down" side to collecting imitation data. Another strategy is to use imitation tasks in combination with another method of collecting expressive language information so that the validity of the information can be cross-checked from one method to the other.

> Imitation tasks may be particularly helpful with clients who have poor intelligibility because you will know what the client is attempting to say.

The Cloze Technique

This is really a fill–in type of task and is commonly used to elicit expressive language. The examiner presents a sentence or sentences in which one or more elements are missing. Usually the missing element(s) is at the end of a sentence or a phrase. The grammatic closure subtest from the TOLD–2:P is an example of a cloze technique. For example, a client could be shown a photograph of a child climbing a tree and be told, "Yesterday the boy climbed the tree. Today he _____ . . . ." and the client is expected to complete the sentence by saying, "climbs the tree." The portion of the sentence that is given should provide the client with sufficient cues to produce the grammatical form or structure of interest that has been left out of the sentence. This technique is frequently used when testing adults with suspected language problems and is thought to be a good indicator of stimulability. When testing adults, the cloze technique uses stimuli that vary along the convergent/divergent continuum. Stimuli that produce one or only a few possible responses (e.g., Grass is _____) are convergent and stimuli that have numerous appropriate responses (e.g., I like _____) are considered divergent.

Retelling Tasks

With these, a story or some text is presented to the client either auditorily, visually (e.g., via pictures, videotape, written text, or film), or by a combination of the two. The client is told to listen or watch carefully or to read the presented material, and then to tell the "story" back to the examiner. Of course, the client has received some sort of model representation in a retelling task but usually it is so lengthy that it would be largely impossible for the client to be using imitation skills only to complete it. Sometimes, too, the client is permitted to have accompanying visual stimuli while retelling the story. This reduces the memory loading of the task and makes it more likely that the examiner is eliciting information that only reflects the client's expressive language abilities. The sounds–in–sentences subtest of the *Goldman-Fristoe Test of Articulation* (Goldman & Fristoe, 1986) is an example of a *retelling task*. Delayed recall has been used to distinguish dementing illness from other neurogenic language problems, such as aphasia (Bayles & Tomoeda, 1990). Used that way, problems with specific memory may be determined by comparing immediate with delayed recall.

LANGUAGE SAMPLE COLLECTION

Language sampling is another expressive language task that can be employed to evaluate language production abilities. Because of its widespread use, the next section of the chapter has been devoted to the collection and analysis of language sample data. Although language sampling is a frequently used method of obtaining data for the evaluation of children's language abilities, typically it has not been part of adult language assessment. That may now be changing, however, due to the proliferation of studies of adults with neurological deficits—traumatic brain injury (TBI) and dementia, to name two—where language sampling procedures have been used with some success to diagnose and treat these patients. Language sample analysis is valuable because it can provide a clinician with a very rich window into the client's language competencies. Although some clinicians may view language sample collection and analysis as too time consuming for their employment setting, we believe that it is important to find a way to collect some information in this venue.

Language Sampling Techniques

A spontaneous language sample is a set of utterances produced by clients usually without being elicited by the examiner, and collected and analyzed by clinicians to help determine language production abilities. Our clinical goal is to collect a sample that is "representative" of the client's entire language repertoire. We recognize that we cannot gather every possible utterance a client can produce, so instead we hope to collect a sample of at least 50 and preferably 100 or 200 utterances that will cover the range of possible forms and structures we would find if it *were* possible to collect every single possible utterance.

Some clinicians attempt to collect samples that are chiefly monologues; others prefer to collect samples from naturalistic conversations. Regardless of which focus is selected, language samples should not contain imitated or rote-learned passages for much the same reason that imitation tasks, in general, are limited in usefulness (Miller, 1981). The examiner should also avoid eliciting too much of the sample through question asking because responses to questions tend to contain diminished length and complexity. An open-ended request like, "Tell me about your favorite TV program" is better than a question like, "What is your favorite TV program?" Language samples that are largely comprised of answers to specific questions, memorized passages, and imitation may either underestimate or overestimate the client's true language capabilities and so they should be avoided. Similarly, samples collected in highly structured settings (e.g., putting together a puzzle with a conversation partner) will yield more limited language information than samples collected in a less structured context (e.g., having the child choose an activity of interest).

Typically, the examiner constructs situations in which the client can choose the topic and range of the conversation. For young children, provocative toys (e.g., a truck with a missing wheel, a doll with a missing limb) and unfamiliar objects (i.e., items that the child may not have previously seen or have a name for) are made available for play because they often elicit interaction from the client (e.g., "What's that?" "How did that get broken?"). Toys that support "scenario" or role play are also useful for this purpose (e.g., dollhouse, camper). Older children may prefer pictures and an interview format (Evans & Craig, 1994), while adults may need little prompting beyond some general, open-ended requests/questions like, "Tell me what you like to do in your spare time," to elicit a lengthy sample for analysis. Most clinicians are aware that individuals with language disorders tend to be reticent. Therefore, collecting language samples from these clients may require more time, patience, and planning than would be the case with clients whose language systems are intact.

We may also choose to use different types of discourse in collecting the sample. In addition to the quasi-monologues that speech-language pathologists often collect, *narratives, expository text*, and *conversation* are three examples of discourse type that could be utilized in language sample collection. For example, a clinician may want to collect a sample that reflects a client's understanding of story structures, and so a *narrative* sample will be collected. To this end, a clinician can provide the client with the title of a story, a topic, or the first line of a story. In a series of story creation tasks, Stein and Glenn (1979) presented schoolage children with the first line of three different stories, for example, "Once there was a boy named Alan who had many different toys." The children were told that they could make their stories as long or as short as they liked, but that the stories should contain all the things a good story should have. Another option is to give the client very little direction beyond telling him or her to make up a story on any topic. Often, clinicians help put younger clients on the right track by telling them to start their stories with the phrase, "Once upon a time . . . ." This serves as a cue, so that even if the direction "tell me a story" does not make sense, "once upon a time" is often a sufficient reminder of what a story means and how to begin it. Of course, for this cue to work as intended, we are assuming a background in literacy learning, and not all of the children we evaluate will have this background.

A sample of *expository* discourse provides an explanation to the listener, and sometimes a clinician may ask a client to produce some expository discourse as part of sample collection. We may ask a child to explain to us how airplanes fly or how to make the best peanut butter and jelly sandwich. Explanation topics should be chosen carefully according to the client's age and cultural background. For example, one of our recent graduates who was from Japan wanted to collect expository text samples from a group of schoolchildren there. She came up with a topic that gave her subjects very little trouble when she asked them to tell her how to prepare for an earthquake. With the frequent incidence of earthquakes in Japan, there is a high degree of public awareness of earthquakes, their disaster potential, and public preparedness. Thus, this is a procedure that each Japanese schoolchild must know something about. On the other hand, for many adults in the United States, topics like explaining how to grocery shop efficiently and how to parallel park may be useful if expository discourse tasks are selected.

There are considerable problems in trying to write down the sample during the interview itself. Not only is it difficult to write down the utterances and context notes quickly enough (except in a situation where a clinician works with clients who have minimal language output), but there is a tendency to write down sentences that are more complete than those the client actually produced or to otherwise incorrectly recall utterances. As a result, in most examining situations, the interview is audiotaped or videotaped for later analysis. Videotaping presents a better opportunity for recording a sample because it preserves the sample's contextual information along with the language content. That is, it is important to know what preceded a client's utterance, both linguistically and nonlinguistically, so that the appropriateness of a client's utterances can be determined.

Elicitor Effects

It is reasonable to assume that some features of a conversation depend on the relationships between the people involved in the conversation. When the focus is on the conversation of a client, we give some attention to the other person(s) in the conversation, whom we call the "coconversationalist." As already mentioned, clinicians need to guard against providing too much input, thereby unnecessarily biasing the client's sample. Samples collected with parents or other family members, like spouses or siblings, may also be biased because a particular coconversationalist may typically dominate conversations with the client or, conversely, may always be a passive coconversationalist. If only one coconversationalist is used for data collection, the picture of the client's expressive abilities that emerges may reflect only one type of conversation interaction. One solution to this problem is to collect several smaller language samples in different settings where the coconversationalists vary (Fey, 1986). Some may be familiar to the client and some may be unfamiliar. Some may be older or younger than the client so that the coconversationalist's language competence may sometimes match and sometimes be dissimilar to the client's. This way the clinician can determine if the client can demonstrate a number of different styles of language use or if the client has one pervasive language use style that is relatively unaffected by the different demands placed by coconversationalists who are more assertive in conversation than others or who may need more information and less sophisticated language. Fey's (1986) system of classifying language use in conversational contexts emphasizes the importance of determining how a client actually uses the language he or she is capable of using.

Language Sample Analyses

Analyses of a language sample can delineate information about semantics, morphology, phonology, pragmatics, or syntax. Historically, syntax and morphological measures have been the most widely used analysis types, with MLU probably being the most commonly used measure of sentence length, and Developmental Sentence Scoring (DSS; Lee, 1974), being a popular measure of sentence complexity (see Figure 6–5).

Each of these measures provides a quantitative index of the child's level of grammatical development. These quantitative mea-

MEASURE	DESCRIPTION
MLU (Brown, 1973)	A measure of the average number of morphemes per utterance where an utterance consists of a simple sentence. MLU is a general index of grammatic development in the range between 1.01 and 4.49.
DSS (Lee, 1974)	A measure of grammatical development that scores a sentence based upon the presence of certain grammatical forms. Forms that are later developing receive higher values than early developing forms. Thus, the DSS score increases as more advanced grammatical forms are used.

Figure 6–5. Descriptions of mean length of utterance (MLU), a commonly used measure of sentence length, and developmental sentence scoring (DSS), a common measure of sentence complexity.

sures, when used in conjunction with the normative data available for them, can be used to evaluate the child's development status. There are several excellent resources for discussion of clinical language sample collection and analysis, among them: Barrie-Blackley et al. (1978); Retherford (1993); Miller (1981); and Hughes et al. (1997), with the last focusing on analysis of narrative transcripts. You are encouraged to consult these references for a detailed explanation of a number of different analysis procedures as well as for information about the theoretical underpinnings of sample collection.

Clinicians select from among the available language sample collection procedures for a number of different reasons. For example, a clinician may know a priori that a client's ability to use language efficiently and successfully in conversation is often compromised. Rather than use a language sample analysis procedure that only codes syntactic structures, the clinician may choose to use a procedure that takes into account the functioning of the client's utterances in terms of topic maintenance or topic initiation (pragmatics), for example. Analysis of topic maintenance or topic initiation would not require a sample of complete sentences but would require that the language sample be collected in a conversational context and coded for method of topic management (e.g., topic initiation, topic management). Other sampling procedures might be selected because of the extent or type of normative data provided by the author(s) of the procedure. For example, if an analysis provided normative data for 8-year-olds, this sampling instrument might be a more attractive "fit" for a particular clinical situation.

A number of language analysis procedures are available in computerized form, for example, *Systematic Analyses of Language Transcripts* (SALT) (Miller & Chapman, 1985) and *Computerized Profiling* (Long & Fey, 1998), among others. By coding and inputting the samples in prescribed ways, these computer programs tally different dimensions of language production. Depend-ing on the particular program used, some calculate standard measures like MLU, DSS, and provide clinicians with a less laborious task than traditional analysis of language samples by hand. Often, context notes can be included directly into the sample so that none of the information that would be helpful in interpretation of the sample is separated from the analysis.

You should recognize that, even if computerized programs are used for language sample analysis, you, and not the computer, are responsible for understanding the underlying analyses that are being applied to the samples. Without an understanding of how the language sample analyses are applied and calculated, it is unlikely that you will be able to determine which analysis type to apply, how to interpret changes in the analysis from calculation to calculation, and how to figure out if the results obtained from the computer may be indicative of a program or coding error.

See Table 6–1 for a summary of language sample collection and analysis strategies for the preverbal child, preschool child, school-aged child, adolescent, and adults.

Table 6–1. Language sampling across the life span.

Age Range	Suggested Sampling Activities	Look for:	Helpful References
Infants and Toddlers (Preverbal to Emerging Language; approximately 0 to 2 years of age)	• Observation of the child with the primary caregiver(s). • Use a variety of familiar and unfamiliar toys; place some just out of reach or make them otherwise inaccessible without assistance from an adult. • Coggins & Carpenter (1981) suggest a sample of 45 minutes duration.	• Evidence of responsiveness on the part of the caregiver(s) to the child's initiated bids. Compare styles of interactions. Does the infant provide clear signals of interest in interaction? • Evidence of developing communicative interactions, e.g., protoimperatives and protodeclaratives. • Evidence of nonlinguistic comprehension strategies, e.g., "imitation of on-going actions," versus evidence of true word comprehension. • Evidence of the child's repertoire of volitional vocalizations and speech sounds; precursors to word use. • Evidence of real word use: (1) resemblance to an adult word, (2) consistent phonetic form, (3) used in consistent context. • Analysis of early words in terms of pragmatic function and semantic categorization.	Rossetti (1990) Coggins & Carpenter (1981) Bates (1976) Chapman (1978) Proctor (1989) Owens (1996) Dore (1974); Bloom (1973); Nelson (1973)
Preschoolers (approximately 2 to 5 years of age)	• Collect several language samples with different coconversationalists in different settings and with different degrees of structure. 50–200 utterances are usually recommended. • Use materials that lend themselves to the creation of scenarios, e.g., dollhouse, toy farm.	• Evidence of assertiveness and responsiveness in conversations and their different proportions relative to the different samples collected. • Evidence of age-appropriate syntactic structure and use of grammatical morphemes as per mean length of utterance and Developmental Sentence Scoring, for example.	Fey (1986) Brown (1973) and Miller (1981) for MLU analysis; Lee (1974) for DSS, and Retherford (1993)

(continued)

Table 6–1. *(continued)*

Age Range	Suggested Sampling Activities	Look for:	Helpful References
Preschoolers *(continued)*	• Use open-ended requests for information that do not constrain response length and complexity, e.g., "Tell me about . . ." • Use a variety of familiar and unfamiliar materials and follow the child's lead. • Although conversation samples are most often used, you can also use prompts for personal narratives, scripts, and story retelling. Be sure to use a lot of visual support materials.	• Evidence of a \ ety of vocabulary words in the sample, e.g., Type–Token Ratio, as per Templin (1957). • Evidence that the child is accommodating language to his/her listeners via responses to or requests for clarification, presuppositional skills; question comprehension is evident by appropriate responses made to questions asked. • Evidence of observation of turn taking rules; little if any "simultalk" occurs. • Child can maintain a topic for several turns.	Brinton & Fujiki (1989)
School–age children (approximately 6 to 12 years of age)	• Provide prompts for personal narratives, fictional stories, and scripts with visual support, e.g., "Make up a story about something that's not real." • Use of interview questions as per Evans & Craig (1992): (1) What can you tell me about your family? (2) Tell me about school. (3) Tell me about what you like to do when you are not in school. • For older children, collect both written and oral samples. • Collect samples of classroom discourse from both ends of the formal-informal continuum.	• Evidence of a cohesive discourse structure: What is the overall structure of the discourse and how adequate is it? • Use of later-developing syntax forms: postmodification of nouns, coordinate conjunctions, adverbial clauses, infinitives, complements, and subjunctive modals. • Evidence of more sophisticated sentence repair strategies or use of alternation rules when faced with communication breakdowns.	Hughes, McGillvray, & Schmidek (1997); Roth & Spekman (1986) Scott (1988); Nippold (1998); Weiss & Johnson (1993) Damico (1991); Westby (1994)

(continued)

Table 6–1. *(continued)*

Age Range	Suggested Sampling Activities	Look for:	Helpful References
Adolescents (junior high school and high school age)	• Use activities that require story creation or retelling either with or without visual support. • Collect a sample of expository discourse. • Elicit samples of both oral and written discourse. • Use written materials to prompt conversations, e.g., a provocative newspaper article.	• Evidence of perspective taking and acknowledgment of others' perspectives and opinions. • Greater finesse should be expected in terms of discourse cohesion and structure. • Comparison of cohesion in samples where information is shared versus not shared with the audience.	Hughes, McGillvray, & Schmidek (1997)
Adults	• Story generation and story retelling without visual stimuli; context not shared. • Fable retelling, proverb interpretation, picture descriptions; use of picture sequences, cartoon stimuli.	• Sentence complexity, completeness of episode structure, proportion of core information presented (in recall); proportion of revisions, words per minute.	Nicholas & Brookshire (1993), Chapman (1997); Chapman, Ulatowska, Franklin, Shobe, Thompson, & McIntire (1997); Chapman, Levin, & Culhane (1995); Ulatowska, Chapman, Highley, & Prince (1998)

INTERPRETATION OF INFORMATION

For quite a while now we have been talking about the ways in which we go about gathering information concerning the client's language performance. Remember, however, that all of this information gathering is done for a purpose: to determine in what areas the client is having problems with language and the particular character of these problems. To draw some conclusions with respect to these issues, we must begin to interpret the information we have gathered. Much of what we will talk about here builds on information covered in Chapter 1 on the interpretation of clinical measures. As you may recall, there are three common interpretive approaches that are often used: *norm-referenced, criterion-referenced* and *client-referenced.* Each of these approaches may be used in determining whether or not your client has a language disorder.

Norm-Referenced Interpretation

The norm-referenced approach is often used when it appears that we are dealing with a developmental language disorder. Recall that a norm-referenced interpretation involves the comparison of your client to some group of individuals referred to as the normative group. Further, norm-referenced interpretation involves a quantitative statement regarding how the person stands within the normative group through the use of standard scores or percentiles (see Chapter 1). Since developmental language disorders seem to involve impairments in the rate of development, we often base our decision about a child's language status with regard to where the child is in this growth process versus where we would expect the child to be. Thus, language impairment is determined by a discrepancy between the client's expected language status and the levels of achievement we obtained from our observations.

Two different approaches can be used as a basis for our expectations for clients and these approaches lead us to compare the client to different normative groups. The first approach seems rather obvious: we use the client's *chronological age* as the basis of our expectations and, therefore, we compare our client to other individuals of a similar chronological age. One rationale for this approach is that our society bases its expectations on the age of the person. For instance, children are expected to enter elementary school at around 6 years old, and they are expected to be able to perform much like an adult by age 15 or so. A child who presents with language skills substantially below those of his age peers is likely to have difficulties meeting these expectations.

In contrast to the use of chronological age, some have argued that we use the child's level of *nonverbal development* or the adult's level of *nonverbal ability* as the basis for determining our expectations. However, the relationship between nonverbal processing and language functioning in adults is less clear than in children. In the case of a child, the level of language development, based on standardized measures, is compared with nonverbal intelligence, and the child is considered to have a developmental language disorder if the verbal development and performance are substantially poorer than nonlanguage development and performance. Therefore, a child's language development should follow cognitive development, and when it does not, we have evidence for language impairment. The rationale for this approach has rested on the belief that language development is dependent on cognitive development. In recent years this diagnostic standard has received criticism from several sources (Lahey, 1989; Cole et al., 1990). Adults with brain lesions may have differences between verbal and nonverbal skills, in either direction, with verbal skills being lower or higher than nonverbal skills. This information is used to understand the basis of the communication problem and develop appropriate treatment goals. In some instances when working with adults, nonverbal skills are used to suggest potential for improvement but in a guarded manner. The rationale for this approach has rested on the belief that language development is dependent on cognitive development and that language and cognition are inextricably linked in adults. Regardless of which standard you use for basing your language development expectations, if you decide to use a norm-referenced approach to the determination of language impairment, then you will need to select measurement methods that provide the appropriate norms for your client.

Criterion-Referenced Interpretation

Criterion-referenced standards for measurement interpretation compare the client's performance to a performance standard based on what is considered by some authorities to be minimally adequate. For example, soon your clinical work will be evaluated and your supervisor will decide whether you are doing "acceptable" work. It is very likely that this judgment will be based on her beliefs about what kind of clinical work is necessary for appropriate service to the client. In so doing, this supervisor is using a criterion-referenced grading system. Criterion-referenced decisions for the determination of language impairment may be used for either developmental or acquired language disorders. Based on discussions with primary grade teachers, a speech-language pathologist may decide that first grade children should be able to express themselves in simple but grammatically acceptable sentences, to follow a set of basic commands, and to retell a simple short story. Failure by a child to do any of these things could result in a determination of a language disorder. Likewise, we know that adults should be able to carry out routine conversational activities. An adult who demonstrates several failures in the maintenance of a conversation because of an inability to either formulate ideas or to comprehend things said may be judged to have a language disorder on the basis of these criterion-referenced standards.

Client-Referenced Interpretation

Client-referenced standards use the client's own performance as the basis for making a decision regarding a language disorder. This type of standard is frequently used as the basis for evaluating acquired disorders. Although we rarely have formal language measures on clients prior to their acquiring a language disorder, we can obtain a reasonable sense of how a person was doing prior to a stroke or head injury. Some of this information may come directly from an informant such as a spouse, but we can also make some inferences about the person's language status based on the client's occupation and education. Using this information, we can compare our observations of the client's current performance with levels of performance we believe to have existed prior to the brain injury. A substantial decline in language performance may be viewed as evidence of an acquired language disorder.

Arriving at a Conclusion: Is There a Language Disorder?

Using one or a combination of the interpretative methods described above, you should be able to arrive at a conclusion as to whether or not the client has a language disorder. In making this decision, you will no doubt use your observations of the person's performance on both structured and informal language tasks. Further, you will draw on your knowledge of the client's background in interpreting the kinds of communication demands this person faces and the language abilities you have observed. Based on this information and the ways in which you can interpret it, you will ultimately need to answer the question: Is this person likely to have difficulties in his or her life because of the language skills he or she now possesses or will have in the future? If the answer is "yes," you have concluded there *is* a language disorder.

Determining Areas of Strengths and Needs

The observations we have made about a client's language status should allow us to go beyond a simple statement that he or she has a language disorder. At the same time that we are considering the information obtained from our language evaluation for the purposes of determining the presence of an overall problem, we are also looking for patterns of strengths and needs. Here we see an obvious place for us to use a client-referenced approach to interpretation, because we will be comparing one area of language performance to another within the same person. As we noted earlier, some language assessment instruments are comprised of a set of subtests that cover several different areas of language performance. These test batteries are usually designed so that the client's scores can be arranged to form a profile both of strengths and of areas in which the client demonstrates some needs. In other instances, the profile of performance will be derived from information obtained from different tests.

The use of profiles to display a client's strengths and needs requires that the measures obtained be converted into a common format. For instance, if you have obtained an MLU score for a child and also have a receptive vocabulary measure based upon the PPVT-III raw score, you will not be able to compare these two numbers because they are counting very different things. The typical solution to this problem has been to use norm referencing. Thus, for example, the client's raw scores on the two measures above would be converted to standard scores, such as percentiles, based on the client's chronological age. In this way, all the scores are comparable in that they represent where the client stands in the normative population for MLU and receptive vocabulary. This should be a very familiar process to you since you no doubt took the SAT or the ACT as a high-school student. These tests both have subtest areas and when you received your results, you were given a simple profile having to do with your scores in each area. If it was the SAT that you took, you may have learned that you did better in the quantitative subtest than the verbal. The scores you were looking at were standard scores in each case, where the mean was 500 and the standard deviation was 100.

Notice that in our effort to identify a client's strengths and needs we are using two interpretive systems at once. We are using norm-referenced standard scores to make each test comparable so that we can then make a client-referenced interpretation of strengths and needs. A note of caution needs to be added here about using norm-referenced scores from different tests to identify areas of strengths and needs. What we want to do is identify the strengths and weaknesses of our client. The norm-referenced standard score translates the client's performance in two areas reflected by raw scores into two scores of relative standing. If we are to compare these scores of relative standing, it is important that the norms come from comparable groups; otherwise, the differences in the scores will not reflect differences within the client, but rather differences between the two normative groups. In our example of comparing a client's MLU and PPVT-III performance we will need to use two different normative groups to convert our scores to standard scores. Many people use norms provided by Miller and Chapman (1981) to interpret MLU values, whereas we use norms provided by the developers of the PPVT-III to interpret performance on this test. The same children were not in both normative groups, however. If one normative group was linguistically more advanced than the other group, the standard scores we obtain from these groups will not be comparable. As a result, when we convert our client's raw scores into standard scores, we may find differences that are not due to strengths and needs within the client, but rather, are due to differences in the normative populations. This problem can be solved by using measures that are normed on the same population, as are often provided by some of the test batteries.

DETERMINATION OF CONCOMITANT FACTORS

Language problems do not exist in a vacuum. Instead, we must assume that there are factors that have influenced and in some cases caused the problem. We will refer to these factors collectively as *concomitant factors*. These factors might be biological, psychological, and/or environmental in nature. In considering these factors, we want to know not only what things might be working against the client's language status, but also what might be working for the client's language performance. To think about this issue, you will need to develop a scheme that allows you to think about what might influence the client's language status. Many of these concomitant factors will be shared between developmental and acquired language disorders; however, their impact on language performance or their relevance to this performance may be different. Therefore we will talk about these two forms of language disorders separately.

Examining for concomitant factors requires that you have a theory about what can influence language performance.

Concomitant Factors in Developmental Language Disorders

By now you no doubt have had some course work concerned with language development, and it should come as no surprise to you that there is a lot we do not know about the factors that influence language development. Specifically, we do not understand, as well as we probably someday will, how to weigh an individual factor's influence on the presence of a language disorder for an individual child. This forces us to work with partial knowledge, but the clinical world often requires that we do the best we can with what we do know.

One concomitant factor that must be considered when thinking about developmental language disorders is *hearing*. We know that a child needs to hear language in order to learn oral speech and language. Thus, any time we find a child having problems with language development, we want to know if there is a hearing loss. This is one of the concomitant factors that can directly cause a language problem. Further, by treating the hearing loss either medically or with a hearing aid, and thus reducing the child's hearing impairment, we should improve the child's ability to learn language. Notice here that it is just as important clinically for us to know that the child has normal hearing as it is for us to know that the child has a hearing loss. It is the child's hearing status, not just the presence of a hearing loss, that is important to us. Many of our language measures assume that the child heard what we said. Unless we know the child's hearing status, we will not be able to be sure our test results are valid.

Another concomitant factor we want to know about is the child's *home environment.* We know that children need to be exposed to language in order to acquire it. At this time we do not know what circumstances are absolutely necessary for adequate language learning. We can say, however, that better rates of language development are found in homes in which the parents talk with their children about things the child is doing and saying. This coincides with a pattern of language interaction that is often found in mainstream American households where children are viewed early on as viable communication partners and thus included frequently in conversations even when they are minimally competent to hold up their own end of the conversation (van Kleeck, 1994). There are probably only a very few children who present language disorders because they have been denied even minimal levels of language exposure; however, there are probably many children whose unfavorable home environment is compounding their language learning problem. Unfortunately, we have few ways, short of visiting the home, to learn about the rearing environment. It is possible, though, to talk with parents about the ways they talk with their child and, as well, in some clinical settings you can observe the parent interact with the client. There are no clear guidelines as to when you would want to conclude that the environment is contributing to the problem and is likely to conflict with the course of therapy. At this point, however, you should recognize the need to think about the child's opportunities for language exposure and their potential impact for good or ill on the child's language development.

Language development and use are influenced by and influence the cognitive functions of concept development, memory, attention, problem solving, and many other mental systems. The relationship between language and cognition is sufficiently complex that we are unlikely to be able to make strong claims about a child's cognitive skills causing deficits in language development. Many clinicians have made the reasonable assumption that children with developmental language disorder who have normal or above normal nonverbal intellect will fare better with respect to language progress than those who have subnormal nonverbal skills. If this is true, even though you might not attribute the language impairment to the cognitive status of the child, you may employ this information in making predictions about the child's future progress. Recently, there has been some evidence that the beneficial influence of higher cognitive ability on language development is not necessarily true (Cole et al., 1990). More research will be required before we will know how or under what circumstances the child's nonverbal cog-

The hearing status of the child with a language impairment must always be determined.

nitive abilities limit or promote language development. Thus, just as with the issue of language exposure, you will need to keep this factor in mind, and as new information becomes available, you can determine how you will use it in your clinical decision making.

There is one concomitant factor with which many parents of children with developmental language disorders will be concerned. This factor is *brain dysfunction* or *brain injury*. For many of the children you will see who have language problems, you will find that they have normal hearing, they seem to have been provided with sufficient exposure to the language of their community, and they have adequate nonverbal cognitive skills. Through a process of elimination one could argue that, for these children, there is something about their brain that must be causing them to have language problems. Others have argued that this conclusion is based solely on negative evidence, and that this negative evidence is not sufficient to claim that we know that the child has a neurological problem. There are a number of ways in which neurological problems are determined and the speech-language pathologist does not make that particular diagnosis. However, speech-language clinicians should know when to refer a child to the appropriate professionals (neurologists and/or neuropsychologists) for neurological examinations. And therefore, SLPs need to be familiar with the tools used by those professionals. To determine the presence of neuropathologies a variety of different brain imaging techniques can be used, such as the computerized tomography (CT) scan or the magnetic resonance imaging (MRI) technique, both of which are available at most hospitals. As well, there are a number of functional tests such as electroencephalography (EEG), evoked potentials, and nerve conduction studies that neurologists use to document the presence of a neuropathology. Finally, both neurologists and neuropsychologists use a variety of behavioral measures to infer the presences of neurological disease. Some recent research evidence is suggesting that at least some children with developmental language problems may have some subtle differences in their brain structure. This evidence comes from imaging studies of the central nervous system that require very expensive equipment and unusual expertise. Currently, this type of examination is not done as a part of routine clinical examinations of clients with developmental language disorders. As a result, most of the time we are unable to know whether or not a child has any unusual brain characteristics. We said earlier that parents will ask about this issue. When this topic comes up, what do you say? The best answer is the truth, and usually this is that we do not know whether there are subtle brain differences and there is at this time no good way of answering the question.

On the other hand, there may be evidence of brain damage not requiring such sophisticated examination methods. For example, if the client demonstrates certain neurological signs, such as very poor motor skills, or evidence of seizures, you should refer the client to a neurologist. You should also refer the client to a neurologist if you have evidence that he is regressing in language status. Recall that developmental language problems involve limitations in the rate of language growth, but we do not expect these individuals to lose skills that they have developed. If this is happening, there may be an active disease process occurring and the client should be seen by a neurologist.

The concomitant factors we have just discussed are the principal ones having to do with developmental language disorders. There are others that you may also want to keep in mind—for instance, the client's attitudes and concerns about the problem, the presence of behavioral or emotional problems, or the presence of other health factors. These things and many more all may have an impact on the client's general status and may influence the decisions you make.

Concomitant Factors in Acquired Language Disorders

As indicated earlier, the concomitant factors in acquired language disorders are similar to those already mentioned for children with developmental disorders, but there are a few important differences. Among the similarities are *hearing, home environment*, and *cognition*. As with the child, hearing status is important. This is particularly true for older adults who frequently suffer sensorineural hearing loss as a function of growing older. As with the child, it is important to know if the client has a hearing loss or normal hearing in order to best interpret the results of our language testing.

Also similar to the child is the need to know something about the home environment. Thus, when assessing adults we should gain enough information about the home environment to determine the presence of factors that may facilitate or impede communication. With adults we also need to gain information about the work environment to determine the needs and factors at work that may exacerbate the client's problems.

As is also the case with children, the interrelationship between language and cognition must be considered in the evaluation of adult language skills. In some instances one may need to consider that the basis of the language problem is in the cognitive domain. For instance, a number of the communication problems seen in individuals with traumatic brain injuries may stem from cognitive problems such as memory loss or poor attentional abilities. Moreover, many persons with right hemisphere involvement have high-level language problems such as an inability to make logical inferences that may go beyond verbal stimuli. Thus, knowledge of nonverbal skills is an important aspect of understanding acquired language disorders.

In the case of acquired language disorders, sensory modalities other than hearing loss may be disturbed as a function of aging or brain injury. For instance, assessment of visual status is as important as assessment of hearing. Since we frequently test reading and writing ability in adults with acquired language problems, knowledge of visual status is critical. As well, changes in vision can affect the interpretation of any stimulus (e.g., object or picture) placed before the client and thus change performance. Visual changes to be aware of in adults with acquired problems include sensory changes as a result of the aging process as well as visual function change as a result of neurologic insult. Common types of problems related to neurological lesions include visual field deficits (i.e., patients may be blind in a portion of their vision) and color, depth, or form perception problems. Tactile and proprioceptive sensory changes may also occur following brain damage and these need to be considered in interpretation of performance on language tests.

Another important concomitant factor when evaluating adults is the motor ability of the client. Many persons with brain injuries suffer paralysis of all or part of their body. Thus, movement of body parts may be impaired, making interpretation of pointing responses difficult. The clinician will need to find ways to assess language that do not rely on a fine motor response. In other words, the reliability of the client's motor response must be carefully considered in evaluation of adults with acquired language problems. In addition, most adults with aphasia have concomitant motor speech problems. For instance, individuals with lesions of the left frontal lobes and aphasia frequently have apraxia of speech as well. This makes delineation of the language and speech components of the overall communication problem difficult.

A particular problem with adults with acquired language problems has to do with the emotional status of the client. Many neurologic problems result in changes in emotion and personality. Thus, the person may not be motivated to cooperate during an evaluation or may be inappropriately angry or euphoric (catastrophic response). In addition, because the individual has suffered a potentially life-threatening event and is coping with a host of other physical problems, he or she may be less motivated to engage in communication testing. For instance, the person with a concomitant paralysis is often more concerned with an arm not working than with difficulty talking.

Finally, as is the case with children, the presence of other behavioral, health, or financial factors may impact on the client's current and future communication ability as well as the ability and willingness to seek appropriate special services. For this reason, all concomitant factors should be considered by the clinician.

PREDICTION OF THE COURSE OF THE LANGUAGE PROBLEM

As we talked about the identification of concomitant problems we began to talk not only about the client's current status with regard to language, but also the client's future status. In fact, one of the principal uses of the information gathered about concomitant factors is in predicting the future course of the problem. You will discover that clients and their family members are very interested in your answer to this question. In most instances the client's current status is well known to them and, therefore, your determination that the client has a language problem is not surprising. What they do want to know, however, is how the client will be doing in the future. Many clients with developmental or acquired language disorders will improve in their abilities over time, whether treated or not. However, even if they improve, they may never achieve normal status. Often, then, the question is how much improvement can be expected and can this outlook be improved by therapy? Our answer will depend, in part, on whether the disorder is developmental or acquired.

One of the important clinical services you can provide is to help the client and family build reasonable expectations for the future.

Predicting the Course of Developmental Language Disorders

As usual, the best guide to the future is the past. Thus, a child who presents evidence of very poor language development at age 4 is likely to continue to show very poor language development in the future, whereas the child with marginally normal levels of language development is likely to continue at this level. These predictions can be made assuming that none of the concomitant factors influencing language change. However, if we believe some of these concomitant factors have had a negative impact on the child's language development and we believe this negative influence can be removed, for example, through the use of hearing aids, then our prognosis will be more positive.

There is one group of children whose prognosis is particularly challenging. These are toddlers and young preschool children who are showing signs of slow language growth. Because of the fact that even normally developing children show uneven rates of language growth, we have difficulty determining whether a more persistent language problem will exist or whether they are going to "catch up" with their normal peers. The problem for us then is determining whether a young child with poor language skills will continue to have such a problem. Fortunately, this problem has received the attention of researchers and we now have some ways of improving our guesses. One of the most consistent positive signs for potential language development is the child's language comprehension abilities. Children whose language delays are limited to expressive language only are more likely to do better with respect to long-term language growth than those who have problems in both receptive and expressive language usage. This provides a good example of how the information you obtain in the assessment of language and, in particular, the client-referenced interpretation of strengths and weaknesses can be used to aid in an important clinical decision.

So far we have considered predicting the course of the language problem without intervention. We also must predict whether the client will improve with therapy and determine with which type of treatment the child is most likely to succeed. Our professional ethics dictate that we will provide therapy only when we believe that the client will benefit from it.

In the case of a young child, cooperativeness during the evaluation can be a predictor of how easily the client will be incorporated into the treatment setting. With young children, the transition into treatment may require more time and patience and a delay in the addition of activities that are structured and less playlike. So, if a child demonstrates some eagerness to participate in activities planned by the clinician during the evaluation and a willingness to try tasks that are obviously difficult or impossible to complete correctly, the clinician has obtained some valuable information: the client is a risk taker, at least where new skills are concerned, and fear of failure may not impede the forward progress of therapy. Therefore, it is a good idea for the clinician to plan some activities during an evaluation that are clearly beyond the client's easy capability. These provide an opportunity for the clinician to observe the client's perseverance and willingness to be wrong on the road to learning how to be right.

The Prognosis of Acquired Language Disorder

Patients who have an acquired language disorder as a result of neurological damage will usually present considerable variability with respect to their language status, as well as other behavioral characteristics over the course of their recovery. This is particularly true for those who have suffered from a stroke or traumatic event. For most of these patients, there is a period immediately after the insult during which many neurophysiologic events are occurring in response to the trauma. In particular, there will be swelling of the brain tissue, referred to as edema. During this early phase of recovery, you will often observe much poorer language function than you will later on. As the edema and other physiological responses to the trauma resolve, we can expect some return of language function. The challenge for us is to determine how much recovery can be expected.

When working with adults with acquired language problems, judgments about prognosis should be made with extreme caution, particularly in the early stages following neurologic insult. Although some clinicians suggest that age, gender, education level, and premorbid intelligence (to name a few) are predictors of outcome, recent data do not support these claims. Likewise, more research is needed on type, size, and site of lesion information in relation to prediction of outcome, particularly in the adult epoch. Only one standardized test, the *Porch Index of Communicative Ability* (PICA; Porch, 1968), purports to have prognostic value. However, numerous concomitant problems, including physical problems, rate of physiological recovery, emotional problems, cognitive impairments, and client motivation, impede our ability to accurately and reliably predict eventual language outcome. Prognosis, then, is a continually changing activity and we constantly need to assess and update our information.

In the later stages (at least 1 year postinsult), when the client's abilities in all areas have begun to stabilize, prognosis can become more accurate. This lack of ability to forecast outcome is often frustrating for clients and family members and these individuals will require our most supportive efforts during this time.

Another important piece of information that should be obtained during an evaluation involves the degree to which the client can monitor his or her language performance. That is, if it becomes obvious to the clinician at the time of the evaluation that the client can identify the language target and can accurately evaluate the acceptability or unacceptability of his or her attempts at producing the target, then the clinician knows that the rehabilitation process, in the case of an acquired language problem, or the habilitation process, in the case of a developmental problem, has begun. Often, monitoring skill is demonstrated by the client's ability to self-correct. Learning to monitor or make accurate judgments about one's own language is an essential component of the therapeutic process. In a sense, the clinician's goal is to make therapy and the clinician's participation obsolete by teaching the client how to become his or her own clinician. If the clinician's input for judging client productions is not needed or only needed intermittently, then the clinician has some evidence of a positive prognosis.

Conveying Diagnostic Information to the Client and Others

Clients should receive at least some information at the end of an evaluation session. It is true that additional testing sometimes must be scheduled for another test session and that after an initial meeting with a client it is not possible to tell the client very much about his or her problem. However, clients should be told where things stand and given any impressions the clinician may have formulated at that time. If there is a plan to obtain more information, the client must be informed concerning the status of that plan. Depending on the age and cognitive and/or language status of the client, it is sometimes appropriate for the clinician to convey outcomes of the evaluation to a person other than the client or other than to the client alone. And, in the case of a young child with a significant language disorder, it is important to remember that parents may not be able to process all of the diagnostic information we could give them in one setting. We should be sensitive to their need to process many of the details of their child's status over subsequent visits.

Options for Treatment

Depending on the amount and type of information a clinician is able to glean from the language evaluation, plans can be made following the evaluation to set up a treatment schedule. A number of different variables will enter into the recommendations for that schedule. Clinician availability, as well as the availability and willingness of the client to participate, are two immediate factors that will need to be addressed. When caseloads are crowded, clinicians may need to place a client on a waiting list until a space becomes available for receiving clinical services. If the client presents with a severe or profound disorder, cases may need to be reprioritized, with clients who have been on the caseload for a while and who have not made significant progress receiving a hiatus in their treatment schedule to make space available for new, needier clients. This may be one of the more difficult decisions that you have to make and can only make fairly when results from in-depth reassessments are collected and evaluated (Fey, 1988).

TRANSITION FROM ASSESSMENT TO TREATMENT

What Can Assessment Data Tell You About the Plan of Therapy?

It is wise to view test battery planning as more than an avenue to get results from standardized tests and nonstandardized probes. That is, in addition to providing numerical support for inclusion or exclusion from treatment, language evaluations should also be designed to answer questions about client capabilities and preferences for different therapy materials, provide tasks employed to elicit productions or facilitate learning, and result in the gathering of behavior baselines.

To that end, different types of materials should be used during evaluations to determine their meaningfulness to the client. One example of this is using the evaluation to determine whether three-dimensional or two-dimensional stimuli or both could be employed as therapy materials for a particular client. For some young children, presumably those who have had limited experience with books, the use of three-dimensional stimuli (objects) will be more appropriate for use in therapy. For these children, the use of two-dimensional stimuli (pictures) may be less meaningful, especially if the pictures are line drawings. Likewise, with adults diagnosed with acquired problems, line drawings may be too abstract and three-dimensional stimuli may need to be used to facilitate testing. Photographs may serve as a viable middle ground between line drawings and objects, providing an acceptable method for presentation of two-dimensional prototypes. That is to say that when limited experience with books is suspected, photographs may present enough of an accurate replica to allow the child to respond. When working with adults, the prototypicality of a given stimulus item may need to be considered since some clients may have difficulty with less prototypical items (e.g., use a *robin* instead of a *wren*).

Similarly, the evaluation should be utilized as a testing ground for the different task types that could be used in therapy. As noted above in the discussion of the different task types that have been utilized for assessing receptive and expressive language, some tasks are more demanding than others because they provide more or less cuing and other support for the individual completing them. Remember that the tasks illustrated in Figure 6–3 were arranged according to which contexted support could be utilized. If the clinician can establish which tasks are feasible for use with a client from information gleaned at the time of the evaluation, this information can be utilized in therapy planning.

The collection of baseline measures as part of an evaluation or a period of diagnostic therapy will inform you as to the extent of the client's learning for a set of probable therapy goals. That is, goals that will be addressed in therapy rarely reflect targets that are entirely absent from a client's repertoire. It is more likely that the targets are partially learned and inconsistently used. With the help of baseline measures that probe the scope of the target's current use, you can better set appropriate levels of expectation for the client's performance once therapy begins. For example, the client who has demonstrated inconsistent use of plural markers (60%), is more likely to achieve a 90% criterion level earlier (all other factors being equal) than the client who has shown no evidence of any plural marker production. For the latter client, setting a criterion of 50% usage as therapy begins would be more appropriate.

How Reassessment Differs From Initial Assessment

It is important to reevaluate treatment programs periodically to determine whether any changes are occurring and, if they are, if they are occurring rapidly enough or in as far-ranging a manner (generalization) to recommend ongoing treatment. This is another purpose of assessment. Reassessment will probably focus both on the specific goals being addressed in therapy and on overall changes to the language system that treatment may have brought. As speech-language pathologists we are very much aware that the natural human cognitive tendency to generalize to new settings and new instances of the language target is the basis of the treatment we provide. That is to say, we know that we cannot provide all possible examples in therapy. Instead, we present a representative sample of all the possible examples of therapy targets and hope that we are teaching a general rule that allows the client to expand what he or she has learned to all other possible examples. Reassessment allows us to figure out how close we are to dismissing the client from therapy and it should also help us to troubleshoot the therapy procedures we are using to determine whether adequate progress is being made (Fey, 1988). Where adequate progress is not being made, this troubleshooting should provide suggestions for the aspects of therapy that need changing to enhance therapy efficiency. For example, reassessment may indicate a lack of generalization stemming from the selection of too few or too many examples for rule learning. Also, adults with a language disorder may not be ready for treatment after a first evaluation but change enough to warrant intervention later. Thus, periodic reevaluation is highly recommended for adult brain-injured clients. Frequent reassessments are also recommended with the infant-toddler population, given the high degree of variability in their performances and potential for rapid growth and change.

REFERENCES

Barrie-Blackley, S., Musselwhite, C., & Rogister, S. (1978). Clinical oral language sampling: A handbook for students and clinicians. *A monograph of the National Student Speech and Hearing Association*, Danville, IL: Interstate Publishers and Printers.

Bates, E. (1976). *Language in context*. New York: Academic Press.

Bayles, K., & Tomoeda, K. (1990). Delayed recall deficits in aphasic stroke patients: Evidence of Alzheimer's dementia? *Journal of Speech and Hearing Disorders, 55,* 310–314.

Bloom, L. (1973). *One word at a time: The use of single-word utterances before syntax*. The Hague: Mouton.

Brinton, B., & Fujiki, M. (1989). *Conversational management with language–impaired children: Pragmatic assessment and intervention*. Rockville, MD: Aspen Publishers.

Brown, R. (1973). *A first language*. Cambridge, MA: Harvard University Press.

Campbell, T., & Shriberg, L. (1982). Associations among pragmatic functions, linguistic stress, and natural phonological processes in speech-delayed children. *Journal of Speech and Hearing Research, 25,* 547–553.

Carrow, E. (1974). *Carrow Elicited Language Inventory*. Austin, TX: Learning Concepts.

Carrow-Woolfolk, E. (1985). *Test of Auditory Comprehension of Language* (TACL-R). Allen, TX: DLM Teaching Resources.

Chapman, R. (1978). Comprehension strategies in young children. In J. Kavanaugh & W. Strange (Eds.), *Speech and language in the laboratory, school, and clinic* (pp. 308–327). Cambridge, MA: MIT Press.

Chapman, S. (1997). Cognitive-communication abilities in children with closed head injury. *American Journal of Speech-Language Pathology, 6,* 50–58.

Chapman, S., Levin, H., & Culhane, K. (1995). Language impairment in closed head injury. In H. Kirschner (Ed.), *Handbook of neurological speech and language disorders* (pp. 387–414). New York: Marcel-Dekker.

Chapman, S. B., Ulatowska, H. K., Franklin, L. R., Shobe, J. L., Thompson, J. L., & McIntire, D. D. (1997). Proverb interpretation in fluent aphasia and Alzheimer's disease: Implications beyond abstract thinking. *Aphasiology, 11,* 337–350.

Coggins, T., & Carpenter, R. (1981). The communicative intention inventory: A system for coding children's early intentional communication. *Applied Psycholinguistics, 2,* 235–251.

Cole, K., Dale, P., & Mills, P. (1990). Defining language delay in young children by cognitive referencing: Are we saying more than we know? *Applied Psycholinguistics, 11,* 291–302.

Crain, S. (1982). Temporal terms: Mastery by age five. *Papers and Reports on Child Language Development, 21,* 33–38.

Crystal, D. (1987). Towards a "bucket" theory of language disability: Taking account of interaction between linguistic levels. *Clinical Linguistics and Phonetics, 1,* 7–22.

Damico, J. (1991). Clinical discourse analysis: A functional approach to language assessment. In C. Simon (Ed.), *Communication skills and classroom success: Assessment and therapy methodologies for language and learning disabled students* (pp. 165–206). Eau Claire, WI: Thinking Publications.

Dore, J. (1974). A pragmatic description of early language development. *Journal of Psycholinguistic Research, 4,* 343–350.

Dunn, L., & Dunn, L. (1997). *Peabody Picture Vocabulary Test-R* (PPVT-III) (3rd ed.). Circle Pines, MN: American Guidance Service.

Evans, J., & Craig, H. (1994). Language sample collection and analysis: Interview compared to freeplay assessment contexts. *Journal of Speech and Hearing Research, 35,* 343–353.

Fey, M. (1986). *Language intervention with young children.* Needham Heights, MA: Allyn & Bacon.

Fey, M. (1988). Dismissal criteria for the language impaired child. In D. Yoder & R. Kent (Eds.), *Decision making in speech-language pathology.* Toronto: B.C. Decker, Inc.

Gardner, M. (1979). *The Expressive One-Word Picture Vocabulary Test* (EOWPVT). Novato, CA: Academic Therapy Publications.

Goldman, R., & Fristoe, M. (1986). *Goldman-Fristoe Test of Articulation.* Circle Pines, MN: American Guidance Service.

Goodglass, H., & Kaplan, E. (1981). *Assessment of aphasia and related disorders* (2nd ed.). Philadelphia, PA: Lea & Febiger.

Hughes, D., McGillvray, L., & Schmidek, M. (1997). *Guide to narrative language: Procedures for assessment.* Eau Claire, WI: Thinking Publications.

Kaplan, E., Goodglass, H., & Weintraub, S. (1983). *The Boston Naming Test.* Philadelphia, PA: Lea & Febiger.

Lahey, M. (1989). Who shall be called language disordered? Some reflections on one perspective. *Journal of Speech and Hearing Disorders, 55,* 612–620.

Lee, L. (1974). *Developmental sentence analysis.* Evanston, IL: Northwestern University Press.

Leonard, L., Prutting, C., Perozzi, J., & Berkeley, R. (1978). Nonstandardized approaches to the assessment of language behaviors. *Asha, 20,* 371-379.

Long, S., Fey, M., & Channell, R. (1998). *Computerized profiling* (MS-DOS Version 9.0). Cleveland, OH: Case Western Reserve University.

McNeil, M., & Prescott, T. (1986). *The Revised Token Test.* Baltimore, MD: University Park Press.

Miller, J. (1981). *Assessing language production in children: Experimental procedures.* Baltimore, MD: University Park Press.

Miller, J., & Chapman, R. (1981). The relation between age and mean length of utterance in morphemes. *Journal of Speech and Hearing Research, 24,* 154–161.

Miller, J., & Chapman, R. (1985). *Systematic analyses of language transcripts (SALT): A computer program to analyze free speech samples* (IBM version). Madison, WI: Language Analysis Lab, Waisman Center.

Nelson, K. (1973). Structure and strategy in learning to talk. *Monographs of the Society for Research in Child Development, 38* (1–2, Serial No. 149).

Newcomer, P., & Hammill, D. (1997). *Test of Language Development: Primary (TOLD-P:3)* (3rd ed.). Austin, TX: Pro-Ed.

Nicholas, L., & Brookshire, R. (1993). A system for quantifying the informativeness and efficiency of the connected speech of adults with aphasia. *Journal of Speech and Hearing Research, 36,* 338–350.

Nippold, M. (1998). *Later language development: The school-age and adolescent years* (2nd ed.). Austin, TX: Pro-Ed.

Owens, R. (1996). *Language development: An introduction* (4th ed.). Boston, MA: Allyn and Bacon.

Panagos, J., Quine, M., & Klich, R. (1979). Syntactic and phonological influences on children's articulation. *Journal of Speech and Hearing Research, 22,* 841–848.

Porch, B. (1968). *Porch Index of Communicative Ability (PICA).* Palo Alto, CA: Consulting Psychologists.

Proctor, A. (1989). Stages of normal noncry vocal development in infancy: A protocol for assessment. *Topics in Language Disorders, 10*(1), 43–56.

Prutting, C. (1979). Process: The action of moving forward progressively from one point to another on the way to completion. *Journal of Speech and Hearing Disorders, 44,* 3–30.

Records, N., & Tomblin, J. B. (1994). Clinical decision making: Describing the decision rules of practicing speech-language pathologists. *Journal of Speech and Hearing Research, 37,* 144–156.

Retherford, K. (1993). *Guide to analysis of language transcripts* (2nd ed.). Eau Claire, WI: Thinking Publications.

Rossetti, L. (1990). *Infant-toddler assessment: An interdisciplinary approach.* Boston, MA: Little, Brown & Co.

Roth, F., & Spekman, N. (1984). Assessing the pragmatic abilities of children: Part 1. Organizational framework and assessment parameters. *Journal of Speech and Hearing Disorders, 49,* 2–11.

Roth, F., & Spekman, N. (1986). Narrative discourse: Spontaneously generated stories of learning disabled and normally achieving students. *Journal of Speech and Hearing Disorders, 51,* 8–23.

Sattler, J. (1988). *Assessment of children* (3rd ed.). San Diego, CA: Jerome M. Sattler, Publisher.

Scott, C. (1988). Spoken and written syntax. In M. Nippold (Ed.), *Later language development: Ages nine through nineteen* (pp. 49–55). Austin, TX: Pro-Ed.

Stein, N., & Glenn, C. (1979). An analysis of story comprehension in elementary school children. In R. O. Freedle (Ed.), *New directions in discourse processing* (Vol. 2, pp. 53–120). Norwood, NJ: Ablex.

Tomblin, J. B., Records, N., & Zhang, X. (1996). A system for the diagnosis of specific language impairment in kindergarten children. *Journal of Speech and Hearing Research, 39,* 1284–1294.

Tyler, L. (1992). *Spoken language comprehension: An experimental approach to disordered and normal processing.* Cambridge, MA: MIT Press.

Ulatowska, H., Chapman, S., Highley, A., & Prince, J. (1998). Discourse in healthy old-elderly adults: A longitudinal study. *Aphasiology, 12,* 619–633.

van Kleeck, A. (1994). Potential cultural bias in training parents as conversational partners with their children who have delays in language development. *American Journal of Speech-Language Pathology, 3,* 67–77.

Wechsler, D. (1974). *Wechsler Intelligence Scale for Children—Revised.* New York: Psychological Corporation.

Weiss, A., & Johnson, C. (1993). Relationships between narrative and syntactic competencies in school–aged hearing-impaired children. *Applied Psycholinguistics, 14,* 35–59.

Westby, C. (1994). The effects of culture on genre, structure, and style of oral and written texts (pp. 180–218). In G. Wallach & K. Butler (Eds.), *Language learning disabilities in school-age children and adolescents.* New York: Merrill-MacMillan College Publishing Company.

CHAPTER

7

Speech Sound Disorders

Ann Bosma Smit, Ph.D.

Difficulties in producing speech sounds can cover a very wide range, from the speech errors that are the result of a cleft palate to the severely unintelligible speech of certain deaf speakers. This chapter is one of the "basic parameter" chapters mentioned in the Preface. It serves as an introduction to the issues surrounding disordered speech production, and its focus is on the types of disorders illustrated in the following examples:

- a young woman who distorts the /r/ slightly (a phonetic error). In her case, the exact nature of her distortion may be obvious only to a trained listener, and the distortion may not interfere with either her communication or her success on the job.
- a teenage boy who produces /s/ and /z/ laterally (a phonetic error). This distortion is typically a very prominent one, and it may interfere with communication to the extent that it calls a listener's attention to the medium (speech) and away from the message.
- a girl in second grade who was born with cerebral palsy that resulted in weakness and incoordination of the speech production mechanism (developmental dysarthria). She communicates orally, but her speech is effortful and is intelligible only with careful listening.

Speech sound disorders include a very diverse set of communication problems.

- a man who has suffered a cerebral vascular accident (stroke) resulting in significant weakness in the oral and laryngeal systems. The stroke has left him able to produce speech only with great difficulty (adult-onset dysarthria). The speech he can produce is obviously labored and is very difficult to understand.
- a boy aged 2 years, 7 months, who is entering preschool and who is extremely reluctant to talk and whose speech is virtually unintelligible to listeners who are not familiar with him because of many systematic errors, such as omitting sounds (phonological disorder). His speech is surprisingly effortful, and he appears to use very short utterances, although his comprehension of complex commands appears to be intact (possible developmental verbal apraxia).

These examples illustrate that we can have speech sound production disorders for a number of reasons: failure to learn the sound system of the language (phonological problems), difficulties making the necessary movements because of neuromotor impairments (dysarthria), difficulties with sequencing the movements needed to produce speech sounds (apraxia), or difficulties producing the sounds of speech due to other structural problems (such as cleft palate). Some of these difficulties are discussed in greater detail in other chapters of this book.

Each of the clients mentioned above is an example of one of the traditional diagnostic groupings, which are based on what we understand the etiological (causal) factors to be. These diagnostic groups can occur in relatively pure forms, for example, a dysarthria without complications of hearing loss, aphasia, or loss of intelligence. However, as a speech-language pathologist, you will find more often that the client exhibits one or more complicating factors. For example, a child who simplifies many words by leaving out sounds may also have mild oral-motor difficulties, and/or difficulties in speech perception, and/or general difficulty in language use.

The range of severity that may be found in clients with disorders of spoken communication is very wide, ranging from mild to profound. And the degree to which the disability is handicapping also varies considerably.

The challenge to you as the speech-language pathologist who must assess the communication abilities of these clients is to determine the scope of the speech sound difficulties, to assess any concomitant communication difficulties, to determine which potential etiological factors are involved, to determine the likely effects of this communication disability, to determine the prognosis (outlook) for change with and without intervention, to make recommendations concerning treatment, and to make referrals to other professionals as needed.

At this point, a word about other populations is appropriate. Two other groups that typically exhibit marked communication disorders are (a) persons with severe/profound involvement of any age and

(b) the 0–3 population. Although many of the concepts in this chapter will be appropriate for toddlers who are already producing words, whenever there is severe developmental delay, the larger issue is whether oral communication will even be possible. For such clients, the diagnostic process will be much more oriented toward cognitive and linguistic function and in some cases, feeding and swallowing. For example, a child of 1 year, 4 months who is exhibiting few communicative intentions, and who rarely engages in eye contact, is at serious risk for language and communication disorders. Another example would be a 15-year-old with a progressive neurological disorder who has regressed to the cognitive level of a much younger child, has started to choke on food, and is becoming unintelligible. This client should receive a dysphagia assessment and may be considered a candidate for alternative/augmentative communication (AAC). Any assessment of speech sounds would be oriented toward functional communication. The interested reader may refer to Chapters 15 and 16 and also to the Recommended Readings at the end of the chapter for information about these areas.

> In the 0-to-3 and severe/profound populations, concern about speech sound production takes a back seat to concerns about cognition, functional communication, and even feeding difficulties.

A FRAMEWORK FOR DIAGNOSIS

The starting point for our diagnosis of a client is a set of concepts that describe levels of functioning. These concepts were introduced in Chapter 1, and they include *impairment, disability,* and *handicap.* Briefly, *impairment* is the loss or abnormality of any function or structure that we think is basic to normal speech sound production. Many of the potential impairments appear to have a causal relationship to impaired speech sound production. For example, weak oral musculature would represent a type of impairment, as would difficulties in speech perception.

At another level, we find *disability,* which is a reduction in the ability to communicate effectively using speech sounds. Disability can refer to completely unintelligible speech. Disability can also refer to intelligible but obviously defective speech.

Finally, the term *handicap* represents the effect that the disability has on a person's life. For example, a stroke resulting in severe dysarthria is handicapping for a woman whose speech is so unintelligible that very few persons understand her. She is at a disadvantage because she has trouble making her wants, needs, and ideas known. Less severe difficulties can also be handicapping, as in the case of a third-grader whose classmates tease him about his babyish speech.

As a practical matter, speech-language pathologists usually begin their evaluation with estimates of disability, and they investigate the components of that disability. They also evaluate potential sources of impairment, judge the degree to which the situation is handicapping, and determine a prognosis after evaluating prognostic indicators. At the end of the diagnostic process, they make recommendations based on all of their findings.

> Impairment: "Patrick has difficulty retroflexing the tongue."
>
> Disability: "Patrick substitutes [w] for /r/."
>
> Handicap: "Aw, don't listen to Patrick. He still says *wabbit!*"

We can think of the diagnostic process as including five parts to the clinical question we need to answer:

1. *To what extent is this client limited in ability to communicate using the sounds of speech?* At this point, we are trying to estimate the *degree of disability* in oral communication, and for this task we use listener judgments, quantitative measures of connected speech, and standardized tests, as well as less formal measures.

2. *What characteristics of this client's speech and language contribute to this limitation in ability to communicate orally?* The goal of answering this question is to determine the *components of disability* in oral communication. For example, perceived unintelligibility in a young child may be related to extensive use of phonological processes, to the presence of phonetic errors, and to concomitant difficulties in voice, resonance, prosody, or fluency. The content, form, and use of the child's language may also be related to the overall disability.

3. *For this particular client, what potentially related variables are evident?* This question looks at *impairment of function*. These concomitant impairments may be present in our client if the client has chronic otitis media, if the status of the speaking mechanism is compromised, if cognitive and language abilities are reduced, if there is a history of medical difficulties, or if there is a history of abuse or neglect.

4. *To what extent is the difficulty in oral communication likely to have psychosocial, educational, or vocational consequences?* When we explore this question, we are estimating the *degree of handicap* experienced by our client. To do this, we might use the reports of parents, teachers, and significant others in the client's environment, as well as our own judgment of the degree of handicap.

5. *What positive and negative prognostic indicators characterize this client?* To answer this question about *prognosis,* we may use information from the client's medical, developmental, and psychosocial history. We may examine the client's response to stimulability tasks, and we may also evaluate variability of errors.

Our Goal—The Comprehensive Diagnostic Statement

Our goal is a comprehensive diagnostic statement that lays out and interprets all the issues relating to the communication difficulty.

The goal of our evaluation is to develop a comprehensive statement in terms of the answers to the five–part question we have asked. We assume that all relevant factors will be mentioned in our statement. Furthermore, the statement will be followed by recommendations, and we assume that the recommendations will address all factors for which we are able to initiate change.

Of course, we will cover some areas of this evaluation in greater depth than others, depending on the traditional diagnostic category of which our client is a member. When we are evaluating an adult who has had an injury resulting in the neuromotor difficulties we call dysarthria, we will certainly assess his respiration and phonation in considerable detail. In the case of a young child whose speech sound difficulties have no known etiology, we most likely would assess respiration and phonation only in a cursory way, but we would spend a large portion of our assessment time documenting her patterns of speech sound use.

AN EXPANDED VIEW OF DIAGNOSIS

Estimating the Degree of Disability

As we begin to think about the ways we assess disability, it is important to keep in mind that some aspects of communication may be affected *by* the speech sound difficulties and others may be affected *in addition* to the speech sound difficulties. These aspects all combine to produce a communication disability. We also need to keep in mind that disability includes not only difficulty in conveying a linguistic message, but can also refer to speech that is obviously defective or distorted, although still understandable. In such cases the speech draws undesirable attention to itself, attention that may even interfere with communication of a message.

To estimate the degree of disability in oral communication, we may use one or another *index* (indicator) of the client's ability to communicate using speech (Figure 7–1). These indices may be estimates of intelligibility (how understandable the client is), or they may be estimates of perceived severity or defectiveness. We may use categorical scales ("speech is intelligible only to familiar persons") or we might decide to use a percentage scale ("the client's speech was judged to be intelligible about 75% of the time"). Finally, we can use equal-interval rating scales that are anchored at both ends ("on a scale of 1 to 6, with 1 being most intelligible and 6 being least intelligible, the intelligibility of this client's speech was ranked 3").

Global Listener Judgments of Disability

Listener judgments are of two types. In the first instance, a person in a child's everyday environment, perhaps a parent, makes an estimate of how much is understood in that environment. Or we may ask that person to estimate how limited the client is in her ability to communicate in daily living. The second type of listener judgment of disability is made by the clinician. It may be based on taped or face-to-face conversational samples. These judgments may use either numerical rating scales or categorical scales.

Global listener judgments, especially those made by parents or close associates of the client, have very high face validity because

Using descriptive categories*
Sound errors are occasionally noticed in continuous speech.
Speech is intelligible although noticeably in error.
Speech is intelligible with careful listening.
Speech intelligibility is difficult.
Speech usually is unintelligible.
Speech is unintelligible.

Using percents (Example)
"Speech was estimated to be about 80% intelligible if context was known, and about 50% intelligible if context was not known."

Using a scale with equal-appearing intervals
Normal speech   1 2 3 4 5 6   Most severely disordered speech

*Categories taken from Fudala (1970).

Figure 7–1. Some indices that describe the degree of deficit as reflected in intelligibility or severity ratings.

Global listener judgments reflect the client's ability to communicate in the everyday world.

they are derived from the client's life and reflect her ability to communicate on a daily basis. A global judgment made by the clinician also has considerable validity because it usually reflects how the client communicates with someone who has no previous acquaintance with her.

Incidentally, it is important to attend to a parent who tells you that no one, not even the parent, readily understands a child whom you are evaluating. Lack of intelligibility is one of the most important criteria used to determine how urgent it is that a child receive intervention services. Certainly, the child who is unintelligible and who cannot make her wants and needs known is seriously handicapped.

Quantitative Measures of Disability in Speech Sound Production

The speech-language pathologist has a number of ways to quantify intelligibility or severity of speech difficulty. Some of these measures are based on a recorded conversational speech sample. One measure that is often used to quantify intelligibility is the percent of words that the transcriber can understand or figure out. A well-known measure to quantify severity in children with phonological disorders is the percent of consonants that are correct (Shriberg & Kwiatkowski, 1982). In the assessment of dysarthria caused by brain damage, you might want to use a multifactorial index of the efficiency of communication that looks at both accuracy of consonants and rate of speech (Yorkston & Beukelman, 1981a). A comprehensive discussion of quantitative measures like these may be found in Kent et al. (1994).

There are other ways to quantify intelligibility and severity besides those based on taped conversational samples. For example, there are numerous published tests that the clinician can use to assess speech in a formal way, such as the *Goldman-Fristoe Test of Articulation* (Goldman & Fristoe, 1986) or the *Assessment of Phonological Processes* (Hodson, 1986). Most formal tests require the client to name pictures or objects while the clinician transcribes the client's production of specific target phonemes in each word. Most such tests result in a total score or a standard score that can be compared to normative data (at least for children). The degree to which a child does not meet the norms for his age group is an index of severity of disability. In the assessment of adult dysarthria, there is a well-known procedure for presenting randomly chosen word lists and sentence frames for the client to produce (Yorkston & Beukelman, 1981b). Judges who do not know the specific words the client is producing then try to write down what the client said. The resulting score can then be compared with normal performance, which is ordinarily 100% intelligible.

The types of quantitative measures discussed here have less face validity than global listener judgments because they allow the clinician plenty of processing time, and they are usually based on word-by-word transcriptions or glosses. However, these measures are used because they appear to be accurate measures of severity or intelligibility, because they appear to be related to the global measures, and because they are sensitive measures to use in evaluating change in a

There are several quantitative ways to measure degree of disability.

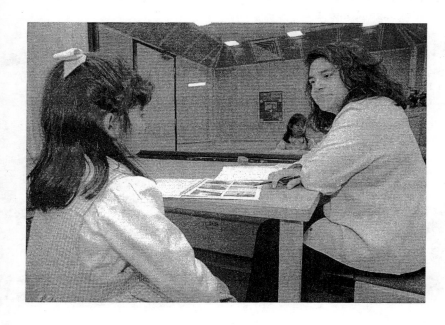

client's speech over time. Moreover, such measures can provide valuable information that cannot be obtained from global judgments. For example, formal tests typically sample all the consonants in English, not just the consonants the client chooses to attempt in a conversational sample, so that the speech-language pathologist has a more complete picture of the client's sound system.

Determining the Components of Disability

Components of disability are those aspects of spoken communication that contribute directly to disability. For example, in a preschool child, the presence of many error patterns may make a large contribution to poor intelligibility. In an adult dysarthric, labored speech with weak articulator contacts may be the primary contributor to perceived severity of the client's speech. Other components may not be related specifically to articulatory production but to voice, resonance, prosody, or fluency. Finally, language (content, form, and/or use) may contribute to disability. For example, an adolescent with phonological errors may also show pragmatic errors by shifting from topic to topic with little warning to the conversational partner. These abrupt shifts in topic contribute to the listener's judgment that intelligibility is reduced.

Depending on how the client presents, we may just screen in some areas and perform extensive evaluation in others.

The ways in which we assess the components of disability vary, depending somewhat on the traditional diagnostic grouping in which our client fits. Sometimes we may simply screen in one area by listening carefully to the client, while for other clients we may need to do an extensive evaluation in that area. Nevertheless, every evaluation should include attention to the client's articulation or phonology (or both), to prosody, to voice, to resonance, to fluency, and to language (content, form, and use).

Components of Disability—Articulation and Phonology

When a client is referred for evaluation because of poor intelligibility or because of obvious phonetic errors (distortions), we expect to evaluate this area extensively. If the client has many consonant substitutions, or if she appears to distort specific speech sounds, we may well administer one of the published tests of speech sound production and report the nature of the errors. We would also tape a conversational sample to determine the nature of the errors in conversation and the frequency of occurrence of those errors.

When young children have poor speech intelligibility, we expect them to exhibit many of the phonological processes that we know are typical of unintelligible speech. We can think of these typical phonological processes as patterns of speech sound errors. For example, a child might omit all final consonants in words, or the child might produce most velar consonants as alveolars. For such children, we would use both formal tests of phonology and our analysis of a conversational sample. From these two kinds of observations, we can derive several inventories, a list of phonological processes the child uses, and a determination of whether any of the child's productions are unusual or idiosyncratic. (This approach is similar to the one outlined by Stoel-Gammon and Dunn, 1985, Chapters 4–6.)

The most important inventory is the phonetic inventory, which is a listing of all the different sounds a child uses in two or more positions in words, regardless of what the adult target sounds are. For example, Sammy, a child of 3 years, 1 month has the phonetic inventory shown in Table 7–1, which includes φ (this symbol is called *phi*, and it represents a voiceless bilabial fricative).

Sammy's phonetic inventory is extremely restricted and is comparable to that of a child of about 18 months. Sammy uses only one final consonant, no clusters, and very few fricatives, all of which should have been attempted by age three, although they are not always correct at that age. It is obvious that Sammy has very little flexibility in attempting to say the words of his language, which contain a much greater variety of sounds.

The second inventory we might construct is called a phonemic inventory, in which we examine what the child does for each adult phoneme target. A part of Sammy's phonemic inventory is shown in Table 7–2. This table shows us that even in this small part of the phonemic inventory, Sammy collapses a number of adult distinctions. For example, he uses [t] for both adult /t/ and adult /k/. And he does not use most final consonants, so that there is the potential for many of his words to be homophones (words that sound the same). For example, his version of *bath* and *bat* would sound the same: [bæ].

Our third inventory is a listing of all the word shapes used by the child, using C to stand for consonants and V for vowels. In Sammy's case, the word shape inventory is extremely limited: V, CV, CVm, CVCV. In contrast, the English language has a much larger variety of word shapes, including clusters and multisyllabic words.

The last inventory in our analysis is the list of phonological processes the child is using. There are many ways to obtain this list, including formal tests, formalized analyses of conversational speech, and

> With children who have a phonological disorder, three types of inventories become important: the phonetic inventory, the phonemic inventory, and the syllable/word shape inventory.

Table 7–1. Sammy's phonetic inventory of consonants.

Initial		Final
w		
m	n	m
p	b	
t	d	
φ	f	

Note: φ is a voiceless bilabial fricative.

computerized analyses. Typically, the speech-language pathologist looks for regularities in the pattern of errors. Many test forms and analysis systems are arranged in a way that facilitates this search. For example, in Figure 7–2 you can see portions of two formal tests that facilitate your search for patterns of errors. One of these, the SHAPE, also provides a series of overlays to help determine the phonological processes used.

You can also determine phonological processes without using a formal test instrument—you can simply examine the phonemic inventory you have prepared. For example, even in the small portion of Sammy's phonemic inventory, shown in Table 7–2, it is possible to identify phonological processes very easily: Sammy is obviously using the processes of fronting (producing velars as alveolars) and final consonant deletion (omitting all final consonants except /m/).

Our final step is to determine if any of the processes or characteristics of a child's production are unusual or idiosyncratic. For example, Sammy's use of *phi* as an alternate to [f] is quite unusual. Unusual phonetic or phonological processes persisting beyond a few weeks suggest that the child has taken a wrong turn on the path to adultlike phonology.

When we are assessing the speech of clients from diverse cultural and dialect groups, we need to be careful to sort out which aspects of communication are within normal limits for the client's dialect or language group, and which aspects represent disorder or delay. For example, although /r/ is pronounced in Standard English every-

Table 7–2. A portion of Sammy's phonemic inventory.

Initial		Final	
Adult Target	Sammy's Version	Adult Target	Sammy's Version
w	w		
m	m	m	m ~ ø
n	n	n	ø
p	p	p	ø
b	b	b	ø
t	t	t	ø
d	d	d	ø
k	t	k	ø
g	d	g	ø
f	φ ~ f	f	ø
v	b	v	ø

Notes: φ is a voiceless bilabial fricative, ø is the null (omission) symbol, and ~ means "alternates with."

Bankson-Bernthal Test of Phonology

Phonological Process Inventory

Assimilation	Fronting	Final Consonant Deletion	Weak Syllable Deletion	Stopping	Gliding	Cluster Simplification	Depalatal-ization	Deaffrication	Vocalization
tæt tæ	kæ	kæ tæ							
det tet gek	de det	ge de							
	tʌp tʌ	kʌ tʌ							
	tændi					kæni kædi			
gɔg dɔd	dɔt	dɔ							
		bɛ							
		bo							
dot do		go do							
gʌŋ dʌ	dʌŋ dʌ	gʌ dʌ							
	tau								
		kræ				twæb tæb kwæb fræb kæb			

Target Word/ Phonetic Transcription	Word Correct	Transcription of Child's Production	Modeled
1. cat kaet	☐	_____	☐
2. gate get	☐	_____	☐
3. cup kʌp	☐	_____	☐
4. candy kændi	☐	_____	☐
5. dog dog	☐	_____	☐
6. bed bed	☐	_____	☐
7. boat bot	☐	_____	☐
8. goat got	☐	_____	☐
9. gun gʌn	☐	_____	☐
10. cow kau	☐	_____	☐
11. crab kræb	☐	_____	☐

Smit-Hand Articulation and Phonology Evaluation

Initial Stops	Final Stops
/p-/ _____ __ 46 pipe	/p-/ _____ /3 47 pipe 50 cup
/t-/ _____ __ 23 teeth	/t-/ _____ /3 5 cat 17 goat 40 hat
/k-/ _____ /3 4 cat 49 cup 56 cake	/k-/ _____ /3 10 duck 37 sock 57 cake
/b-/ _____ /3 32 bib 41 bag 64 bed	/b-/ _____ __ 33 bib
/d-/ _____ /3 1 dog 9 duck 14 deer	/d-/ _____ __ 65 bed
/g-/ _____ /2 16 goat 59 gum	/g-/ _____ /2 2 dog 42 bag
Subtotal (Max: 6) ___	Subtotal (Max: 6) ___

Figure 7–2. Excerpts from two examples of formal tests that assist the clinician in determining which phonological processes the child uses. In the first example, the **BBTOP** (*Bankson-Bernthal Test of Phonology*; *Bankson & Bernthal*, 1990, reproduced with permission from Applied Symbolix), each target word is placed next to a grid showing the kind of error that each relevant process would represent. In the second example, the **SHAPE** (Smit-Hand Articulation and Phonology Evaluation; Smit & Hand, 1997) is an analysis form that helps the clinician arrange the data so that multiple examples of the same sound are together and so that members of the major sound classes are listed together. This facilitates the finding of patterns of errors.

where it occurs, there are several dialects of English in which /r/ occurring at the end of a word can be pronounced as a vowel, as in /fɔə/ (four); these dialects include Vernacular Black English, Bostonian dialect, and Southern dialect. Furthermore, in the United States there are many people whose English is influenced by a first language, such as Spanish or Chinese. Like Vernacular Black English, these variants of English may differ from Standard English in quite systematic ways, especially with respect to consonant systems.

It is important to differentiate sound patterns that may be characteristic of the client's dialect from sound patterns that indicate delay/disorder.

Consequently, a characteristic that would be considered an error in Standard English may well be typical of the language of the client's community. Chapter 2 contains additional information about this important topic.

On the other hand, we must be careful that we attribute only appropriate features of a client's speech to dialect or language background, so that we do not miss real delay or disorder. And for children, the whole picture is sometimes complicated by competing demands that the child's speech fit into the community mold for social reasons and into the "school" mode (closer to Standard English) for educational reasons. Needless to say, this area of practice can become politicized; nevertheless, the focus must remain on the communication needs of the client.

Components of Disability—Other Speech Factors

Problems with speech sound production often coexist with other speech or language deviations, and these other deviations can make their own contribution to the communication disability. Deviations in prosody (stress, rate, intonation, and use of pauses) are often present with speech sound disorders, especially in clients whom we suspect have a verbal apraxia (difficulty in sequencing the movements of speech). At present there are standard ways to transcribe stress patterns of words and to determine rate of speech, but there are no commonly used ways to transcribe or evaluate sentence intonation contours. However, the clinician should pay attention to whether the client marks the ends of declarative clauses or sentences with downward inflection, whether intonation contours and pauses correspond to syntactic units, and whether questions and emphatic statements carry appropriate intonation contours.

Other components of communication disability include voice, resonance, fluency, and language ability. Each of these topics is discussed in detail elsewhere in this volume. However, we need to be aware that each of these factors can contribute to perceived unintelligibility, perceived severity, or both.

Determination of Potentially Related Impairments

There are many factors that may be related to the presence of speech sound disorders in persons who do not have any obvious physical difficulties in the oral mechanism. Some of these are variables that may bear a causative relationship to speech sound disorders, while others may predispose the client to develop a disorder if other factors are present. Potentially related variables include the status of the hearing mechanism; perceptual abilities; integrity of the respiratory, laryngeal, and oral systems; status of general cognitive abilities; and the general health of the client. Potentially related variables also include the presence or absence of behavioral difficulties and information about the developmental history of the individual, including any hospitalizations. Interestingly, language ability may represent not only a component of the perceived disability, but also a potentially related factor, because language difficulties suggest a general problem in symbol use.

As a speech-language pathologist you need to be aware that sometimes we are very limited in what we can deduce about how variables may be related to speech sound disorders. For example, if we attempt to assess speech perception, and the client performs very well on the test that we have chosen, it is appropriate to say the client's speech perception skills are excellent (assuming a valid test). However, if the client performs poorly, we must be more cautious in our statements, because tests of speech perception are notoriously subject to confounding variables. In such cases there is always the possibility that we have simply not been clever enough to find a way to let the client show us her skills.

Potential Impairments—The Auditory Mechanism

Severe-to-profound hearing loss has an obvious causal relationship to speech difficulties in persons who are deaf. In addition, mild-to-moderate hearing loss, past or present, and a history of otitis media may predispose a child to develop phonological delay or disorder, but probably not to develop the well-known characteristics of "deaf speech." Some discussions of these groups are presented in Chapters 17 and 18.

Potential Impairments—The Oral Mechanism

Obvious defects in the oral mechanism, such as cleft palate, are clearly related to characteristic speech errors, such as nasal emission on consonants. Other structural deviations, such as a very high hard palate, are not known to be related to any speech difficulties.

More important than minor structural deviations is the neuromotor integrity of the speech mechanism. Recent evidence suggests that subtle deficiencies in oral strength and coordination may be related to developmental verbal apraxia, a severe-to-profound impairment of speech in children. It is certainly possible that mild oral-motor impairment may be related to less severe phonological difficulties as well. Finally, in both adults and children we would want to note the presence of any groping movements of the articulators because of their known relationship to apraxia of speech. See Chapters 5, 12, and 14 for more information about these relationships.

Potential Impairments—Speech Perception

It is intuitively appealing to assume that a client's ability to discriminate speech and categorize speech sounds is critical to accurate speech production; however, this statement is probably true only for clients whose errors are not developmental. That is, current research findings suggest that in young children, speech perception

Many impairments influence speech sound production.

and production skills may develop in parallel. Unfortunately, even in older clients, speech perception is notoriously difficult to test without interference from other variables. Consequently, as was indicated earlier, it is much more difficult to interpret errors in performance than it is to interpret good performance. For example, if you show children a set of four pictures, such as *bee, beet, bead,* and *bean,* and ask them to point to the one you say, even some children who say all these words accurately will make "perception" errors. Because these children do produce the words accurately, it is likely that some other variable influenced their errors in this test.

On the other hand, there are clients who do very poorly on perception tasks and who truly do not say sounds accurately because they do not perceive them accurately. Consequently, if your client gives every indication that she is not able to perceive differences in speech stimuli you present, then this client most likely will not make progress in remediation unless you provide perceptual training.

Potential Impairments—Cognitive Status

We usually relate phonologica evelopment to cognitive development rather than to chronological age.

In children with developmental delay, the status of cognitive development may aid in the interpretation of the findings from your analysis of the child's phonology. For example, if Sammy's phonological status is that of an 18-month-old and his cognitive functioning is at a similar level, then Sammy may be doing as well as can be expected in phonological development. In other words, we peg phonological development to mental age rather than to chronological age.

We should note that even if Sammy's cognitive development and phonological development are comparable, we still have obligations to Sammy (and to other children with developmental delay). First of all, we need to ensure that Sammy is communicating critical needs and wants in ways that his caregivers understand. Second, we need to counsel the caregivers to provide an environment that is rich in speech and language input, and to provide this stimulation in ways that Sammy can make use of (such as talking about the here and now, using short utterances, and using considerable repetition). Third, we need to monitor Sammy to make sure that subsequent phonological development keeps pace with other aspects of development.

Another possibility is that a child's phonological status is less developed than his cognitive status would suggest. In such cases, intervention is warranted because we assume that the child's phonology and ability to communicate can be brought up to a level commensurate with mental age. Of course, this assumption would be modified if there were negative prognostic indicators in other domains such as oral-motor or psychosocial.

In adults, cognitive status continues to be an important variable, whether we are dealing with developmental delay or with a cognitive deficit due to acquired neurological damage. In such clients, the importance of this variable lies in the area of prognosis and in determining what type of intervention we will recommend. Additional discussions of the importance of cognitive status are in Chapters 6, 11, 12, and 16.

Potential Impairments—Language Abilities

Because a child's phonological system is one part of the larger linguistic system, we can expect interactions with other aspects of that system. For example, because there is a strong relationship between syntactic errors and severity of the phonological disorder, we expect to have to deal with both in our treatment, although some studies suggest that treating just one area improves the other as well. Another language area of particular interest is the relative status of receptive versus expressive language. Many children with phonological disorders show deficits in expressive language (especially in grammar and in oral vocabulary), but they have receptive language that is within normal limits. When receptive language is better than expressive, we assume that with intervention the child can eventually achieve an expressive language and phonological level that is commensurate with her receptive language level.

Other language difficulties often coexist with speech sound disorders.

On the other hand, the child with a phonological disorder who shows both receptive and expressive language delays poses a different problem. This child may be better served by making sure the child has functional communication through speech and by incorporating phonological intervention into a broader intervention for the general language deficit.

Potential Impairments—Psychosocial Factors

Both intrapersonal and interpersonal factors can have an impact on communication and on intervention. For example, clinical depression is relatively common in persons who have had a stroke affecting communication. One result of this depression is that the client may not be interested in putting forth his best effort at communication, or he may be unwilling to attempt certain diagnostic tasks.

Psychosocial factors can influence both speech sound development and the prognosis.

Children with speech sound disorders only rarely show clinical depression, but other psychosocial variables are relevant to your assessment. For example, the child who is teased about her speech, or who experiences considerable parental pressure to speak correctly, may become reticent and may be reluctant to experiment with new sounds. And, of course, a child who has experienced deprivation and abuse may show any number of behavioral consequences, including impaired communication.

Potential Impairments—The Client's History

The client's medical and developmental history help us to interpret our other findings. Premature birth, especially if the baby has a very low birth weight, may be associated with subsequent delays in development. Perinatal distress, or adverse events at about the time of birth, such as anoxia, may be related to a specific neuromotor impairment, or they may produce an overall delay in speech and language. If a child is slow to achieve developmental milestones such as sitting unaided, walking, and producing the first word, this suggests an overall delay, and phonological development should be evaluated accordingly. Finally, a hospitalization or severe illness in childhood may have general delaying effects.

In the case of adult-onset speaking difficulties, the nature and the extent of neurological or other impairment will influence your findings. These factors may also be important in determining a prognosis. For example, if you are evaluating a client who has multiple sclerosis (MS), and if his speech shows primarily components of incoordination, you may recommend treatment focusing on rate and stress patterns rather than on strengthening the oral musculature. At the same time, the prognosis for improvement in the client with MS must be guarded because MS is a progressive illness.

Estimates of Handicap

The limitations in ability to communicate that we discussed above usually constitute a handicapping condition in aspects of the client's life. For example, children with speech disorders may be regarded less favorably by their peers than are children without such disorders. Or adults with cerebral palsy may believe that they are stigmatized by their speech.

Handicap is the interaction of disability with the env   nment.

The person with a speech sound disorder sometimes experiences handicap in education. For example, the child with a severe phonological disorder may volunteer to answer a question in class, but if the teacher knows that he and the rest of the class will not understand the child, he may be reluctant to call on her. Or the adult with an obvious speech disorder may be counseled out of certain fields or experiences.

Finally, the client may experience a handicap in choosing or pursuing a vocation. For example, a man who is the foreman in a crew of electricians may not be able to return to his former position following a stroke that leaves him dysarthric. Sometimes even a mild degree of disability may have serious vocational consequences. A woman with a lateral lisp who wants to become a courtroom lawyer will find that the lateral lisp is an obstacle to achieving her goals, in spite of the fact that the lateral lisp is a far less severe problem than dysarthria.

Obviously, estimates of handicap are based to a considerable degree on the judgment of the speech-language pathologist. Often the very fact that a client has been referred by someone else for evaluation suggests that a handicap exists. Sometimes sensitive questioning of the client will reveal feelings of being stigmatized or devalued because of the speech disorder.

In the early days of our profession, one of the ways in which a communication disorder was defined was this: An individual had a communication disorder if either the person himself or anyone in his environment thought that he had one. Today, we tend to neglect this definition in most of the areas covered by speech-language pathologists, except for voice and fluency disorders. However, it is also true in the area of speech sound disorders that we need to pay attention to the opinions of the client and the client's caregivers or associates. After all, it is from the client's social interactions, and from the reactions and opinions of others, that handicap arises.

You should be aware that investigating this area sometimes poses dilemmas for us. For example, we may feel overwhelmed by the seeming callousness with which a client has been treated, apparently on the basis of having a speech sound disorder. On the one hand, we try to find ways to improve the client's speech, but on the other hand, we may wonder if our time could be more profitably spent trying to change society's attitudes about handicap. Frequently, of course, we must do both.

Evaluating Prognostic Indicators

Prognostic indicators are characteristics or factors that can influence the client's progress over time in ability to communicate. Certainly we know that stating a prognosis is always an educated guess on our part. And because of the ethical standards of our profession, the speech-language pathologist must be careful not to promise, or to be seen as promising, a specific outcome. Rather, we usually make statements that many clients with certain specified characteristics achieve the predicted level of functioning.

A prognostic statement is a cautious prediction about the outcomes with and without intervention.

You will notice that several prognostic variables were mentioned under other sections of the evaluation. It should not be surprising to find prognostic variables mentioned in both places, because if a factor represents an impairment that is implicated in delayed development or caused a deficit, then that factor can continue to exert a negative influence unless it is alleviated or removed.

When we discuss prognosis, we usually specify the predicted outcome assuming that intervention is provided. Alternatively, we may give two prognostic statements, one assuming intervention, and another assuming no intervention. In the case of a child with a phonological disorder, we may develop a prognostic statement as follows:

■ The prognosis for Jimmy to become intelligible to most listeners within a 2–year period, with treatment, is good. Without treatment the prognosis is fair-to-poor.

Prognostic Indicators—Severity

One of our first prognostic considerations is the severity of the speech sound disorder. When the disorder is severe, it can affect the prognosis in two ways. First of all, the eventual outcome may not be as positive as it would be in the case of a mild or moderate disorder. Second, the amount of time needed to reach a particular outcome may be longer. This is not to say that a mild disorder always has an excellent prognosis; probably every practicing speech-language pathologist has experienced the frustration of working with a client with a mild disorder that did not improve much in treatment. Rather, the degree of confidence with which we can predict a limited outcome is greater when the disorder is severe.

Prognostic Indicators—Characteristics of the Client

Several personal variables can influence the projected outcome. These include motivation, consistency, stimulability or response to trial intervention, and medical, developmental, and therapeutic history.

Motivation as a Prognostic Variable. The client's motivation, or the desire to make a change, appears to be a variable that is particularly important for adults and for children beyond about 9 or 10 years of age. For younger children, we typically supply the motivation in the form of positive reinforcement and activities that keep the client's interest. In older children and adults, motivation is important, but it is also a "slippery" variable, in part because it is very much influenced by the clinician's ability to structure the treatment to provide success for the client. Motivation is also "slippery" because it depends in part on other events and conditions in the client's life. For example, the adolescent client with distorted /s z ʃ tʃ dʒ/ may have difficulty attending to treatment because his parents are at the point of divorce.

Stimulability or Response to Trial Intervention. Stimulability is the ability to improve sound production under conditions of focused stimulation. Trial intervention is a short period of treatment during which the client's ability and potential to make changes is assessed. In adults, both stimulability and improvement during trial intervention are positive prognostic indicators. In young children with phonological disorders, stimulability is considered a prognostic indicator for improvement, both with and without intervention.

Variation in Production. Inconsistency and contextual variation refer to two types of variability noted in the client's spontaneous speech production. Many clients exhibit little variation in the way they produce specific targets, and we say that their errors are "consistent." However, other clients show variability or "inconsistency" in their speech. For some of these clients, there is no apparent pattern to the inconsistency. For others, we can determine that there are particular phonetic contexts in which the client usually produces an accurate sound (contextual variation). The chief value of finding these occasional correct productions is that they can provide the starting point for treatment for that target. In other words, the existence of correct variants is a mildly positive prognostic indicator.

> Many clients show considerable variation in their production of error sounds in connected speech.

Medical, Developmental, and Therapeutic History. As we discussed earlier, medical and developmental history can be important for both children and adults. If earlier medical or developmental problems are still present, we may be skeptical about the probability of improvement. However, if they have been resolved, the prognosis is more positive. Medical history is especially important in cases of adult-onset neurological problems. For example, a client's history of one or more chronic, serious medical conditions would suggest a relatively poor prognosis.

Therapeutic history may also be an important variable in some cases. If a client has had several years of intervention for the same speech sound difficulties that you have documented in your evaluation, and has made little progress, then the prognosis for improvement with more intervention is relatively poor. The exception might be if the type of intervention the client received appeared to have been inappropriate for the types of speech sound difficulties you have documented.

Other Prognostic Variables

In addition to considerations of the status of the client, there are two other areas that we explore when determining a prognosis. The first of these is the existence of social or familial support for the client. Children who are candidates for treatment usually live with their family or are in a foster situation. Ordinarily there will be support and encouragement for the child's efforts and for changes the child will be making. However, in seriously stressed or dysfunctional families, you can expect that intervention for the child may have to take a back seat to the resolution of other major difficulties in the family's life. In fact, family counseling may be one of your recommendations in such cases, because the child will not be able to make progress in communication until the family's difficulties are resolved.

Clients of any age will need social support and resources.

Adult clients may not have family nearby, but it is a positive prognostic sign when the client clearly has the support of a social group, whether or not that group is made up of family. On the other hand, clients without such a support group will have to rely on their own internal resources and on interactions with the speech-language pathologist to support them in the work of intervention.

A second consideration is the resources available to the client. Resources in this case refer to the availability of services and the financial support to pay for them. If a community offers a variety of services and makes sure that they are available to all, then the client's prognosis is relatively positive. If, on the other hand, the client lives in an area where services are few and far between, and the client will not be able to get to them, the prognosis is less positive. If financial support is not available to pay for services, the clinician may try to find support for the client or may refer the client to a social worker.

THE COMPREHENSIVE DIAGNOSTIC STATEMENT

The goal of these assessments is the development of a comprehensive diagnostic statement about the client's communication difficulties, which will include statements of how the relevant variables contribute to the chosen index of conversational speech. A logical and recommended format for this statement would be the following:

- General diagnostic statement, including the speech-language pathologist's overall severity rating
- Estimates of disability in speech communication
- Statement of the components of the disability
- Statement of potentially related impairments
- Estimate of degree of handicap imposed by the disability
- Statement of prognosis

Statements of this sort may be called "clinical impressions" or "clinical summary."

A comprehensive diagnostic statement interprets your findings for the client and family as well as for other professionals.

The recommendations should address the variables for which the speech-language pathologist can initiate change. For example, if the client is a dysarthric adult and one component of the disability is a weakened respiratory system, we may refer him for further medical examination, and perhaps physical therapy.

An example of such a comprehensive diagnostic statement might be this statement about Russell, a 20-year-old college freshman with a history of treatment for speech sound disorders (phonological processes). You have determined that he exhibits mild weakness in the oral musculature, and you suspect a very mild form of cerebral palsy, although no such medical diagnosis appears in his records:

- "Russell exhibits difficulties in speech sound production that are moderate to severe for a person of his age. He exhibits phonological process use that is typical of much younger persons, complicated by very mild oral neuromotor weakness that may have been present since birth. (GENERAL DIAGNOSTIC STATEMENT)
- Russell's conversational speech is judged by the clinician to be about 80% intelligible with careful listening, and his percent of understandable words in a conversational interaction is 87% (in a sample of 100 different words). (INDICES OF DISABILITY)
- The most important components of Russell's reduced intelligibility appear to be (a) frequent omissions of sounds (deletion of final and intervocalic nasals and obstruents) in connected speech, (b) weak articulation of the sounds that are produced, together with (c) vocal intensity that is frequently inadequate. (COMPONENTS OF DISABILITY)
- Russell exhibits very mild weakness of the mandible, lip, and tongue musculature affecting primarily the tongue tip; he also reports that his mother told him that he had feeding difficulties in the first year of life. He reports no history of otitis media or of severe illness during childhood. Hearing was screened and found to be within normal limits. Russell reports that in his college classes that do not require a speak-

ing component, he is getting grades of B and C. (POTEN-TIAL RELATED IMPAIRMENTS—ARTICULATORY MUS-CULATURE, AUDITORY SYSTEM, MEDICAL HISTORY, LANGUAGE AND COGNITION)

■ Russell was referred to this clinic by one of his classroom instructors, and Russell himself states his concern about the effects of his speech on his ability to make friends; conse-quently, it appears that Russell experiences both academic and social limitations because of his speech. (ESTIMATES OF HANDICAP)

■ The prognosis for improvement with intervention is fair. One positive indicator is that Russell is readily stimulable for improved articulatory precision and for production of all deleted consonants. Another positive indicator is that al-though vocal intensity in conversation is often inadequate, Russell can generate increased intensity in conversational speech with little apparent effort and can sustain it for at least 30 seconds. On the other hand, the fact that Russell has already experienced extensive intervention but has not main-tained the skills he needs for adequate oral communication is a poor prognostic indicator. (PROGNOSTIC STATEMENTS)

■ Recommendations for Russell include the following:

1. A 3-month course of trial intervention focused on strengthening articulatory contacts and on intelligible production of utterances longer than 2–3 words.

2. During this period of trial intervention, the clinician should be in communication with Russell's instructors for both monitoring and counseling purposes.

3. Russell should consult with a neurologist to confirm that the oral motor weakness is not progressive."

EMPHASES IN DIFFERENT DIAGNOSTIC GROUPS

Although the focus in this chapter has been on the common aspects of evaluation for speech sound disorders, you should expect to tai-lor your evaluation to the client's general diagnostic group, while maintaining the flexibility to alter those emphases if necessary. And, of course, you will plan a very different evaluation for a child from the one you would plan for an adult.

When a child exhibits a phonological delay or disorder, you will pay close attention to the developmental history and to the caregiv-er's account of the dynamics in the home relating to the child. You will plan to elicit and analyze more than one speech sample, perhaps one from conversation during a play period and another from a for-malized assessment instrument. You will probably do a screening examination of the oral mechanism, in part because it is difficult to elicit certain oral movements from very young children. And because

Because of the wide range of speech sound disorders, the evaluation will include different emphases for different diagnostic groups.

phonological disorders often coexist with language disorders, you will assess language in several domains.

If the client you are assessing makes phonetic errors, such as a lateral lisp, you may plan to use a formal, published test that elicits all the consonants of English. You will assess stimulability and document any inconsistency or contextual variation. You may evaluate speech discrimination abilities. You will consider whether the current status of the child's dentition or dental occlusion plays a role in the phonetic errors. Finally, because clients with phonetic errors are often children of school age, you will consider issues of motivation and social support.

If the client with phonetic errors is an adult whose speech patterns are of long standing, you will carefully address prognostic factors such as motivation and stimulability. After all, an adult has been "practicing" these speech patterns for almost a lifetime, and the prognosis may be considerably poorer than for younger children.

When your client appears to have a verbal apraxia, your evaluation will include an emphasis on detailed examination of the functioning of the oral mechanism, as well as on the characteristics of the client's speech. You will carefully evaluate prosody. If the client uses gesture extensively, you will document that fact. In the case of children, you will want to know if the child has previously had treatment and what the results were.

If your client is dysarthric, you will concentrate on an appraisal of the speech and respiratory mechanisms, as well as the client's speech characteristics. Prosody is an important variable. Medical history is also very important, in part because it will document the location and extent of brain damage, and in part because it is important in determining a prognosis.

SUMMARY

The goal of this chapter has been to provide you with a framework for your evaluations of persons who have speech sound disorders. The range of speech sound disorders is very large, perhaps the largest of any of the communication disorders that we study. Nevertheless, the same principles are appropriate for each: describe the disability and its components, estimate the extent to which the disability is handicapping, determine the components of that disability, investigate potentially related variables or impairments, determine a prognosis, and make appropriate recommendations. Now it is up to you, the speech-language pathologist, to flesh out the framework for your own evaluation of an individual client.

REFERENCES

Bankson, N. W., & Bernthal, J. E. (1990). *Bankson-Bernthal Test of Phonology.* Chicago, IL: Applied Symbolix.

Goldman, R., & Fristoe, M. (1986). *Goldman-Fristoe Test of Articulation.* Circle Pines, MN: American Guidance Service.

Fudala, J. B. (1970). *Arizona Articulation Proficiency Scale: Revised.* Los Angeles, CA: Western Psychological Services.

Hodson, B. W. (1986). *Assessment of Phonological Processes—Revised.* Danville, IL: The Interstate Printers and Publishers, Inc.

Kent, R. D., Miolo, G., & Bloedel, S. (1994). The intelligibility of children's speech: A review of intelligibility procedures. *American Journal of Speech-Language Pathology, 3,* 81–95.

Shriberg, L. D., & Kwiatkowski, J. (1982). Phonologic disorders III: A severity metric. *Journal of Speech and Hearing Disorders, 47,* 256–270.

Smit, A. B., & Hand, L. (1997). *Smit-Hand Articulation and Phonology Evaluation.* Los Angeles, CA: Western Psychological Services.

Stoel-Gammon, C. & Dunn, C. (1985). *Normal and disordered phonology in children.* Austin, TX: Pro-Ed.

Yorkston, K. M., & Beukelman, D. R. (1981a). Communication efficiency of dysarthric speakers as measured by sentence intelligibility and speaking rate. *Journal of Speech and Hearing Disorders, 46,* 296–301.

Yorkston, K. M., & Beukelman, D. R. (1981b). *Assessment of intelligibility of dysarthric speech.* Tigard, OR: C.C. Publications.

RECOMMENDED READINGS

Arvedsen, J. C., & Brodsky, L. (Eds.). (1993). *Pediatric swallowing and feeding: Assessment and management.* San Diego, CA: Singular Publishing Group.

Reichle, J., Piche-Cragoe, L., Sigafoos, J., & Doss, S. (1988). Optimizing functional communication for persons with severe handicaps. In S. N. Calculator & J. L. Bedrosian (Eds.), *Communication assessment and intervention for adults with mental retardation* (pp. 239–264). Boston, MA: College-Hill Press.

Sparks, S. N. (1994). Assessment and intervention with at-risk infants and toddlers: Guidelines for the speech-language pathologist. In K. G. Butler (Ed.), *Early intervention II.* Gaithersburg, MD: Aspen Publishers, Inc.

Yorkston, K. M., Beukelman, D. R., & Bell, K. R. (1988). *Clinical management of dysarthric speakers.* San Diego, CA: College-Hill Press.

CHAPTER

8

Stuttering

Patricia M. Zebrowski, Ph.D.

As a student clinician, and again as a professional in the field, you will most likely see children and adults who have been referred to you for "stuttering." Your specialized training in speech-language pathology will make you uniquely qualified to help people who stutter. You will no doubt find your work with these individuals to be interesting and sometimes perplexing, but almost always challenging and rewarding as well. In this chapter, you will learn how to diagnose stuttering and its associated speech and nonspeech behaviors. But as you will see, analyzing the speech behaviors that characterize stuttering is only part of the story. Stuttering is one of the most intricate and least understood of all speech disorders. It begins in early childhood and is believed to result from the interaction of a number of risk factors, such as age at onset, positive family history of stuttering, and phonological status, which are thought to be present in some, but not all, people who stutter. Finally, the factors most likely interact in different ways across individuals, to produce the same end product—stuttering. The perpetuation of early stuttering into more chronic forms of the disorder is believed to be related to a complex interaction among such variables as the integrity of overall communications skills, learning, both the reactions and responses of listeners to stuttering, and the speaker's response to these listener reactions. Therefore, speech-language pathologists must know how to diagnose and treat not only the *observable* speech behaviors associated with stuttering, but also the *unobservable* thoughts, attitudes, and feelings about stuttering reflected by the client and his significant others. Hopefully, you will gain an appreciation for the unique relationship between and among these factors, and how they affect the assessment process.

We will begin with a discussion of how to differentiate "stuttering" from "disfluency," as well as how to examine the behaviors associated with each to determine both the need for and initial focus of therapy. The pronouns she and he will be used throughout the chapter to refer to the speech-language pathologist and the client, respectively. This format is not meant to be exclusionary in any way, but was used to facilitate the flow and "readability" of the chapter. The pronoun assignment was chosen to best represent each population; that is, most speech-language pathologists are women, and most people who stutter are men or boys.

UNDERSTANDING "STUTTERING" WITHIN THE CONTEXT OF DISFLUENCY AND FLUENCY

When is stuttering "stuttering"?

Stuttering is a disorder of speech *fluency*. Speech fluency can be described as the forward-moving flow of ongoing speech (see Conture, 1990a, 1990b; Williams, 1978). It is the way in which a speaker connects the sequential sounds, syllables, words, sentences, and phrases he produces as he is talking. When a person moves from one sound to the next, or connects one word or sentence to the next in a relatively smooth, undisturbed fashion, his speech sounds "fluent." On the other hand, when a person disrupts or interrupts these smooth sound-to-sound or word-to-word connections, his speech can be described as "disfluent" (the prefix *dis* means *without*). Most speakers produce disfluent speech from time to time. Therefore, disfluency itself is not abnormal or unusual. However, there is a *type* of disfluent speech, which when produced in (relatively) frequent amounts, is considered to represent "stuttering," and not the disfluent speech of normal talkers.

DISFLUENCY TYPES: PRODUCTION AND PERCEPTION

Are there different types of disfluency?

Our goal is to describe and measure disfluent speech objectively, both for diagnostic reasons (Is he stuttering or is he *normally* disfluent?) and designing treatment (What is he doing when he stutters, and what does he need to do to speak more easily?). To accomplish this, it is helpful to consider a scheme for classifying the different types of speech disfluencies people have been observed to produce. The following section offers such a scheme.

Within- and Between-Word Disfluencies

The speech disfluencies that people produce can be classified into two broad categories: within-word and between-word disfluencies. Figure 8–1 provides examples of both disfluency types.

Disfluency Type	Examples
Within-word speech disfluencies	
a. Sound/syllable repetition	"He is ruh-ruh-running home."
b. Audible sound prolongation	"Mmmmore cake, please."
c. Inaudible sound prolongation	(lips closed, no accompanying voice) "Buy some milk, please."
Between-word speech disfluencies	
a. Monosyllabic whole-word repetition	"I-I-I can't do that." "He-he-he is a big boy."
b. Multisyllabic whole-word repetition	"She really-really is here."
c. Phrase repetition	"I was-I was going to invite them." "They are-they are fun people."
d. Interjection	"I will, you know, be late."
e. Revision	"She is-she was here." "Please stay-please go."

Figure 8–1. Examples of various types of speech disfluencies (after Conture, 1990a and Williams et al., 1968).

Within-word speech disfluencies are the result of a speaker disrupting the connection or transition between sounds *within* a word. The person repeats a sound or a syllable in a word more than once, and so does not smoothly move away from that sound and into the subsequent one (*sound/syllable repetition*) or the person interferes with the fluent production of a word by drawing out or prolonging an individual sound within a word for an abnormally long period of time (*sound prolongations*). When that happens, he disrupts the smooth sound-to-sound movement which characterizes normally fluent speech. He may also prolong voicing and/or turbulent noise, as in production of /s/, for example (*audible sound prolongation*), or no voicing or noise is heard (*inaudible sound prolongation*).

Between-word disfluencies are those in which the smooth transition *between* words is in some way disrupted. In general, there are more readily observable examples of between-word than within-word disfluencies in speech. One may interfere with the linking of words by repeating an entire word in a particular phrase or sentence more than once (*whole-word repetition*). An entire phrase can also be repeated (*phrase repetitions*). Sometimes a speaker will insert individual syllables or routine, nonmeaningful words or phrases *between* adjacent words in a sentence (*interjections*). Finally, one can revise what he is saying (*revisions*), sometimes to the extent that he doesn't complete the message.

Disfluencies Produced by People Who Stutter

The majority of people who stutter begin doing so during their pre-school years (Bloodstein, 1995). Over the years an important research focus has been to describe and compare the speech disfluencies produced by children who stutter and those who do not. Much of what we know about the disfluent and stuttered speech of children was obtained through either parents' answers to interview questions or their written responses on questionnaires. In addition, several investigators have collected speech samples from stuttering and nonstuttering children and analyzed them.

Results from these studies have essentially shown that the speech disfluencies of stuttering and nonstuttering children are similar in *kind*, but different in *degree* or frequency. Specifically, both groups of children produce all types of disfluencies, both within- and between-word. As a group, however, children who stutter produce *more* disfluencies in general (are more disfluent), and specifically produce *more* within-word disfluencies than their nonstuttering peers. As we will discuss later in this chapter, we use this consistent observation, along with other available information, to help us make decisions about which children are *most likely* stuttering or at risk for stuttering, and which are not.

Listener Judgments of Disfluent Speech

One of the earliest theories about what causes a young child to begin producing stuttered speech described stuttering as a speech problem essentially "created" by listeners. In his "diagnosogenic" theory of the onset of stuttering, Wendell Johnson proposed that stuttering in children was the result of listeners' (and specifically, parents') negative evaluations of a child's *normal* disfluencies (Johnson, 1959). Although the basic premises of the diagnosogenic theory have been challenged by numerous clinicians and researchers, the theory is significant because it highlighted the importance of listener contributions to the problem of stuttering. As a result, numerous studies have been conducted to examine the ways in which people perceive and judge various characteristics of disfluent speech.

Results from these investigations have shown that listeners tend to use frequency and type of speech disfluency to make judgments about (1) whether a disfluency is "stuttered," "not stuttered," or "normal" and (2) whether a speaker is "stuttering," a "stutterer," or "normally speaking." Further, listeners use the same characteristics to make judgments about the severity of stuttering.

As one might expect, the more instances of disfluency a speaker produces, the more likely listeners are to judge that person to be "stuttering" or a "stutterer." In addition, the higher the frequency of disfluency, the more severe listeners tend to judge the individual's disfluent speech. Studies that have examined the relationship between disfluency type and listener judgment have shown that listeners most frequently judge *within-word* speech disfluencies to represent stuttered speech or stuttering, while *between-word* disfluencies are most frequently regarded as not stuttered or normal. For the most part, *repetitions* of sounds, syllables, and, to some extent, words, are the disfluency types most often labeled as stuttering. Sound prolongations are also generally regarded as stuttering, but less frequently so. Finally, between-word disfluencies (interjections and revisions) are typically judged to be "not stuttered" or "normal" by listeners.

Production and Perception: Putting It Together

Taken together, results from studies of production and perception tell us that the *type* of disfluency a person produces (within-word), and the *frequency* of disfluency are two objective indicators of who is stuttering and who is not. Further, this *interrelationship* between the characteristics of the speech of children who stutter, and listener judgments of their speech, most likely holds important consequences for the development of stuttering. For example, if a child produces a relatively high frequency of sound/syllable repetition, it is likely that his parents or other significant others will consider him to be "stuttering" or "a stutterer." As a result of this judgment, parents may give the child negative feedback about his speech. Finally, as a response to adverse reactions to repetitions of sounds and syllables, the child might develop the habitual use of inappropriate speech production strategies to attempt to change or keep from producing these repetitions (Conture, 1990b; Zebrowski & Conture, 1989). This proposed relationship between stuttered speech and listener reactions to stuttering, as well as the speaker's responses to both, suggests that these factors should be examined during an evaluation.

STUTTERING ASSESSMENT IN CHILDREN

The assessment of any speech and language problem, including stuttering, is the first step toward solving the larger problem of how to provide treatment. When we are dealing with children, the first objective of our assessment procedures usually is to determine whether or not a problem exists. In this way, the evaluation objectives for children differ importantly from those we might set for adults. Specifically, with children we must determine whether they are stuttering, at risk for stuttering, or are normally disfluent. On the other hand, adults referred for a stuttering evaluation are probably not wondering whether or not they stutter, but are most likely looking for information about the nature, severity, and extent of their problem, and the likelihood that they can be helped.

How can we tell whether a child is having a fluency problem?

There are many pieces in the diagnostic puzzle.

Figure 8–2 is a schematic representation of the four main questions that need to be answered in the assessment of stuttering in children, along with objectives for achieving each. These questions are: (1) Is this child stuttering or at risk for developing a stuttering problem? (2) Will the child experience recovery from stuttering; will he "outgrow" it? (3) Is treatment needed and recommended? and finally (4) What should be the focus of therapy, or the kind of treatment approach taken? As Figure 8–2 shows, you will need to accomplish six objectives to satisfactorily answer these questions. These objectives are related to different questions, and allow you to gather information on several fronts. The information you obtain can be viewed as pieces, that fit together to complete the puzzle of stuttering diagnosis.

Question 1: Is the Child Stuttering or At–Risk?

We start here by describing and measuring speech (dis)fluency through focused observation of the child's conversational speech, as well as administration and scoring of formalized techniques, procedures, and rating scales. Obtaining a sample of the child's speech while he is talking to his parent(s) will also allow you to observe any verbal or nonverbal reactions and responses the parent(s) may have to the child's disfluent speech. When appropriate, you also need to talk with the child to find out his beliefs and attitudes about talking and speech disfluency, as well as his thoughts about his own speech. Finally, you must interview the parents or primary caregivers to obtain a family history and information about stuttering onset, as well as the nature of any change in the child's stuttering which has occurred since then. While talking with parents, you can also identify their concerns, attitudes, and beliefs about disfluency and stuttering, both in general and specific to their child. Through achieving the following objectives, you will obtain the information you need to answer this first question.

Objective 1: Describing and Measuring Speech Disfluencies

There are no standardized tests to help you to decide which children are stuttering and which are normally disfluent. For that reason, you need to base your decision partially on objective measures taken from the speech of these children, considered along with results from some commercially available assessment techniques, procedures, and rating scales.

The first measures discussed are usually obtained from samples of the child's conversational speech. To acquire a representative sample of the child's spontaneous speech and language, you will need to ask the parents or caregivers to engage in conversation with the child, while you observe (if possible in an adjoining observation room.)

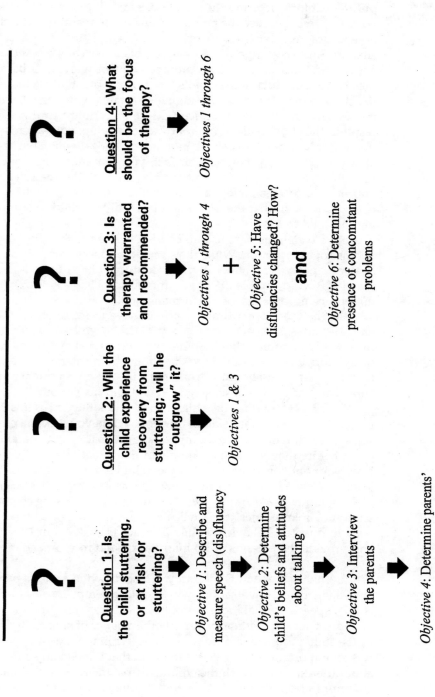

Figure 8–2. Questions to be addressed in the diagnosis of children who stutter.

Make sure to provide age-appropriate materials for the parents to use as conversational "props." These can include small toys, Playdoh, puzzles, Colorforms, and the like. Books and drawing materials do not work well, because the parents often end up reading to the child or encouraging the child to read, or the child draws and colors silently. Similarly, large or noisy toys (this latter category includes Legos and blocks), as well as puppets, do not work well because they can either obscure the child's face or can potentially be used by the child to make noise (e.g., banging on a table with Legos), which makes listening to speech difficult. More importantly, puppets can result in the child using a different way of talking, one that may be fluency-enhancing. You can tell parents that they do not have to talk about the provided materials; in fact, you can encourage them to talk about anything they want to. However, if the materials are appropriate for the child's age, as well as interesting to him, the chances are high that the play materials will be useful in stimulating the child to talk.

As you watch the parents and child talk, attempt to collect several types of information. While the size of the speech sample you collect and analyze can and will vary, Conture (1990a) has suggested that a 300-word sample of conversational speech is a sufficient size for observing a range of performance. Obviously, the larger the sample, the more opportunity you will have to make observations and measures of speech disfluency. Further, your measures will most likely be more reliable. While you may be able to simultaneously videotape and audiotape the parent-child interaction for further analysis, you should also attempt to make preliminary measures "on-line" while observing the child and his parent(s).

The ability to analyze the child's speech (dis)fluency *as it is being produced* is an important skill to develop. When you assess a child's speech, it is important to give immediate feedback to the parents or client before they leave to go home. In this situation, most parents want your opinion about whether their child is stuttering before they leave his examination. Even though measures made from video and/or audiotaped samples (with the luxury of reviewing segments several or many times over) will likely be the most accurate, you need to quantify behavior on-line in order to make your diagnosis and provide the parent(s) with information and recommendations.

Frequency of Speech Disfluency. Once the child and his parents are engaged in conversation, you should attempt to describe the child's speech by making a variety of measures. The first one, frequency of speech disfluency, reflects the *amount* of speech disfluency the child produces, regardless of type (within- or between-word). It is an important diagnostic measure, in that it tells you something about the extent to which the child disrupts the flow of speech and communication. In addition, overall frequency of disfluency is the measure which clinicians typically use to document *broad* improvement in therapy.

Usually, you report an average and range of disfluency so that you can form an impression about the variability of disfluent speech. Frequency is expressed in percent and can be measured by either counting the number of disfluent syllables per total syllables produced in a sample, or by counting the number of disfluent words per total words produced. The unit of measure (either syllables or words) is not as important as the consistency with which it is used; that is, if you express frequency in percent disfluent syllables, you need to do so consistently when describing the client's speech throughout subsequent evaluations and treatment of that client.

During your evaluation, you can calculate frequency as the average number of disfluent words in 100 words spoken, expressed as a percent. Count the number of disfluent words in *at least one* 300-word sample, and compute the average and range of disfluency produced (Conture, 1990a). Results from studies of the speech of young stuttering and nonstuttering children have shown that, in general, children who stutter produce *more* speech disfluencies overall than children not diagnosed to be stuttering.

Types of Speech Disfluency and Their Distribution. (See Figure 8–1.) In recent years, the proportion of different disfluency types produced has been considered a more sensitive indicator than frequency in differentiating children who stutter from those who are normally disfluent. Further, analyzing the type(s) of disfluencies a child most frequently produces can help you to understand what the child *is doing* to interfere with talking, how the child's disfluencies have changed over time, and how these changes might be related to coping or "compensatory" speech production strategies the child has developed. In this section, we will discuss type as it might help you to answer the question "Is the child stuttering, or at risk?"

One consistent observation has been that stuttering and nonstuttering children produce the same *types* of disfluencies, but in different proportions. Studies comparing the disfluent speech of young stuttering and normally disfluent children have shown that children who stutter produce more *within-word* speech disfluencies (sound/syllable repetitions and sound prolongations) than their nonstuttering peers (Johnson, 1959; Kelly & Conture, 1992; Yairi & Ambrose, 1992a, 1992b; Yairi & Lewis, 1984; Zebrowski, 1991). This holds true regardless of age, even for preschool children who are very close to stuttering onset. Further, children who stutter typically produce *at least* 3 within-word speech disfluencies in 100 words of conversational speech, while nonstuttering children produce *fewer* than 3 in 100 words.

These research findings, along with our own and others' clinical experiences, have led us to consider children who produce 3 or more within-word speech disfluencies in 100 words of conversational speech to be either stuttering, or at risk for developing stuttering. Obviously, this observation plays an important role in your diagnosis, but it is only one piece of the puzzle. Further, the likelihood or probability that a child is stuttering or at risk increases with increases in the proportion of within-word disfluencies (> 3) per 100 words produced, or parent(s) or primary caregiver(s) concern that the child is stuttering or a "stutterer."

You need to document the types of speech disfluencies the child demonstrates and their proportions through analysis of the same 300-word sample from which you've measured frequency. Individual proportions are determined by dividing the number of instances of a specific disfluency type (e.g., sound prolongation) by the total number of disfluencies produced in the sample, and are expressed as percentages of the total. As with frequency of disfluency, you will need to make "on-line" observations of disfluency types and their distributions so that you will be able to make a diagnosis at the time of the evaluation. Then, prior to writing your diagnostic report, you can review the video and/or audiotaped recording of the same conversational sample, and make the measures again.

Duration of Within-Word Speech Disfluencies. The duration of individual moments or instances of within-word disfluencies has long been considered a diagnostic indicator of the presence and severity of stuttering. For one thing, duration can reflect the degree of difficulty the child exhibits in making smooth transitions between sounds and words. In general, children who stutter produce sound/ syllable repetitions and sound prolongations averaging one-half second or so in duration (500 ms), and ranging from one-quarter of a second (250 ms) or less to approximately 1½ seconds (1500 ms).

Duration should be measured, then, as another way to describe or characterize the ways in which the child disrupts the smooth, forward flow of speech. Further, clinical observations indicate that a decrease in the duration of instances of stuttering is often the earliest sign of progress in therapy (Conture, 1990a; Conture & Caruso, 1987). During your evaluation, you can use a digital stopwatch to make on-line measures of *at least* 10 within-word speech disfluencies. By measuring 10 stutterings, you will be able to obtain a mean duration and a range, from low to high. You can use these duration measures to describe the problem further but, as we'll discuss later, you can also use them in determining stuttering severity through conventional rating scales and instruments.

Speaking Rate. There is clear evidence that, with regard to the rate of their *fluent speech only*, children who stutter do not speak significantly faster or slower than nonstuttering children (Kelly & Conture, 1992). We have found, however, that the measurement of *overall* speech rate (i.e., the rate of speech when all pauses and disfluencies are included) is helpful for a number of reasons. First, there is an *inverse* relationship between overall speech rate and both stuttering frequency and duration. That is, the more disfluent or stuttered speech the child produces, or the longer the duration of stutterings, the fewer words per minute he will be able to produce. Therefore, speech rate will be slower. You can measure speech rate, then, to gain a better understanding of how disfluencies and stuttering are affecting the *amount* of speech output a child is able to produce, and thus are interfering with communication. Second, you can compare this measure with a later rate measure obtained when and if the child receives therapy. It seems likely that speech rate will increase as a child becomes either more fluent, or shows a decrease in duration of stutterings.

There are several ways to measure speech rate in the clinic and laboratory, some regarded as more accurate and precise than others. You can sample the child's speech rate by counting the number of words he produces in 10 separate, randomly selected 10-second intervals. Overall rate can be calculated for each sample by dividing the number of words by the time in seconds (10 in this case), and multiplying by 60 (seconds), yielding the number of words produced in 1 minute. You can then compute the average rate and range, in words per minute, of all 10 samples.

Associated Speech and Nonspeech Behaviors. Often, a child shows visible or audible physical behaviors while he is repeating or prolonging sounds or syllables. These are called **associated behaviors**, and are also sometimes referred to as **secondary** behaviors. Associated behaviors can take many forms, and some children and adults who stutter develop highly complex and idiosyncratic ones.

Associated behavior is another piece.

The most common *nonspeech*-related associated behaviors include eye movement (lateral, up-down, and blinking, closing or widening), head movement, and torso and limb movement. Some typical *speech*-related associated behaviors are audible exhalations or inhalations immediately prior to the instance of stuttering, pitch rises during the production of a stuttered disfluency, visible physical tension in the lip, cheek, jaw or neck muscles, and nostril flaring. Even the youngest children who stutter, and those who are within weeks or months of stuttering onset, have been observed to produce associated behaviors.

Associated behaviors are thought to reflect the child's *awareness*, at some level, that he is doing something "different" when he stutters. At most, they are thought to be associated with the child's attempts to cope with, compensate for, or in some way change his speech disfluencies. (See Conture and Kelly, 1991, for a discussion of why young stuttering children might produce associated behaviors.) An additional view might be that associated behaviors are related to the things the child does to try to keep from stuttering (Williams, 1979).

During your evaluation, you should document the number and variety of associated behaviors produced by the child. For some children, the appearance of associated behaviors is the first indication of a beginning awareness of the problem. Further, associated behaviors are sometimes the only evidence of awareness you will be able to observe, especially for young children who are unable or unwilling to talk to you about their speech and their concerns about disfluency. Finally, normally disfluent children typically *do not* produce associated behaviors when they are disfluent, so the presence of associated behaviors can help to differentiate stuttering from nonstuttering children.

Severity. Severity is a dimension of stuttering that is often described. It is also the most familiar way in which speech-language pathologists, and listeners in general, characterize stuttering (Bloodstein, 1995). You can talk about a child's stuttering in terms of its frequency of occurrence, type, and duration, but almost always parents and other professionals will ask, "Yes, but how *severe* is the problem?" Thus, even though severity is not as useful in *clinical* terms for describing the nature and characteristics of a child's individual stuttering problem, it is *very* useful in that it helps you to communicate about stuttering in terms familiar to most.

Severity involves making a global judgment of the *degree* of the child's stuttering problem, and describing this degree with the terms "mild," "moderate," or "severe" (or a combination of terms, when a problem is thought to border on a category; for example, "mild-moderate"). Listeners use the frequency, type, and duration of disfluency, along with the appearance of associated behaviors, to make subjective judgments of severity.

One way to make the measure of severity more objective is to use commercially available or published rating scales. Both the *Iowa Scale for Rating Severity of Stuttering* (Johnson et al., 1978) and the *Stuttering Severity Instrument for Children and Adults* (SSI; Riley, 1994) are severity rating instruments which you can include as part of your diagnostic protocol. Both instruments will allow you to assign either a number or a numerical score to a composite profile of the child's disfluent speech (based on either observations or direct measures of frequency, type, duration, and associated behaviors). The numerical ranking (as in the case of the Iowa Scale) or score (as in the SSI) is associated with a level or degree of severity ranging from "no stuttering" to "severe" and "very severe stuttering."

As reported by Ludlow (1990), Riley (1972) demonstrated a high rank correlation (.89) between severity ratings obtained through the Iowa Scale and the SSI. In addition, in a study examining the diagnostic records of 100 children who stutter, Conture et al. (1990) observed significant correlations between measures of stuttering frequency and scores on both the Iowa Scale and the SSI. Although not without their problems, the convenience, ease of use, and concurrent validity of both the Iowa Scale and the SSI make them useful parts of an assessment battery.

Adaptation and Consistency of Stuttering. Adaptation and consistency of stuttering are two well-known phenomenon which have been observed in both adults and children who stutter. **Adaptation,** or the **adaptation effect**, is the tendency for the frequency of disfluency to *decrease* during successive *oral* readings or speakings of the same material. **Consistency,** or the **consistency effect**, refers to the tendency for disfluencies to be produced on the *same words* during successive oral readings or speakings of the same material. Both effects are exhibited by people who stutter *as a group*; that is, some adults and children who stutter do not show either adaptation or consistency when reading the same passage several times in a row.

Adaptation and consistency are other pieces of the puzzle.

Adaptation and consistency should be measured for a number of reasons. First, if a child adapts or if he is consistent, you have additional evidence that his performance is similar to that of other children who have been diagnosed to be stuttering; that is, his stuttering behavior is predictable. In addition, you can use the results of adaptation and consistency tasks to answer the fourth diagnostic question: What should be the focus of therapy? For example, if the child consistently stutters on bilabial sounds (/m/, /p/, and /b/), perhaps an early focus for treatment would be to teach the child appropriate strategies for smoothly moving into or away from those sounds at the single-word level. If a child does not adapt, or is not consistent, you might view this as an indication that he is not like other stuttering children as a group, but instead may be either at risk for stuttering or normally disfluent. A second, and related possibility, is that the child will be essentially fluent while successively reading or speaking the test passage or sentences. This might suggest that it is fairly simple to elicit fluent speech from the child, or that he has not yet come to expect to stutter on particular sounds or words.

You can measure both adaptation and consistency by asking the child to read or repeat a short passage or series of sentences five times in succession (with no pauses or conversation in between repetitions). For school-aged children, age-appropriate passages of about 50 words or so are fine. For younger children, you can use sentences developed by Neelly and Timmons (1967) specifically for this procedure. If the child can read, instruct him to read the entire set of sentences, from top to bottom, "over and over until we tell him to stop." If reading the sentences presents difficulty for the child, or if he is a nonreader, tell him to "Say these sentences just like I do," and in that way elicit the repetitions from him.

Adaptation is calculated by subtracting the number of disfluencies in the fifth reading (or repetition) from the number of disfluencies in the first reading, and dividing by the number of disfluencies in the first reading. The degree of adaptation is expressed in percent. An adaptation measure of 50% or higher indicates that the child exhibits the adaptation effect; the higher the percentage, the more he has shown adaptation. Conversely, a score below 50% indicates that the child has not significantly reduced the frequency of disfluency over five readings or repetitions.

Consistency is calculated by comparing the disfluencies produced in the first three readings or repetitions only. Three **consistency indexes** (Johnson et al., 1978) are calculated: 1–2 (comparison of reading one and two), 1–3 (comparison of reading one and three), and 2–3 (comparison of reading two and three). The index for each comparison is computed by dividing the proportion of disfluently produced words in one reading *which are also produced* in a second reading, by the number of disfluently produced words in the second reading. So, the equation for the 1–2 comparison (readings one and two) would be the percent of disfluent words in reading one also disfluent in two, divided by the number of disfluencies in reading two. If an index is 1.0 or higher, the child is consistent in the location of his disfluencies within the passage or sentence. The higher the index (> 1.0), the more consistency the child exhibits.

Stuttering and Communicative Demand. The Stocker Probe Technique (Stocker, 1980) is a formal procedure that will allow you to observe the child's disfluent speech as it relates to increasing levels of communicative demand or responsibility. In this procedure, the child is asked five questions about each of 10 different common objects. The questions range from low to high with regard to the demands for creativity, intelligibility, and fluency that the child needs to use to respond successfully. The assumption is that for children who stutter, there is a strong relationship between these demands and fluency; that is, the higher the demand, the less fluent the response. Such a relationship has not been observed in normally disfluent children (Stocker & Usprich, 1976; Weiss & Zebrowski, 1992). You can use the Stocker Probe primarily to see if such a relationship exists for the child; if so, then this observation is one more piece of evidence that the child is stuttering or at risk fot stuttering. In addition, the way the child responds to the varying levels of demand can indicate where to start in therapy. If the child is essentially fluent when responding to relatively low level probes such as answers to questions ("Who would you buy it for?"), but is consistently disfluent for higher level probes ("Make up your own story about it."), then you might start teaching fluency strategies within these less demanding contexts, therefore increasing the probability for success.

> Communication demand is another piece.

Objective 2: Determine the Child's Beliefs and Attitudes About Stuttering

In addition to measuring and describing the child's speech (dis)fluencies, you need to find out something about the child's level of awareness and concern about his disfluent speech. As previously discussed, for young children who are unable or unwilling to "talk about talking," you will need to look for associated behaviors to provide some indication of awareness. You will need to do the same for older, school-aged children, but you should also spend some time during the evaluation talking with the child about his speech. Williams (1985) and Zebrowski and Schum (1993) provided some detailed descriptions of how to talk with children who stutter and their parents.

The main purposes of your discussion with the child at the time of the diagnostic are to find out (1) what he believes "stuttering" is, (2) why he thinks he talks this way, (3) what, if anything, he does to "help himself" when he talks, and finally, (4) does his talking worry him or bother him in any way? The best way to start the discussion is by asking the child, "Why do you think you came here today?" and let his response point the way for additional probing. For example, if the child says he does not know why he came, then you can *gently* ask him if he can think of "any reason" why he might be visiting that day. Do not lead the child or put words in his mouth. If he continues to say he doesn't know, then an alternative line of questioning should be used, beginning with the instruction to "Tell me about your talking," followed by specific questions such as "Are you a good talker?" "What do you like about your talking?" and "What would you like to change about your talking?"

If the child does not respond to your questions or prompts, then the discussion should end. If, on the other hand, the child reports that he came for a particular reason ("I don't talk well," "I stutter," and so on), then the next question should be something like, "What does that (stuttering, kind of talking, speech) sound like? Why don't you show me." From there, the conversation should move to a discussion of why he thinks or believes he talks this way, what he does to help himself, and what bothers him the most about his speech.

You need to be careful at this point to avoid commenting on the correctness or incorrectness of the child's thoughts and beliefs. This discussion is primarily to help you gather information and form impressions about the child's beliefs, not to provide the child with a tutorial on the problem of stuttering. When, and if, the child begins therapy, you can be a source of information. During the evaluation, however, you should be an active listener, letting the child talk and making sure you frequently check your understanding by reflecting back to the child what was said. In our experience, children who stutter, even younger ones, often form beliefs and possess attitudes about their stuttering that may lead to the development of speech behaviors which serve to either suppress or change their disfluencies.

The speaker's attitudes about talking is another.

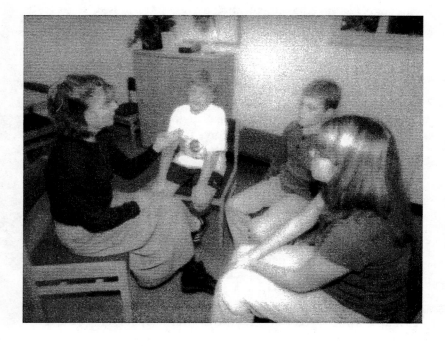

Recently, Brutten (1985) has developed, and De Nil and Brutten (1991) have obtained norms for, a test that assesses the attitudes children who stutter possess about talking and stuttering: *Children's Attitudes About Talking—Revised* (CAT). The CAT contains 32 statements about talking which the child reads and decides are either "true" or "false," based on how closely each statement represents the way he feels. The clinician can then compare the child's responses to those of a group of 70 stuttering and 271 nonstuttering children ranging from 7 to 11 years of age. For school-aged children, using the CAT helps to gauge a child's attitudes and beliefs when he is unwilling or unable to discuss them. In addition, the test statements included in the CAT can be used as a guidelines for interview questions or discussion topics when probing for information about the child's attitudes, beliefs, and concerns about his speech.

Objective 3: Interviewing the Parents

When evaluating stuttering in children, it is essential to interview the parents or primary caregivers. The main purposes of the parent interview are to obtain a history of the child's speech (dis)fluency, as well as to find out the parents' major concerns and beliefs about their child's disfluent or stuttered speech. Just as children themselves frequently develop theories about why they stutter, so do their parents possess beliefs and hypotheses about what either caused or maintained their child's disfluent speech.

The interview should be similar to any you might conduct with parents. That is, background information about the child's overall development should be obtained, as well as the child's speech and language, health, educational, and social-emotional history. In addition, a specific history of the presenting problem should be obtained, along with information about the incidence of stuttering within the family. It is also important to know whether affected family members exhibited recovery from stuttering during childhood. As discussed later in this chapter, this information can help you to assess the likelihood that the child will recover without treatment.

You should ask the parents when the problem was first noticed, by whom, and the manner and degree in which it has changed since it began. It is important that parents *describe* what the child's speech disfluencies looked and sounded like at the time they were first noticed and at present; however, it is even more helpful if the parents *show* you examples of the child's disfluencies at both points in time. From the parents' model, you can obtain a clearer picture of whether or not the child's disfluencies have changed over time with regard to frequency or type, and this may be a factor in predicting recovery. Further, asking the parents to show (as opposed to describe) examples of their child's speech can help you to gauge their willingness to produce stuttering. A parent who is unwilling to produce disfluent speech is likely to be very uncomfortable with disfluencies. In addition, you can compare the parents' model to your clinical observations of the child's speech disfluencies. A large discrepancy (e.g., the parents imitate effortful sound prolongations with many associated behaviors, while you observe the child producing mainly "easy" sound/syllable repetitions) often indicates that the parents' perceptions and the child's productions may be out of sync, a situation that might contribute to the perpetuation of the problem, and which points to the need for the speech-language pathologist to provide parent counseling.

Parents' beliefs and concerns about the *cause* of their child's stuttering often take one of three forms, which include (1) there is something physically (but as yet undetected) wrong with the child, (2) there is something psychologically or intellectually (again, undetected) wrong with the child, or (3) the parents have done or failed to do something which caused the stuttering (see Zebrowski and Schum, 1993, for a detailed discussion of this issue). Of course, any or all of these variables might be related to a particular child's stuttering to some extent but, if so, they are most likely related to the continued perpetuation, development, or exacerbation of the problem, and not necessarily its origin. That is, they are *contributing*, but not *causal* factors. The presence of such beliefs about what caused stuttering to emerge can influence the ways in which the parents interact with the child, and therefore they need to be identified and addressed by the clinician. For details about obtaining and reporting case histories, refer to Chapter 3.

> Parental behavior may be a piece.

Objective 4: Determining the Parents' (Non)Verbal Reactions to Stuttering

Finally, during the evaluation you need to observe the ways in which the parents react and respond to the child's instances of disfluency and stuttering. As described earlier, you should collect a sample of the child's speech while he talks with his parents during the first 10–15 minutes of the evaluation. During this time you should also watch the interaction between the child and his parents, paying particular attention to the parents' rate of speech and the duration of their turn-switching pauses (the length of time the parents wait before responding, after the child has finished an utterance), as well as their nonverbal and verbal behaviors during and after the child produces a disfluency (overtly commenting about the child's speech, providing directions for "how to" talk, eye contact and facial expression, body movement and positioning). You should also observe the *quantity* and *quality* of the speech and language the parents use while talking with the child, along with the amount of interruptions produced by both the child and the parents.

As discussed earlier, although there is no evidence that any of these parent (or child) behaviors *cause* children to begin stuttering, it has been speculated that they might *contribute* to either the continued development of stuttering in children, or its recovery.

Question 2: Will the Child Exhibit Recovery From Stuttering? Will He Outgrow It?

Determining the likelihood of unassisted recovery is important.

A key question in the diagnosis of young children who stutter relates to the frequently observed phenomenon of unassisted or spontaneous recovery. That is, a sizable proportion of very young children who stutter show complete recovery without receiving therapy. A number of retrospective and longitudinal studies (Andrews & Harris, 1964; Yairi & Ambrose, 1992a, 1992b; Yairi et al., 1996) have yielded recovery estimates ranging from 32–80%, a wide range by anyone's judgment. Although unaided remission of stuttering is obviously good for the child and his family, it adds another layer of complexity to the tasks of stuttering diagnosis and prognosis. The fact is that when parents invariably ask "Will my child 'outgrow' it (the stuttering)?" we cannot offer a definitive, conclusive answer. There are no absolute predictors of which children will recover and which will not. Neither research nor clinical observation has uncovered characteristics of the child or his environment that incontrovertibly predict that the child's stuttering will either cease or persist. So, we are left with a frequently occurring phenomenon that we cannot predict, with a relatively high cost involved. That is, if we play the odds and take a wait-and-see attitude toward therapy, we run the risk of the child developing a chronic stuttering problem, which may be more resistant to treatment than a case of early stuttering.

What do we do? It is unlikely that we will ever know all we need to know to reliably and absolutely predict recovery from childhood stuttering. We cannot wait for all of the answers before we form clinical relationships with young children who stutter and their families. Therefore, we should carefully use all available information to form well-educated predictions about which young children *are most likely* to recover without direct intervention, and which *are least likely* to do so.

In a recent series of papers, Yairi and associates (1992a, 1992b, 1996) reported the results of a longitudinal study of the development of stuttering in children. Over the course of these investigations, they observed various patterns of stuttering development and *recovery* in a large group of children who were relatively close to the onset of stuttering and who were not receiving stuttering therapy. Yairi and his colleagues were able to examine a variety of factors associated with unassisted recovery from stuttering, and it is possible for practitioners to draw from these observations in their own clinical work. Based on their findings, it appears that the factors most closely associated with stuttering remission or perpetuation in young children are the length of time the child has been stuttering (post-onset interval), the age of the child when stuttering was first observed, gender, family history of stuttering and recovery patterns of affected family members, the decline or stability of sound/syllable and word repetitions over time, and the presence or absence of associated behaviors and coexisting articulation or language problems.

Children who recover from stuttering do so relatively soon after reported onset, usually within 12 to 14 months. The chance of developing a persistent stuttering problem increases as the child continues to stutter beyond 18 months post-onset. In addition, children who recover tend to be those who began to stutter after their third birthday; children who develop chronic stuttering tend to be those who began to stutter quite early, typically prior to 3 years of age. Children are more likely to recover if they are girls as opposed to boys, if they have no family history of stuttering, or if they have a relatively small number of relatives who stuttered but recovered during early childhood. Recovery seems to be somewhat related to a decline in sound/syllable or word repetitions over time; that is, children are more likely to recover if they show a steady decline in these disfluent behaviors very soon after onset. Finally, children are more likely to recover if they exhibit few to no associated behaviors or no concomitant problems in speech articulation or language.

We will be able to gauge the presence or absence of these factors during the evaluation through direct observation of the child and interviewing the parents or primary caregivers. It may be helpful to conceptualize these factors as cumulative; that is, the probability for recovery grows stronger with each variable noted. That being said, it is extremely important to take into account that these factors allow us to only speculate about the *probability* or *likelihood* of the child experiencing unassisted recovery; there are no absolutely valid or reliable predictors. These variables are an additional piece to the diagnostic puzzle.

Question 3: Is Therapy Warranted and Recommended?

If the answer to our first question (Is the child either stuttering or at risk) is "yes," and the answer to the second question (Will the child recover without treatment?) is "probably not," or "unsure," then you will need to answer the third question: Is therapy warranted and recommended? As shown in Figure 8–2, you can develop an answer to this question by evaluating the information obtained for questions 1 and 2. You will also need to *compare* the results from your observation of the child's *present* speech (dis)fluency characteristics (objective 1) with parental reports of those characteristics at the time the problem was first noted (objective 5). The importance of objective 5 is that it allows you to speculate about the *rate* of progression or change of the child's disfluency problem. How much and how fast have the frequency and type of speech disfluency changed since the problem first began? Further, you will need to determine the presence or absence of coexisting speech, language, hearing, or speech-related neuromuscular problems through observation and administration of standardized and informal tests (objective 6). Considering the information provided when you meet objectives 1 through 4, along with the additional information concerning the probability of unassisted recovery (question 2), any changes in the child's disfluencies over time, and the presence or absence of coexisting speech, language, or related problems (objective 6), can assist you in determining the need for therapy.

Objective 5: Determining Change in Speech Disfluencies Over Time

You will need to form an impression of the ways in which the child's speech disfluencies have changed since they were first noticed by the parents, or if they have changed at all. Such changes can be observed in overall frequency (the child is more or less disfluent in general), proportions of different types, duration (instances of stuttering have increased or decreased in duration), presence or absence of associated behaviors, the child's reported awareness and concern about disfluency and stuttering, and the variability of disfluency (e.g., is the child's overall frequency of disfluency stable over time, or does he show peaks and valleys, such that he follows 2 weeks of highly disfluent speech with 3 weeks of essentially fluent talking?).

You can determine *type* of change in two ways. First, during the parent interview, ask the parents to describe any changes they have noted in their child's disfluent speech since the problem first began. Second, ask the parents to *show* you what the child's disfluencies were like when they were first noticed, and then *show* you what they are like at the present time. Then compare these two examples, as well as the parents' example or description of the child's beginning disfluencies, with your observations of the child's disfluent speech during the evaluation. You can attempt to determine *rate* of change by considering these descriptions and observations of change in light of the amount of time the child has been stuttering.

Based on this assessment of type and rate of change, recommend therapy if the child's speech disfluencies have increased in frequency or duration, are more consistent, or if the child has increased the proportion of sound prolongations he produces since the problem first began. In addition, if these changes have occurred over a relatively short period of time, a stuttering problem might exist which is developing at a fast rate. Similarly, if the information you gather suggests a steady decline in the frequency of sound, syllable, and word repetitions and sound prolongations, then indirect therapy with a focus on parent counseling may be most appropriate.

Objective 6: Determine the Presence of Concomitant Problems

It has been shown that a subgroup of children who stutter exhibit coexisting speech and language problems (Louko et al., 1990). Presently, it is unclear how these problems might interact, or whether a child's speech and language problem causes the child's stuttering or vice versa. In particular, some children who stutter display concomitant articulation problems, and it has been speculated that these children might take longer to show progress in stuttering therapy, or might not show as much progress as children without additional problems. In some cases, the child's articulation or language problems interfere more with communication than the child's stuttering, and therefore take precedence for treatment. In other cases, both stuttering and articulation (or language) need to be the simultaneous focus of therapy.

You should routinely assess the child's other speech, language, and related behaviors during your stuttering evaluation. Chapters 6 and 7 provide detailed descriptions of how to assess these behaviors, and you are directed to look there for guidance. Although you should not necessarily conduct a full-scale articulation or language assessment at this time, you should carefully select one or two methods or tests for sampling these communicative behaviors in order to form a general impression of the child's abilities in other areas besides fluency. In addition, you should conduct an oral-peripheral examination to assess structure and function of the speech mechanism. Chapter 5 provides a protocol for conducting such assessment.

If you determine that the child is stuttering or at risk for stuttering, and also shows concomitant problems, you might not recommend stuttering therapy. For example, you might suggest that the child receive *indirect* articulation therapy (if warranted), which *does not* focus on correct, precise or physically tense articulator "placement," accomplished through drill procedures. Or you might recommend that the child receive language-based stuttering therapy, focusing on simultaneous treatment of oral language and fluency skills.

To summarize, if the child produces *at least* 3 within-word disfluencies in 100 words *and* the parents are concerned about the child's "stuttering," or believe he is a "stutterer," you should recommend *some* form of intervention for the child and his family. The case for this recommendation becomes even stronger if the child also conveys concern about his speech. This treatment might take the form of direct parent counseling with indirect treatment for the child, participation in a parent-child fluency group (Kelly & Conture, 1992), parent counseling only, or direct stuttering therapy for the child, in which you explicitly address the differences between fluency and stuttering, and teach the child strategies for producing fluent speech. In addition, for some children the information obtained through objectives 5 and 6 is important in your decision to recommend intervention.

When should we recommend treatment for a child?

Question 4: What Should Be the Focus of Therapy?

If you've decided to recommend treatment, it is important to provide some guidelines for initial therapy focus. Doing so certainly helps you if you are to be the clinician providing therapy. In addition, providing suggestions for treatment emphasis to another clinician (if that is the case) is an important professional courtesy, in that it is not only helpful, but also shows the receiving clinician that we have thought about a particular case beyond the "does he or doesn't he" stage.

As shown in Figure 8–2, you should use *all* the information obtained during the evaluation (objectives 1 through 6) to develop such guidelines or suggestions. As an example, suppose you evaluate a 5-year-old boy who is producing a relatively high proportion of sound prolongations with many associated behaviors and exhibits a concomitant articulation problem. Suppose as well that during the interview the parents of this child expressed the belief that the child stutters because he was the only one of their four children born at home and "the stress was too much for everyone." Finally, when the parents and the child engage in conversation, the parents frequently interrupt and talk simultaneously with the child.

In this case, your recommendations for initial therapy focus might include parent counseling and information sharing, particularly with regard to what is known and not known about the causes of stuttering in children, and the difference between causal and contributing factors in the problem of childhood stuttering. In addition, you might want to discuss with the parents the various ways in which they can modify their verbal interactions with their child. Further, you might recommend indirect treatment for the child, focusing simultaneously on articulation and fluency-enhancing strategies.

The preceding is one example of some possible recommendations. A general rule of thumb for developing suggestions for treatment is to consider all the behaviors and comments produced by both the child and his parents, and to determine which interfere the most with communication, or which need to be addressed before others can be targeted, or both. You will not provide specific therapy plans of course, but in the diagnostic report you should make some broad suggestions for the direction treatment might take.

STUTTERING ASSESSMENT FOR ADULTS

How is stuttering in the child and the adult different?

As previously discussed, for the adult the purpose of assessment is seldom to answer the question, "Is this person stuttering, or at risk for stuttering?" as it usually is for a child. Most adults who stutter have been doing so since they were young children and have been diagnosed as stuttering in the past. That is not to say that the same adults have received consistent therapy, or any therapy for that matter, but the question of "stuttering or not stuttering" has been answered. For this reason, the main question of assessment changes from "does or doesn't he?" to "*how* does he?" or what are the characteristics of the person's disfluent and stuttered speech as well as the stuttering problem?

Figure 8–3 is a schematic representation of the three main questions for the assessment of stuttering in adults, along with objectives. As you can see, the second and third main questions are the

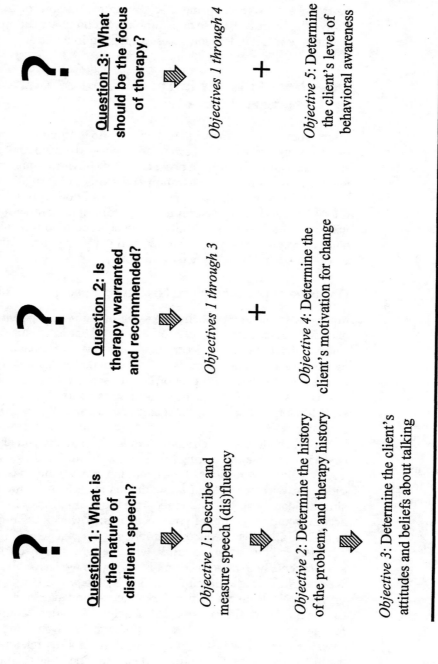

Figure 8–3. Questions to be addressed in the diagnosis of adults who stutter.

same as those for children, and it is only the first that differs. In addition, the objectives are different from those set for children; that is, you want to answer most of the same questions, but you use different information to do so.

The remainder of this chapter will focus on the questions that need to be answered during a stuttering evaluation for adults. As shown in Figure 8–3, these questions are qualitatively different from the ones you ask when you assess stuttering in children.

Question 1: What is the Nature of Disfluent and Stuttered Speech?

Your initial question for adults is *how* they do it. What is the nature of disfluent and stuttered speech? You need to describe and measure speech (dis)fluency through observation of conversational speech, as well as through the administration and scoring of formalized procedures and rating scales or techniques. In addition, you will need to interview the client to determine the history of the problem, therapy history, and to learn his attitudes and beliefs about both speaking and stuttering, as well as his description and demonstration of the things he does to help himself when he stutters.

Objective 1: Describing and Measuring Speech (Dis)Fluency

You need to make essentially the same measures of speech (dis)fluency for adults as you would for children. That is, from a 300-word sample of spontaneous speech, as well as several formal assessment instruments, you need to measure (1) frequency of disfluency, (2) type of speech disfluency and proportion of each, (3) duration of within-word or "stuttered" disfluencies, (4) number and variety of associated behaviors, (5) severity, (6) speaking rate, and (7) adaptation and consistency of stuttering.

You can collect a speech sample for analysis while you engage the client in conversation during the first few minutes of the evaluation. You can also use portions of the client interview, if necessary, to provide you with samples of spontaneous speech. As with children, simultaneously audio- and video tape the evaluation to increase the accuracy and reliability of your measures; however, the importance of on-line analysis needs to be emphasized here.

When talking with the adult who stutters, you need to attend simultaneously to *what* the client is saying, as well as analyze *how* he is saying it. This is a difficult task, and will require a conscious effort on your part. With practice and experience, however, it is a skill that can be mastered. One model that is helpful for such "analytical listening" was described by Adams (1974). It involves using the processes associated with fluent speech production as reference points against which to compare stuttered speech. The basic premise is that

Obtaining a satisfactory speech sample from an adult is usually easy.

in order to speak fluently, a person needs to control the flow of air from the lungs into the vocal tract, as well as to coordinate this airflow with both vocal fold vibration and articulator movement and positioning. When a person produces a sound/syllable repetition or a sound prolongation (stuttering), you will need to make a hypothesis about what this individual *is doing* with his speech production system to produce the disruption in speech. Once the hypothesis of what the person is doing to interfere with fluent talking is made, you will need to develop therapeutic strategies for helping the individual initiate and maintain speech fluently.

For example, suppose during your evaluation you observe that 60% of the client's disfluencies are inaudible sound prolongations. Since these are in the category of within-word disfluencies, it is highly probable that they represent "stuttering." Further, suppose you also observe that this client is producing these inaudible sound prolongations by holding his articulators stationary in a particular position, with no accompanying voice or airflow. To initiate fluent speech, the client will need to initiate airflow and voicing smoothly, while simultaneously moving his articulators to form transitions between sounds. It is your job as a speech-language pathologist to teach the client how to accomplish this.

Objective 2: Determine History of the Problem and Therapy History

As with any referral, it is important to obtain a history of the individual's problem. For adults who stutter, it is important to know when they first started to stutter, and who first noticed it. In addition, you will want to know what the client remembers about the reactions of the significant others in his life to his stuttering (usually parents, relatives, teachers, and childhood friends). You will also want to know how, if at all, the client's stuttering has influenced decisions or choices he has made earlier in his life (e.g., social life and vocational choices). Finally, you will need to find out what the client's perception is of how his stuttering has changed over time. All of this information will help you form an impression about both the significance stuttering has in the client's life and his motivation to change.

During the interview, you will also want to find out the history of any therapy the client received. Specifically, it is helpful to know how often treatment was received, for how long, and what type. If a client has received a good deal of previous therapy, with either little progress or maintenance, you will need to think about possible reasons for this situation. Of course, the best way to begin developing possible explanations for the client's lack of sustained fluency is to ask him why *he* thinks he has not been successful. Conversely, if the client has reached adulthood and has received little to no therapy for stuttering, then you will most likely have to spend a good deal of time in counseling and information-sharing about the nature of stuttering (what we know and do not know). Further, it might be the case that this client's stuttering is more habituated than someone who has stuttered for the same amount of time, but who has a history of therapy (even if sporadic).

Objective 3: Determine the Client's Attitudes and Beliefs

When you interview an adult who stutters, you ask why he *thinks* he stutters, as well as why he *believes* that he does. You should differentiate between thinking and believing, because many times the client has had previous therapy, and so has discussed what is known and not known about the cause(s) of stuttering with his clinician. That often contributes to his *thinking* about why he stutters. However, what a person thinks and what he feels or believes are often not the same. For example, if a client believes that he stutters because of some deep-seated psychological problem, even though intellectually he knows this is not the case, his belief might negatively influence his confidence in his ability to be helped, and your ability to help him.

Related to the client's beliefs about what stuttering is and why he stutters, are the attitudes he has about talking. That is, does he generally like to speak and feel confident in his abilities to communicate, or does he view talking as unenjoyable and himself as a poor speaker? Research with adults who stutter has shown that their attitudes about talking are better predictors of long-term improvements in speech fluency than their overall frequency of pretherapy stuttering (Guitar, 1976; Guitar & Bass, 1978).

Presently, there are several questionnaires available which help to assess the client's attitudes about talking and stuttering. A modified version of the *Erickson Scale of Communication Attitudes* (Andrews & Cutler, 1974) is available, which you can ask the client to fill out either at the beginning or end of the evaluation. The Erickson Scale, similar to the CAT for children, contains a series of statements about communication which the client indicates as either "true" or "false." Norms are available for both stuttering and nonstuttering adults, as well as for stuttering adults posttherapy, so it is possible to compare the client's score with these groups.

Question 2: Is Therapy Warranted and Recommended?

Once you have answered the first question, you need to determine if treatment is needed and whether or not you are going to recommend it. To help you decide whether to recommend therapy, you need to consider the information obtained during the evaluation of your client's speech, as well as your assessment of his level of motivation (objective 4). It's important to know for various reasons that sometimes speech-language pathologists do *not* recommend therapy, even though they conclude from diagnostic information that a client's communication problem warrants intervention.

> Assessing his attitudes and feelings about his stuttering is sometimes not easy.

Objective 4: Determine the Client's Motivation for Change

During the interview, ask the client why he has come for an evaluation at this time; in other words, "Why now?" Many times the reason is related to concerns that others have about his speech, for example, a spouse or an employer. He may not want to enroll in therapy, but attempts to do so as a way of placating or pleasing others. Certainly he may *need* therapy in order to learn how to talk more fluently, but if the speech-language pathologist determines that the client either does not *want* to change the way he speaks or does not want to invest the time and effort needed for therapy, then she may not recommend treatment. Sometimes the client has either made or is attempting to make other changes in his life, for example, a new job or enrolling in college. In such cases, the client may feel that his success in these new endeavors hinges on his ability to speak more fluently. Finally, the client may report that he has "had enough" of his stuttering or has "hit bottom" and is ready to work toward improving his speech. The person who is motivated to change his speech *for himself*, rather than for another person, or because he thinks his speech will interfere with attaining a career or personal goal, may be more likely to maintain his motivation for the long road ahead in therapy.

> A major challenge: to encourage the client to be forthright about motivation for change.

Question 3: What Should be the Focus of Therapy?

As with children who stutter, if you recommend therapy for adults, you should try to make some suggestions for initial treatment focus in the recommendations section of your report. By using all of the information obtained throughout the evaluation, you will be able to make these suggestions. For example, perhaps the client needs to obtain information about the problem of stuttering and what we know about its etiology. Or, he may need some additional counseling for related concerns. Further, at the Wendell Johnson Speech and Hearing Clinic (University of Iowa), we use either a stuttering modification approach or an integration of both "speak more fluently" and stuttering modification approaches. Therefore, we try to assess the client's level of *behavioral* awareness during both stuttered and fluent speech. Is he able to identify *when* he produces a stuttered disruption and *what* he does when he produces instances of stuttering? Similarly, is the client able to identify what he is doing during moments of relatively easy, fluent speech?

You will obtain some information about the client's level of awareness during the interview when you ask him to both describe and imitate examples of what concerns him the most about his speech. In addition, when you ask questions about the situations or conversational partners which are the *most* and *least* difficult for the client, you can make some judgments about the degree of awareness and concern he exhibits about his speech. While the client's verbal descriptions of his speech and related issues provide you with insight into his *cognitive* awareness of his speech and stuttering, an important factor for success in treatment is the extent to which he is aware of the *physical* feeling of both stuttering and fluency.

Objective 5: Determine the Client's Level of Behavioral Awareness of Stuttering

When talking to the client about his stuttering, ask him to show you what he does when he talks which concerns him or what he does when he considers himself to be stuttering. Sometimes the client will be unable or unwilling to show you, but will describe the behavior instead. Similar to the parents of stuttering children, who cannot or will not *show* you what their child does while speaking, an adult client who states that he can't or won't imitate his stuttering might have difficulty objectively analyzing his speech. Further, he may possess such strong negative emotions about stuttering that he is unwilling to produce an example of stuttered speech for any reason. Finally, he might be relatively unaware of the specific characteristics of his stuttering, such that he really can't show you; rather, he might be vaguely aware on an emotional level that "something is happening somewhere" when he speaks and stutters, but he is unable to determine what he is doing while talking and when he is doing it.

One way of determining the client's behavioral awareness of his stuttering is to use a technique that Conture (1990a) has described as "on-line identification." It is easy to do this during the evaluation, and it is helpful in obtaining some impression of the client's awareness of when he stutters. Ask the client either to read a short passage, or describe a picture to you, and either raise his finger or tap the table *as soon as he feels himself using stuttered speech*. Make sure to make the distinction between "hearing" and "feeling" explicit, and between "emotional feeling" ("butterflies-in-the-stomach") and "physical feeling" (kinesthetic or proprioceptive awareness) for the client. Some clients will identify their moments of stuttering *after* they have produced them, some will identify *during* their production, some immediately *before*, and some not at all. Of course, the most helpful time to identify stuttering is immediately before or while producing it. Observe the client's performance in order to make recommendations about where to start in the identification process during the initial stages of treatment.

SUMMARY OF KEY POINTS

This chapter presented the components of a comprehensive stuttering assessment for children and adults. In addition to analyzing the speech and nonspeech behaviors that characterize disfluency and stuttering, it is also important to evaluate the relationship between stuttering and the speaker's beliefs and attitudes about stuttering, as well as the beliefs and attitudes of the client's significant others. Definitions and descriptions of speech fluency, disfluency, and stuttering were provided, along with a discussion of how to differentiate the latter two.

The goal of assessment for children is to obtain information that allows you to answer the questions: (1) Is the child stuttering or at risk? (2) Will the child "outgrow" stuttering? (3) Is therapy warranted and recommended? and (4) What should be the focus of therapy? To address these questions, you will need to describe and measure the child's speech (dis)fluencies along several dimensions, obtain information about onset and family history of stuttering, begin to uncover the child's and parents' beliefs and attitudes about stuttering, observe the parents' responses to the child's stuttering, determine change in the child's speech disfluencies since they were first noticed, and assess the presence of concomitant speech, language, or related problems in the child. For adults who stutter, the information you obtain during the evaluation should help you to answer the questions: (1) What is the nature of disfluent and stuttered speech? (2) Is therapy warranted and recommended? and (3) What should be the focus of therapy? As with children, in order to answer these questions for adults who stutter, you need to describe and measure the client's speech disfluencies. Further, you will need to carefully interview the client in order to determine both the history of the problem and therapy history, his attitudes and beliefs about talking and stuttering, and his levels of both motivation for participating in therapy and behavioral awareness of what he does when he stutters.

REFERENCES

Adams, M. R. (1974). A physiologic and aerodynamic interpretation of fluent and stuttered speech. *Journal of Fluency Disorders, 1,* 35–47.

Andrews, G., & Cutler, J. (1974). Stuttering therapy: The relation between changes in symptom level and attitudes. *Journal of Speech and Hearing Disorders, 39,* 312–319.

Andrews, G., & Harris, M. (1964). *The syndrome of stuttering.* London: Heinman Medical Books.

Bloodstein, O. (1995). *A handbook on stuttering* (5th ed.). San Diego, CA: Singular Publishing Group.

Brutten, G. J. (1985). *Communication Attitude Test.* Unpublished manuscript, Southern Illinois University, Carbondale.

Conture, E. G. (1990a). *Stuttering.* Englewood Cliffs, NJ: Prentice-Hall.

Conture, E. G. (1990b). Childhood stuttering: What is it and who does it? *Asha Reports, 18,* 2–14.

Conture, E. G., & Caruso, A. J. (1987). Assessment and diagnosis of childhood disfluency. In L. Rustin, H. Purser, & D. Rowley (Eds.), *Progress in the treatment of fluency disorders* (pp. 84–104). London: Taylor & Francis.

Conture, E. G., & Kelly, E. M. (1991). Young stutterers' nonspeech behaviors during stuttering. *Journal of Speech and Hearing Research, 34,* 1041–1056.

Conture, E. G., LaSalle, L. R., & Yaruss, S. (1990). *One hundred young stutterers: Making sense of their clinical records.* A miniseminar presented to The Annual Meeting of the American Speech-Language-Hearing Association, Seattle, WA.

De Nil, L. F., & Brutten, G. J. (1991). Speech-associated attitudes of stuttering and nonstuttering children. *Journal of Speech and Hearing Research, 34,* 60–66.

Guitar, B. (1976). Pretreatment factors associated with the outcome of stuttering therapy. *Journal of Speech and Hearing Research, 19,* 590–600.

Guitar, B., & Bass, C. (1978). Stuttering therapy: The relation between attitude change and long-term outcome. *Journal of Speech and Hearing Disorders, 43,* 392–400.

Johnson, W. (1959). *The onset of stuttering* (2nd ed.). Minneapolis, MN: University of Minnesota Press.

Johnson, W., Darley, F., & Spriestersbach, D. (1978). *Diagnostic methods in speech pathology.* New York: Harper & Row.

Kelly, E. M., & Conture, E. G. (1992). Speaking rates, response time latencies, and interrupting behaviors of young stutterers, nonstutterers, and their mothers. *Journal of Speech and Hearing Research, 35,* 1256–1267.

Louko, L. J., Edwards, M. L., & Conture, E. G. (1990). Phonological characteristics of young stutterers and their normally fluent peers: Preliminary observations. *Journal of Fluency Disorders, 15,* 191–211.

Ludlow, C. (1990). Research procedures for measuring stuttering severity. In J. Cooper (Ed.), *Research needs in stuttering: Roadblocks and future directions. ASHA Reports, 18,* 26–33.

Neely, N., & Timmons, R. (1967). Adaptation and consistency in the disfluent speech behavior of young stutterers and nonstutterers. *Journal of Speech and Hearing Research, 10,* 250–256.

Riley, G. D. (1972). A stuttering severity instrument for children and adults. *Journal of Speech and Hearing Disorders, 37,* 314–320.

Riley, G. D. (1994). *Stuttering severity instrument for children and adults—3.* Austin, TX: Pro-Ed.

Stocker, B. (1980). *Stocker Probe Technique for the Diagnosis and Treatment of Stuttering in Young Children.* Tulsa, OK: Modern Educational Corp.

Stocker, B., & Usprich, C. (1976). Stuttering in young children and level of demand. *Journal of Fluency Disorders, 1,* 116–131.

Weiss, A., & Zebrowski, P. (1992). Disfluencies in the conversations of young children who stutter: Some answers about questions. *Journal of Speech and Hearing Research, 35,* 1230–1238.

Williams, D. E. (1978). Differential diagnosis of disorders of fluency. In F. Darley & D. Spriestersbach (Eds.), *Diagnostic methods in speech pathology* (2nd ed.). New York: Harper and Row.

Williams, D. E. (1979). A perspective on approaches to stuttering therapy. In H. Gregory (Ed.), *Controversies about stuttering therapy.* Baltimore, MD: University Park Press.

Williams, D. E. (1985). Talking with children who stutter. In J. Fraser (Ed.), *Counseling stutterers*. Memphis, TN: Stuttering Foundation of America.

Williams, D. E., Silverman, F. H., & Kools, J. A. (1968). Disfluency behavior of elementary-school stutterers and nonstutterers: The adaptation effect. *Journal of Speech and Hearing Research, 11, 622–630*.

Yairi, E., & Ambrose, N. (1992a). A longitudinal study of stuttering in children: A preliminary report. *Journal of Speech and Hearing Research, 35, 755–760*.

Yairi, E., & Ambrose, N. (1992b). Onset of stuttering in preschool children: Selected factors. *Journal of Speech and Hearing Research, 35, 782–788*.

Yairi, E., Ambrose, N., Paden, E., & Throneberg, R. (1996). Predictive factors of persistence and recovery: Pathways of childhood stuttering. *Journal of Communication Disorders, 29, 53–77*.

Yairi, E., & Lewis, B. (1984). Disfluencies at the onset of stuttering. *Journal of Speech and Hearing Research, 27, 154–159*.

Zebrowski, P. (1991). Duration of the speech disfluencies of beginning stutterers. *Journal of Speech and Hearing Research, 34, 483–491*.

Zebrowski, P., & Conture, E. (1989). Judgments of disfluency by mothers of stuttering and normally fluent children. *Journal of Speech and Hearing Research, 32, 625–634*.

Zebrowski, P., & Schum, R. (1993). Counseling the parents of children who stutter. *American Journal of Speech-Language Pathology, 2, 65–73*.

RECOMMENDED READINGS

Stuttering Assessment Issues and Methods

Bakker, K. (1997). Instrumentation for the assessment and treatment of stuttering. In R. Curlee & G. Siegel (Eds.), *Nature and treatment of stuttering: New directions* (2nd ed.). Boston, MA: Allyn & Bacon.

Conture, E. G. (1997). Evaluating childhood stuttering. In R. Curlee & G. Siegel (Eds.), *Nature and treatment of stuttering: New directions* (2nd ed.). Boston, MA: Allyn & Bacon.

Costello, J. M., & Ingham, R. J. (1984). Assessment strategies for child and adult stutterers. In W. Perkins & R. Curlee (Eds.), *Nature and treatment of stuttering: New directions*. San Diego, CA: College-Hill Press.

Curlee, R., & Yairi, E. (1997). Early identification with early childhood stuttering: A critical examination of the data. *American Journal of Speech-Language Pathology, 6, 8–18*.

Gordon, P., & Luper, H. (1992a). The early identification of beginning stuttering I: Protocols. *American Journal of Speech-Language Pathology, 1, 43–53*.

Gordon, P., & Luper, H. (1992b). The early identification of beginning stuttering II: Problems. *American Journal of Speech-Language Pathology, 1, 54–59*.

Ratner, N. B. (1997). Leaving Las Vegas: Clinical odds and individual outcomes. *American Journal of Speech-Language Pathology, 6*, 29–33.

Zebrowski, P. (1997). Assisting young children who stutter and their families: Defining the role of the speech-language pathologist. *American Journal of Speech-Language Pathology, 6*, 19–28.

Characteristics of the Fluent and Stuttered Speech of People Who Stutter

Bloodstein, O. (1970). Stuttering and normal nonfluency—A continuity hypothesis. *British Journal of Disordered Communication, 5*, 30–39.

Johnson, W., & Knott, J. (1937). Studies in the psychology of stuttering: I. The distribution of moments of stuttering in successive readings of the same material. *Journal of Speech and Hearing Disorders, 2*, 17-19.

LaSalle, L., & Conture, E. (1991). Eye contact between young stutterers and their mothers. *Journal of Fluency Disorders, 16*, 173–200.

Van Riper, C. (1982). *The nature of stuttering.* Englewood Cliffs, NJ: Prentice–Hall.

Williams, D. E., Silverman, F. H., & Kools, J. A. (1968). Disfluency behavior of elementary-school stutterers and nonstutterers: The adaptation effect. *Journal of Speech and Hearing Research, 11*, 622–630.

Williams, D. E., Silverman, F. H., & Kools, J. A. (1969). Disfluency behavior of elementary-school stutterers and nonstutterers: The consistency effect. *Journal of Speech and Hearing Research, 12*, 301–307.

Yairi, E. H. (1983). The onset of stuttering in two- and three-year-old children: A preliminary report. *Journal of Speech and Hearing Disorders, 48*, 171–178.

Related Speech and Language Behaviors of Children Who Stutter

Bernstein Ratner, N. (1995). Treating the child who stutters with concomitant language or phonological impairment. *Language, Speech, and Hearing Services in Schools, 26*(2), 180–186.

Schwartz, H. D., & Conture, E. G. (1988). Subgrouping young stutterers: Preliminary behavioral perspectives. *Journal of Speech and Hearing Research, 31*, 62–71.

Schwartz, H. D., Zebrowski, P. M., & Conture, E. G. (1990). Behaviors at the onset of stuttering. *Journal of Fluency Disorders, 15*, 77–86.

Walker, J., Archibald, L., Cherniak, S., & Fish, V. (1992). Articulation rate in 3- and 5-year-old children. *Journal of Speech and Hearing Research, 35*, 4–13.

Attitudes of Children and Adults Who Stutter

De Nil, L. F., & Brutten, G. J. (1991). Speech-associated attitudes of stuttering and nonstuttering children. *Journal of Speech and Hearing Research, 34,* 60–66.

Tests and Measures of Stuttering

Conture, E. G., & Caruso, A. J. (1978). A review of the Stocker Probe Technique for diagnosis and treatment of stuttering in young children. *Journal of Fluency Disorders, 3,* 297–298.

Riley, G. (1981). *Stuttering Prediction Instrument for Young Children.* Austin, TX: Pro-Ed.

Parents' Judgments of Disfluent Speech

Zebrowski, P. (1995). The topography of beginning stuttering. *Journal of Communication Disorders, 28,* 75–91.

Stuttering Treatment

Guitar, B. (1998). *Stuttering: An integrated approach to its nature and treatment* (2nd ed.). Baltimore, MD: Williams & Wilkins.

Stuttering Foundation of America. (1996). *Therapy in action: The school-age child who stutters* [Videotape]. (Available from Stuttering Foundation of America, 3106 Walnut Grove Road, Suite 603, Memphis, TN 38111-0749.)

CHAPTER

9

Voice Disorders

Katherine Verdolini, Ph.D.

PURPOSE OF CHAPTER

This chapter is intended for students of speech-language pathology in early phases of professional training and for practicing speech-language pathologists with limited experience in voice disorders. It is assumed that all readers have completed basic coursework in anatomy and physiology of speech and speech acoustics, and that all have completed or will soon complete a full didactic course in voice disorders.

The chapter's purpose is twofold. The *general* aim is to provide information about important overarching principles of voice evaluation. A second, more *specific* aim is to provide information about how to conduct an elementary voice evaluation. The chapter should serve as a reference for current or future professionals whose main focus is not voice disorders, but who may encounter them in the course of speech-language pathology practice in acute care (hospital) settings, nursing homes, schools, or private consulting. The chapter should further serve as a basic introduction to the principles and practices of voice evaluation for those who intend to pursue in depth study in voice disorders in the future.

The chapter is subdivided into several sections. The first addresses the most fundamental question in any voice evaluation: What is a voice disorder? The second addresses how common voice disorders are and why they are important to individuals and to society. The third section references summary information about causes of the most common voice disorders, as relevant for the discussion about voice evaluation that follows. The fourth section introduces important general principles of any voice evaluation, regardless of which particular measures are used. The fifth section introduces examples of specific assessment procedures, their methodology, and their interpretation. Although the focus of this section is measures that can be made quickly with limited instrumentation, consistent with the requirements of many clinical settings, this section also includes reference to more advanced approaches to voice evaluation to ensure that the reader is aware of them, can consider pursuing them for his or her center, if appropriate, and can knowledgeably refer to other centers for advanced evaluation if warranted. The sixth section provides case examples. The seventh and final section addresses voice disorders in special populations including children, elderly adults, professional voice users, patients with other speech or language deficits, and multicultural issues.

To facilitate your reading, I have listed limited references within the text itself. Most references are listed at the end of the chapter.

SECTION I: WHAT IS A VOICE DISORDER?

This first relevant question in clinical voice evaluation is: What is a voice disorder, anyway? At the simplest level, one could define voice disorder as a persistent abnormality in the sound of the voice. This definition seems obvious, yet it poses a number of problems. For example, what is the point of reference for "normal" that determines the boundaries of abnormality? Is it the quality of voice that can be expected from a lesion-free, disease-free system, or is it the quality of voice that is most typically encountered within the subject's usual cultural environment? Who determines the presence of

> There are several ways to define a voice disorder.

an "abnormality"? Is it a speech-language pathologist (SLP) or other clinician, or is it the speaker under consideration? What about conditions that result in a voice that falls well within normal limits for lesion-free, disease-free individuals, and for the subject's general cultural milieu, but that fails to function well for some social, professional, or other purpose (e.g., auctioneering)? Finally, what about conditions in which voice sounds satisfactory in all regards, but is physically uncomfortable?

These questions raise important issues and point out how the definition of "voice disorder" is not be as obvious as it initially appears. In this chapter I consider a voice disorder a condition in which voice is problematic to the user in social, professional, or other contexts, and for which the SLP or other clinician generally finds some corroborative evidence. By this definition, recognition of a voice disorder extends to situations in which the sound of the voice is acceptable to the speaker but voicing is uncomfortable. The discussion in this chapter is limited to phonation disorders, excluding disorders that primarily involve resonance problems which are considered later in this book (Chapter 14, Peterson-Falzone).

SECTION II: HOW COMMON ARE VOICE DISORDERS AND WHY ARE THEY IMPORTANT?

Voice disorders are common, and they are important. These assertions—discussed in this section of the chapter—tell us why voice evaluations should be conducted and why public and private resources should be allocated to the evaluation and treatment of voice disorders.

In short, voice disorders may be among the most common types of communication disorder, certainly if one considers cumulative occurrence over the life span. Most studies looking at abnormal voice *quality* have indicated that about 3% to 9% of children and adults in the general population are hoarse at any given moment in time—certainly not trivial figures. Self-report clinical epidemiological studies, which more closely reflect the definition of voice disorder used in this chapter, have indicated similar figures. Considering that approximately 25% of the working population in the United States (i.e., about 28,000,000 persons) has jobs that require voice use in some critical fashion (Titze et al., 1997), these figures indicate that something on the order of 1,680,000 employed persons whose job functioning depends on voice experience a voice problem *every day* in this country (assuming 6% of 28,000,000 persons).

Have you ever had a voice problem? Do you know others who have?

Cumulative frequencies of voice disorders over a lifetime have not been formally studied but are certainly much larger. Equally as impressive, about 3% of the work force (840,000) have jobs in which voice is relevant for public safety, including air traffic controllers, pilots, firepersons, and police. Communication impairments due to voice in these subpopulations have potentially sobering consequences for public safety.

Other studies utilizing some form of self-report have identified specific sectors of the population particularly at risk for a voice problem. Consistently, across several continents including North America, Europe, and Australia, teachers emerge as a remarkably high-risk population; for example, in one study, almost 40% of teachers indicated that teaching had negatively affected their voice (Smith et al., 1998). Similarly, studies also indicate a high-risk factor for singers, for whom voice problems may reach rates of 20%–50% or larger at any given moment in time, depending on the study and the type of singing.

One might consider that, despite the figures, voice disorders are not a serious public health concern because they do not impact personal function—or societal economics—in the same way as many other, more visible communication disorders such as traumatic brain injury, progressive neurologic disease, head and neck cancer, or cleft palate. Actually, it turns out that the impact of voice disorders may be significant, from both an individual and societal perspective. Clinical epidemiological studies indicate that about 50%–60% of persons who experience voice problems experience moderate or worse

The physician who specializes in disorders and diseases of the throat is an otolaryngologist.

personal distress and depression, social isolation (particularly the elderly), and professional impairment (Smith et al., 1996) including loss of work days or even loss of job because of the problems. The specific dollar cost to society has not been calculated; however, the numbers are decidedly nontrivial, especially because at least most adults with voice disorders are otherwise high-functioning and employable, if voice can be restored.

The foregoing findings indicate that voice disorders are indeed an appropriate target of clinical focus. Not only do persons with voice disorders deserve our clinical attention; voice problems constitute an area of legitimate concern within the evolving healthcare environment.

SECTION III: WHAT CAUSES VOICE DISORDERS?

Many factors can lead to a voice problem.

Voice disorders can be caused by a number of factors, some physical (organic), some not strictly physical (nonorganic). A complete review of the causes lies well beyond the scope of this chapter, and the reader is referred to primary sources and texts indicated at the end of the chapter. However, at this juncture a brief summary of causes of voice disorders is important because such understanding strongly influences evaluation procedures and certainly the interpretation of evaluation results. Voice disorder causes can be viewed according to many different schemes. Schemes that most directly map onto voice evaluation are, in my experience, those that directly relate to laryngeal structure (Figure 9–1) and function. According to one scheme, which I proposed in the first edition of this book, voice disorders can

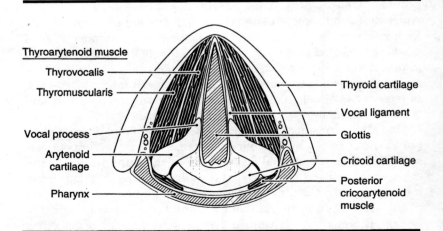

Figure 9–1. Schematic view of the larynx.

be subdivided into (1) those caused by discrete mass lesions of the membranous or cartilaginous vocal folds; (2) those caused by distributed tissue changes within the larynx; (3) those caused by organic movement abnormalities; and (4) those without known organic cause (Verdolini, 1994). Figure 9–2 displays a list of common examples of conditions within each category. For each example, cursory information is provided about the essential physical (or nonphysical) description of the condition, presumed intermediate causes, and typical "chief voice complaints" related by the patient.[1] If this material is unfamiliar to you, look at it carefully because I refer to it frequently in the discussion that follows. Additional sources are Colton and Casper, (1990); and Titze and Verdolini (in preparation).

A final comment before proceeding regards the relationship between laryngeal conditions and voice disorders. The relationship is not perfect (one-to-one). In particular, although various conditions may result in voice changes, the changes are different for different people, and are certainly perceived as different by different people. This is an important principle to remember in considering the complexity of the relationship between structure and function in voice disorders.

SECTION IV: GENERAL PRINCIPLES OF VOICE EVALUATION

Principle 1: The Selection of Clinical Measures Should be Dictated by the Clinical Questions Asked

A common question posed to voice disorder specialists is: How do I perform a voice evaluation? A corollary question is: What instruments should I purchase to set up a voice lab? The most reasonable response to both questions is the same: This depends on what questions you want to answer.

The response seems obvious. Yet, perhaps surprisingly, many of us have the sense that there is "a way" to perform voice evaluations. Not uncommonly, "the way" includes notions that objective measures requiring electronic equipment are somehow inherently superior to other approaches. This bias has in part arisen from the increased availability of sophisticated hard- and software over the past years. In sum, the first general principle of voice evaluation is that fundamentally, *the measures you use in the evaluation of voice disorders should be dictated by the clinical questions you want to answer, not by the technology that is available.*

---

[1]Most voice texts include "vocal abuse" and "misuse" as etiologic categories for a voice disorder. Vocal abuse refers to too much or too loud voice use. Vocal misuse refers to "poor technique." I prefer other terms as outlined here, because I feel that abuse and misuse are circular (lack independent definition), ambiguous, judgmental, and may undermine the clinical process.

Category	Description	Presumed Primary Cause and Possible Contributors	Primary Effect on Voice
Discrete Mass Lesions			
Membranous Folds			
Nodules	Protrusions at midpoint of membranous folds; edematous and/or collagenous	High vocal fold impact force High vocal fold tissue viscosity	Hoarseness
Polyps	Protrusions at midpoint of membranous folds; edematous, possibly vascularized	High vocal fold impact force High vocal fold tissue viscosity	Hoarseness
Cysts	Protrusions along membranous folds, often at midpoint; fluid-filled sacs of epithelium	Glandular blockage	Hoarseness
Papilloma	Laryngeal warts	Virus (presence of vaginal warts in mother, and vaginal delivery)	Hoarseness
Keratosis leukoplakia	White, plaque-like lesions	Irritants (smoke)	Hoarseness
Cancer	White, grainy lesions	Smoke and alcohol	Hoarseness
Posterior Glottis			
Contact ulcers	Protrusions on medial, surface of arytenoids, possibly with contralateral concavity	Gastric reflux "Pressed" phonation Low pitch	Phonatory effort
Distributed Tissue Changes			
Reinke's edema	Distributed edema along membranous folds	Irritants (smoke)	Low pitch in speech
Laryngitis	Distributed inflammation	Bacteria, virus	Hoarseness
Bowing	Persistent bowing of folds (muscular deformation?)	Chronic heavy voice use Elderly age	Weak voice
Sulcus vocalis	Groove parallel to vocal fold margin	Congenital, developmental Heavy voice use	Weak voice
Trauma	(Appearance depends on type of trauma)	Mechanical, thermal, or chemical trauma	Variable
Organic Movement Disorders			
Peripheral paralyses	Limited (medial) movement of affected fold	Local trauma (including surgery) Virus Heart disease	Weak voice
Central paralyses	Resistance to movement	Cerebral cortex lesions (stroke)	"Tight" voice

(continued)

Figure 9–2. Summary of voice disorder categories.

Category	Description	Presumed Primary Cause and Possible Contributors	Primary Effect on Voice
Organic Movement Disorders (continued)			
Extrapyramidal disease (e.g., Parkinson's disease)	Small range of motion	Dopamine deficiency	Monotone voice in speech Weak voice
Nerve–muscle junction dysfunctions (myasthenia gravis)	Rapid fatigue in function	Rapid depletion of chemicals sustaining vocal fold contraction	Rapid voice fatigue
Spasmodic dysphonia	Abrupt adductions during speech (adductory); Abrupt abductions during speech (abductory)	Undetermined	Spasmodic voice
Non-Organic Disorders			
Mutational falsetto	Persistent high pitch in postpubertal male, with normal-appearing larynx	Psychological conflict Learned behavior	High pitch (falsetto)
Ventricular phonation	False (ventricular) vocal folds vibrate and produce sound	Sometimes compensation for poorly functioning true vocal folds	Gravelly voice
Conversion aphonia/dysphonia	Lack of voice (aphonia) or hoarse voice (dysphonia), with normal-appearing larynx	Psychological	No voice or hoarse voice
Muscular tension dysphonia	Persistent posterior glottal gap during phonation, and complaints of voice problems	Simultaneous contraction of laryngeal adductors and abductors	Breathy voice Phonatory effort

Figure 9–2. (continued)

In this vein, what are the clinical questions that we usually want to answer in a voice evaluation? Many possibilities come to mind. One encompassing scheme is indicated in Figure 9–3, in which seven critical clinical questions are asked.

The answers to these clinical questions will come from a variety of sources. These sources include medical reports (primarily from an otolaryngologist, neurologist, internist, and/or primary care physician), your case history, and the specific voice measures that you make. I will describe a typical case history and voice measures in detail shortly. However, first I would like to discuss the clinical questions a bit further, both to provide rationales for the questions and to indicate which general parts of the assessment procedure address them.

Questions	Part of Assessment That Addresses Questions
1. Is there a voice disorder?	Case history
2. If so, how severe is it?	Case history Voice measures
3. What specific voice functions are impaired?	Otolaryngological report Voice measures
4. What factors likely contributed to the onset of the disorder and what are maintaining factors?	Case history Voice measures
5. What is the patient's motivational level to improve the disorder?	Case history
6. What are behavioral treatment recommendations?	Recommendations
7. What is the prognosis for improvement with the treatment plan recommended?	Prognosis

Figure 9–3. Critical clinical questions.

The Questions

Question #1: Is There a Voice Disorder?

Bottom lines: Is the voice satisfactory to the patient's needs? Does the patient regard her voice as normal or "a problem"? Are there any indications of disease?

Consistent with the definition of "voice disorder" in this chapter, the answer to this question ultimately depends on the patient's perspective. As such, the answer emerges from the patient's descriptions of his or her voice and voice complaints and functional impairments, obtained during the case history.

Most often, the patient's identification of a voice problem will coincide with yours. However, sometimes it will not. For example, the patient might be severely hoarse to your ears, and he or she may perform abnormally on a series of voice tests. Yet, the patient may note little or no negative impact on quality of life due to voice problems. In such cases it is questionable that there is a voice disorder, as we have defined it. Hoarseness may even be considered a desirable attribute in some cases, for example with performers whose hoarse or husky voice is a trademark. In the absence of health risks such as suspected cancer, treatment may be inappropriate in such cases. On the other hand, some patients may have a clear voice to your ears, and normal or even superior performance on formal voice tests, and yet describe phonatory discomfort or other voice dysfunctions that negatively impact on quality of life. An example is a patient who experiences throat fatigue after vocally taxing business or social activities. Another patient may be a trained singer who experiences a vague "glitch" between high G# and A. Such patients do have a voice disorder, by our definition, and warrant treatment. The point is that the patient's perspective is the key to determining whether there is a voice disorder.

Question 2: If There Is a Voice Disorder, How Severe Is It (Global Baseline Measure)?

The global severity rating is one of the most pertinent baseline measures in voice evaluation, against which treatment progress will be assessed. Information about global severity will arise from the combination of the patient's complaints (case history) and your direct observations of voice (voice measures).

Question 3: What Specific Voice Functions Are Impaired, and to What Degree Are They Impaired (Differential Baseline Measures)?

Differential baseline measures are those which reflect the functional, perceptual, acoustic, and physiological impairments arising from the specific diagnostic condition at hand. The rationale for such measures is twofold. First, the information is expected to be consistent with the medical diagnosis. In cases where there is a discrepancy, the information can be provided to the physician as a contribution to the ongoing diagnostic process. Second, evidence of improvement in diagnostically specific functions following therapy speaks to therapy specificity, as opposed to general maturational or motivational influences.

Question 4: What Factors Probably Contributed to the Onset of the Disorder, and What Are Maintaining Factors?

These questions are relevant for planning therapy; you will almost certainly want to target factors that contributed to onset and maintenance of the voice problem for the patient. For example, if you find that heavy voice use appeared to cause and maintain laryngeal lesions in a patient, therapy should target training in either voice conservation or voice production modes that can withstand heavy use without injury. Conversely, if history suggests that smoking, alcohol, and drying medications appeared to constitute a significant etiologic factor for lesions, therapy will almost certainly target voice hygiene and specifically hydration. Note that with voice disorders, you will not directly observe many etiologic factors in the clinic during the voice assessment. Rather, you will discern many of them from the case history and/or from the medical report.

Question 5: What Is the Patient's Motivational Level to Improve the Disorder?

Low motivation might suggest that intervention should be relatively brief and treatment goals modest. Strong motivation suggests the appropriateness of "pulling out the stops"; therapy may be longer and more complex, and treatment goals may be more ambitious.

Question 6: What Are Treatment Recommendations?

Information derived from a clinical voice evaluation is not just academic. Its ultimate utility is to formulate specific treatment plans, recommendations, and goals. The physician may make recommendations about pharmaceutical or surgical intervention. You will make recommendations about behavioral intervention (voice therapy). Ideally, a coordinated treatment package will be formulated by both of you together. Recommendations will be based on empirical studies, analytical thinking, and eventually, past clinical experience. Recommendations will also take into consideration the patient's motivational level.

Question 7: What Is the Prognosis for Improvement With the Treatment Plan Recommended?

Predictive statements about the likely outcome of treatment are important for the team working with the patient, and especially for the patient. Prognostic statements may also be required by third-party reimbursers (insurance companies). With some experience, you can usually make prognostic statements on the basis of the combined medical and speech-pathology assessment. Obviously, motivation to change is centrally important.

Principle 2: In Selecting the Specific Array of Measures to be Used in Voice Assessment, the Clinician Should Balance the Relative Importance of Parsimony Versus Exploration for His Clinical Setting

In an ideal world of perfect knowledge, the principle of parsimony should guide the selection of clinical measures. That is, a minimal number of measures should be used to answer the maximum number of clinical questions. The use of a shotgun approach, in which the complete range of possible measures is made, can be conceptually muddy and financially exorbitant for the patient and the clinical service. Consistent with this premise, in this chapter we focus on the targeted and principled evaluation of specific clinical questions. This approach will be most evident in exploring Clinical Question 3 (Figure 9–3): "What specific voice functions are impaired?" Relative to this question, in this chapter a specific assessment framework will be proposed based on the principle of conceptual parsimony and economy.

The examination described here has several components.

Having said as much, I frequently find myself using a different approach in clinical assessment, which might be described as "exploratory" or, in the extreme, "fishing." That is, I find myself using a

broad array of measures sampling not only functions that are expected to be disrupted by specific diagnostic conditions, but also sampling the primary ways that *any* voice *might theoretically* be disrupted, given available knowledge about voice physiology and disorders. The utility of this approach is twofold. First, if we measure only
functions that we know or believe to reflect common voice conditions, we will never break out of our existing framework to identify
new and potentially useful ways of considering voice. If we are set
up to maintain a database of our clinical measures, after a few years
of clinical data collection we can examine the database to confirm
what we know about the conditions, or to update our knowledge
based on findings that would not otherwise have been apparent.
Second, for a specific patient, by using a broad array of measures
that go beyond the obvious expectations for a particular condition,
we may discover some aspect of function for the patient that runs
counter to our expectations. Such findings may contribute to the
diagnostic procedure, treatment, and even treatment outcome.

Quite frankly, my use of targeted versus exploratory assessment
approaches depends on the clinical setting, the presence (or lack) of a
database, and the practical demands of the environment. Other factors
may influence your decision as well. The important point is that you
should make an a priori philosophical decision about the specificity
versus breadth of your voice assessment procedures.

Principle 3: Measures Selected for Voice Assessment Should Be Reliable and Valid

Assuming that you have identified clinical questions that you want
to answer and have made at least a working decision about a targeted versus exploratory approach to assessment, you are now
ready to consider specific measures that you may make in your clinical assessment of voice. The first and most important considerations at this point regard reliability and validity. As indicated in several other chapters, notably Chapter 1 (Tomblin), reliability refers to
the extent to which a measure gives you the same result on multiple trials. In essence, reliability reflects repeatability, or replicability.
Validity refers to the extent to which a measure accurately reflects
the phenomenon it is supposed to examine. Types of validity which
were discussed in Chapter 1, include concurrent, predictive, and
construct validity. In this chapter we are largely concerned with
construct validity. Additionally, we will talk about face validity in a
later section on the functional impact of voice disorders. Some information about various measures' reliability and validity is provided
in this chapter; other information is obtainable from the literature.
Bear in mind that a measure that is made with sophisticated equipment is not necessarily more reliable or valid than simpler measures. Wherever possible, reliability and validity must be demonstrated for any clinical measure that you make. If you do not have

information about a measures' reliability or validity but choose to use it anyway, you must keep this limitation in mind in the interpretation of your results.

Principle 4: Wherever Possible, Results Should be Compared to Formal Norms, and Data Collection Procedures Should Adhere to Procedures Used to Generate the Referent Norms

Clinical data of any sort are only as good as the procedures used to collect them and are only as useful as the norms used to interpret them. In this light, wherever possible, data collection should be limited to procedures that have generated normative data in the literature. A critical corollary is that the same procedures should be used in clinical practice as were used in the normative data collection, and results should be systematically compared to normative results. Several examples will be given in the section that follows on specific assessment procedures.

At this juncture, a further comment is in order about comparing our clinical measures to norms. Where interval or ratio data are involved (i.e., data for which every interval on the scale indicates the same magnitude change as every other interval of the same magnitude on the scale), to compare the patient's data to standardized norms, it is helpful to convert the patient's raw data to standardized z scores. As discussed in Chapter 1, z scores are measures of abnormality. They indicate how many "standard deviations" the patient's performance differs from the norm for healthy subjects. Z scores are computed using the following formula:

The objective is to estimate how the patient's performance compares with that of normal speakers.

$$z = \frac{\text{patient's performance} - \text{normative performance}}{\text{normative standard deviation}}$$

A large z score indicates a large abnormality. A small z score indicates a small abnormality or no abnormality at all. We decide based on our clinical experience and on the literature which z score boundaries we wish to use to delineate normal versus abnormal performance. A z score of "1" is conservative (i.e., it will identify as abnormal even slightly abnormal performance). A z score of "2" leaves more room for accepting a wider range of performances as normal. There are advantages and disadvantages of any z score criteria for normalcy. In brief, a conservative criterion maximizes the identification of any abnormality, but it does so at the risk of identifying some behaviors as abnormal that are, in fact, relatively normal. A demanding z score criterion requires more certain evidence of abnormality, but it does so at the risk of failing to detect some conditions which are, in fact, abnormal.

Principle 5: The Interpretation of Most Clinical Data Lies With a Combination of Measures, Rather Than Single Measures

Almost all the clinical questions we ask in voice disorders are answered not with a single measure but with a combination of measures. Indeed, there is no one-to-one correspondence between "clinical question" and "measurement." Instead, we look for "converging evidence" across measures.

Take, for example, the question: Is there a voice disorder? As illustrated in following sections, the response to this question will arise from the patient's informal reports about his or her condition, from formal questionnaire responses, and from the clinician's impression about functional disruptions due to voice. A further example relates to the question: What specific voice functions are impaired (and to what degree), reflecting the diagnostic condition? In particular this question can be addressed by a profiles approach, in which typical combinations of results or profiles are identified consistent with expectations for different diagnostic conditions. Cases revealing profiles strongly inconsistent with the medical diagnosis may allow the SLP to contribute to the diagnostic process by providing such information to the physician, who then reconsiders the patient in light of the new information. Examples of characteristic profiles for common diagnostic conditions are provided later in the section on case studies.

Principle 6: The Most Important Tool in Voice Evaluation Is Your Brain

With this principle, we come full circle to the first ones that touch on the utility of instrumented versus noninstrumented measures in voice assessment. Just as we select measures in voice assessment based on their ability to answer our clinical questions rather than on their technological sophistication or availability, the most important "instrument" you have for voice assessment is your brain. More specifically, the most important instrument you have is your knowledge of basic voice science, the science of voice injury and repair, and voice measurement science. Your ability, then, to thoughtfully interpret results will complete your capabilities in clinical voice assessment. Although sophisticated instrumentation can enhance your ability to address clinical questions in some or even many cases, any equipment cannot substitute a solid understanding of voice and voice disorders.

Section Summary

In this section, we emphasized important principles of voice assessment, regardless of the specific measures used. These principles are:

(1) select measures that can address your clinical questions; (2) make at least a working decision about whether you will orient towards a parsimonious or exploratory approach in voice assessment; (3) utilize reliable and valid measures; (4) use normative data collection procedures that compare all results to standardized norms, wherever possible; (5) base your interpretation of the results on the combination of measures rather than on any single measure, and (6) use your knowledge about the science of voice and its disorders, your knowledge about the roles and limitations of each measure you use, and your ability to thoughtfully interpret your findings, because these are the most important tools you have in voice assessment. Possession of equipment and sophisticated measurement outcomes without such knowledge produces frail clinical findings, at best.

With the above principles in mind, we proceed to a discussion of measures that can be used to address the clinical questions identified in Figure 9–3. As noted earlier, consistent with this chapter's primary goal of introducing voice assessment procedures to clinicians who are not specialized in voice and who may not have extensive equipment resources, the emphasis will be on principled measures that can be made relatively quickly and inexpensively. More sophisticated measures also will be mentioned to ensure that the clinician is aware of them, can consider using them in her environment, and can make appropriate referrals to other centers as needed.

For the primary, simple measures presented here the required equipment can be purchased for about $50–$200, and includes: (a) a stopwatch, for timed trials (approximately $10); (b) a dB meter for voice intensity measurements (approximately $30 for a simple dB meter that can be purchased at an electronics store); and (c) a pitch pipe (about $15) or a portable electronic keyboard (about $150) for pitch extractions. An audiotape recorder (preferably with a VU meter and counter) and audiotapes are also preferred (starting at about $50). The only "software" that is required is a list of normative procedures and data which are provided in appendices to this chapter (Appendixes 9A–9F).

THE ASSESSMENT

Standard parts of the voice assessment are indicated in Figures 9–4 (Case History) and 9–5 (Data Collection).

Case History

The patient will provide valuable information about the nature and extent of the problem. Listen carefully.

Typical parts of the case history are shown in Figure 9–4. As we have already noted, the case history generally provides information about what may have caused the voice disorder originally and what are the maintaining factors. The case history also provides information about the patient's perceptions of his voice (presence/absence of a voice

CASE HISTORY

Identifying information (age, sex, occupation, or usual activities)

Referral information and diagnosis (e.g., referring physician or other referral; diagnosis)

Patient's complaints
   Open-ended questions
   Ratings of functional impact of voice disorder (Use formal scale)
   Phonatory effort scaling (speech, singing)

Onset and course
   Onset: When?
   Circumstances surrounding onset
   Course since onset

Previous voice and speech history
   Previous voice/speech problems
   Previous treatment
   Previous voice/speech training

Medical information
   Otolaryngological
      Current (conditions, treatment)
      Past (conditions, treatment)
   General medical
      Current (conditions, treatment)
      Past (conditions, treatment, including surgery)

Behavioral and environmental factors that may affect vocal fold tissue
   Smoke (number of cigarettes per day; number of years smoked)
   Alcohol (number and type of drinks per week; number of years)
   Caffeine (number and type of beverages daily)
   Exposure to dry air
   Exposure to chemical irritants

Typical voice use patterns
   Social (past, present, future)
   Family (past, present, future)
   Professional (past, present, future)

Importance of resolving voice problem
(1 = not important; 10 = extremely important)

Figure 9–4. Parts of the voice assessment.

disorder, specific functional impact, and severity). Finally, the case history provides information about how the patient needs to use his voice currently and in the future, and about his motivational level to improve a voice disorder. Critical aspects of the case history are discussed next.

Patient's Complaints (Symptoms)

The patient's complaints are considered "symptoms" (as distinguished from "signs," which are the clinician's observations). Ask the patient to describe her complaints. There are various ways to do this. We can use open-ended questions, such as: "What is bothering you about your voice?" Another, complementary approach is to ask questions about the functional impact of voice. The issue of functional impact has assumed increasing importance within healthcare practice in general. Hospital administrations and healthcare insurers have relatively little interest in "poor membranous vocal fold closure" per se (for example). They are much more interested in functional disruptions due to physical disease or abnormality. The reality may seem harsh. But probably most of us would agree that precious healthcare resources should first be oriented toward conditions that threaten health and survival and that reduce function. In this light, we must see ourselves as advocates for our patients and document functional disruptions caused by voice problems, where such disruption exists. I cannot emphasize enough the importance of this point in voice assessment, and I believe that it will assume even further importance in the coming years.

The easiest way to inquire about functional disruptions due to voice is to simply ask the patient: "To what extent does your voice disrupt professional, social, communicative, physical, or psychological functioning?" Answers may be categorized on a simple ordinal scale ranging from no problem, to mild, moderate, or severe problem. This approach is certainly straightforward. However, the reliability and validity of responses are uncertain. A preferable approach is to utilize a standardized questionnaire format. Examples include the *Voice Handicap Index* (Jacobson et al., 1997) and the *Iowa Quality of Life Questionnaire* (Smith et al., 1996). The first questionnaire is brief and is included in Appendix 9A. The second, which is longer, can be found in its published format (Smith et al., 1996). Studies for both questionnaires have addressed reliability and validity.

A third way to obtain information about symptoms is to ask the patient to indicate how effortful it is to talk and/or sing. The results may provide an important measure of global severity of a voice disorder because phonatory effort is a salient complaint for many or most patients with voice problems. In fact, phonatory effort is one of the few symptoms that are common to almost all patients with a voice problem of any etiology.

In the measurement of phonatory effort, we prefer a direct magnitude estimation method, which is based on published studies assessing its reliability and validity, conducted by Colton and colleagues. To use this method, ask the patient to produce his or her most comfortable voice, even if it does not sound good. (If he is not able to produce comfortable voice at all, you can ask him to imagine it.) Then ask the patient to indicate how much effort he normally uses to produce voice, compared to comfortable effort. The amount of effort in usual speech might be twice as much as comfortable, or three times, or four times. The patient may indicate any multiple; there is no upper (or lower) cap on the scale. Previous research by Colton and colleagues indicated good reliability of the results. The same studies demonstrated a relation of the results to subglottic pressure, which implies physiological effort, as well as to fundamental frequency and intensity, also related to physiological effort. Thus, validity is demonstrated relative to independent measures of physiological effort.

Onset and Course of the Problem

You need as much information as possible about the onset and course of the voice problem. This information generally provides insights about the factors that caused the condition and about factors that maintain it.

Regarding onset, you should ask the patient when he first noted symptoms, and what the surrounding circumstances were. ("When did you first notice problems? Were there unusual circumstances? For example, were you using your voice more than usual, or in a different way? Was there a co-occurring illness?") Long-standing symptoms signal a *chronic* disorder. Recently emerged symptoms may imply an *acute* disorder, assuming the patient is an accurate historian. If onset corresponded to an increase in the amount of voice use, or to a change in voice use patterns, then voice use patterns would seem to have played a role in the development of the disorder. If onset corresponded to a specific illness, then the illness might be relevant. In the absence of remarkable voice use patterns or an identifiable illness, a sudden onset may signal a nonphysical disorder, particularly if the disorder is aphonia.

Regarding the course of the symptoms, we ask about fluctuations in the symptoms and what seems to cause the fluctuations. Again, variations in voice related to voice use patterns imply that these patterns play a role in the maintenance of the disorder. Variations in voice related to illnesses imply the involvement of medical factors.

Previous Voice and Speech History

We need any available information about previous voice problems and about previous voice therapy or training. If the patient had previous voice problems, perhaps the previous problems were never entirely resolved, and the current ones represent a re-exacerbation. An example would be a patient who was hoarse in elementary school, and who received voice therapy for treatment of vocal nodules at that time. The recurrence of hoarseness and nodules as an adult might signal an unresolved susceptibility. If the patient had prior voice training (for the singing or speaking voice), the training might be a building block in the current treatment program. In other cases previous training might be a problem to consider in planning therapy, if the training appears to have contributed to voice problems.

Medical Information

Certainly, we need information about medical status for all patients. This information is especially important for hoarse patients who are in the age range for throat cancer or other significant laryngeal conditions and diseases. This information is also important in understanding the basis for a voice disorder, and possible contributory causes. We obtain medical information from reports made by the otolaryngologist; except in rare cases, word of mouth from the patient or family is not satisfactory. Nor are laryngeal examination findings from another medical specialist (not an otolaryngologist) satisfactory, because for this purpose special training and expertise are required.

Obviously, the speech pathologist depends on important assistance from the otolaryngologist.

As shown in Figure 9–4, we need information about past and present otolaryngological status, other past and present medical or surgical conditions, medication history, and, in the case of suspected or known contact ulcers, gastric reflux symptoms (burning and choking sensations, especially during sleep; acid taste in mouth upon arising).

Behavioral and Environmental Factors That May Affect Vocal Fold Tissue Viscosity or Otherwise Affect Vocal Fold Status

Certain nonphonatory behavioral and environmental factors may produce dry or sticky vocal fold tissue and, as such, may predispose vocal fold tissue to edema-based injuries possibly associated with nodules, polyps, and other conditions. These factors include alcohol and caffeine consumption, smoking, exposure to dry environments, and the use of drying nasal sprays and drying psychotropic medications. We want information about all these factors, and we need as precise answers as possible. For example, you should ask what is the number of cigarettes smoked per day, for how many years?

In addition to these factors, it may be useful to obtain information about exposure to chemical agents, such as ammonia-based cleaning fluids, paint solvents, and so on. Although these are not commonly relevant in causing a voice disorder, occasionally a voice disorder can be directly traced to chemical exposures.

Patient's Typical Voice Use Patterns

We need information about the patient's typical voice use patterns and predicted future voice needs for two reasons. First, information about past and present voice use patterns might point to causative factors for the voice disorder that we want to address in therapy. For example, a physical education teacher who complains of hoarseness may use her voice loudly for several hours a day in a gymnasium or even outdoors. It is easy to think that such voice use patterns may have contributed to the development and maintenance of nodules (for example), and you will want to address these voice patterns in therapy. A second reason to obtain this information is that we need to keep the patient's present and future needs for voice use in mind in planning ecologically valid therapy.[2] For example, a patient with spasmodic dysphonia may need to use her voice daily as a telephone operator. Particularly if she depends on this work activity for income, you may want to plan as quick an intervention program as possible. Another example is a patient with a laryngeal paralysis who is the primary caretaker for an elderly, hearing-impaired person. The level of improvement in loudness required for this patient may be greater than for some other patients.

Importance of Resolving the Voice Problem

The importance that the patient assigns to improving the voice disorder signals the probable motivational level for therapy, which will likely affect the prognosis for improvement. You might ask the patient to rate on a 10-point scale "How important is it to you to resolve your voice problems? 1 = not important at all, 10 = the most important thing in the world."

Data Collection for Direct Voice Measures

The primary reason for making direct observations of voice (voice measures) is to establish global and differential baseline measures of severity. Such measures serve to confirm the presence of a voice disorder and to quantify both overall severity of the problem as a whole and the severity of special functions that are specifically disrupted. Occasionally, the overall picture that emerges of the condition will provide information with possible diagnostic value, which you can relay to the physician. Whether you use these specific measures or others, bear in mind the important principles about measurement selection and interpretation discussed earlier in this chapter.

The data collection sheet shown in Figure 9–5 indicates the types of measures that we will discuss. If you wish, you can use this sheet to collect your measures and to indicate the patient's raw scores. To summarize the data, and to indicate z scores or other summary statements, you might find the form in Figure 9–6 useful.

The Profiles sheet shown in Figure 9–6 displays the organizational framework for direct observations of voice discussed in this chapter. According to this framework, observations about voice can be subdivided into three broad categories: general, acoustic, and physiological.

A method for graphic display of diagnostic findings is useful.

---

[2]Ecologically valid therapy refers to therapy that takes into consideration the demands on voice in the patient's particular work or social environment.

DATA COLLECTION SHEET FOR DIRECT VOICE MEASURES

Patient's Name:_____ Date:_____

Diagnosis:_____ Clinician:_____

General Voice Index
    Functional disruption due to voice (Voice Handicap Index)
        Emotional subscale score   _____
        Functional subscale score   _____
        Physical subscale score   _____
    Phonatory effort (x comfortable)
        Speech   _____
        Singing or other   _____
    Auditory-perceptual ratings
        Voice quality

Grade	_____	(consistent/inconsistent)
Roughness	_____	(consistent/inconsistent)
Breathiness	_____	(consistent/inconsistent)
Asthenia	_____	(consistent/inconsistent)
Strain	_____	(consistent/inconsistent)
Tremor	_____	(consistent/inconsistent)
Nasality (hyper/hypo)	_____	(consistent/inconsistent)

        Speech   _____
        Language   _____

Acoustic Index
    Average F_0 in speech   _____   Pitch   _____
    Semitone pitch range   _____
    Average dB in speech   _____
    Intensity range   _____

Physiological Index
    VF postural closure (arytenoid control)
        L–DDK rate/s   _____
        L–DDK strength   _____
        L–DDK consistency   _____
    VF membranous closure
        S:Z ratio   _____
    Respiratory
        S prolongation   _____

Impressions
    Description of voice; severity
    Diagnosis
    Factors that may have contributed to onset and maintenance

(continued)

Figure 9–5. Data collection sheet for direct voice measures.

Recommendations
    Is voice therapy recommended?
    If so, how often, for what duration each session, for how long?
    What will the focus of therapy be?

Prognosis

Figure 9–5. *(continued)*

General Voice Index

Consistent with our definition of a voice disorder as a condition in which voice causes functional disruption to the patient, usually with some corroboration by the clinician, the General Voice Index includes observations about functional disruptions and the sound of the voice (auditory-perceptual measures). Because phonatory effort is perhaps *the* symptom that is common across most voice patients, a measure of phonatory effort is also included. Functional disruption and phonatory effort measures will actually be derived from the patient's responses, as previously described under Case History. Auditory-perceptual measures will be discussed more fully.

Auditory-Perceptual Measures of Voice. Auditory-perceptual evaluations of voice involve listening to the voice, and describing and/or rating its sound. An important corollary is that sometimes, voice problems interface tightly with motor speech problems and/or nasality problems. Thus, in our auditory-perceptual ratings we must view voice broadly to include not only laryngeal voice quality but also final voice output including resonance and prosody. If frank nasality, prosody, or even speech disorders coexist with a voice problem, this should be noted. Separate data collection procedures discussed elsewhere in this text should then be instituted. If you do not feel competent to pursue these issues, you should refer the patient to another clinician who can address them in tandem with your work on voice.

Sharpen your judgment skills by listening to the voices of people around you and in the public arena.

As a whole, auditory-perceptual evaluations represent a critical aspect of any voice assessment procedure. It would be virtually unthinkable to conduct a voice assessment without them. In fact, in a large study on the use of different measures in voice evaluation, clinicians from various parts of the world indicated that auditory-perceptual measures are among the most clinically useful of all voice measures (Hirano, 1989). It is paradoxical that there is hardly a measure of voice that is surrounded by greater controversy than this family of measures. The primary issues relate to reliability. According to some authors, agreement within and across judges can be quite good even for complex rating systems, if judges have been systematically trained (Sederholm et al., 1993). However, other

VOICE/SPEECH PROFILE SHEET

Patient: Date(s):

Referring diagnosis: Clinician:

		POOR			NORMAL			SUPERIOR	
GENERAL									
VHI									
Functional	40	30	20	10	0				
Physical	40	30	20	10	0				
Emotional	40	30	20	10	0				
Effort	x 4	x 3	x 2		x 1				
Voice									
Grade	SEV (C/I)	MOD (C/I)	MIL (C/I)		NORMAL				
Roughness	SEV (C/I)	MOD (C/I)	MIL (C/I)		NORMAL				
Asthenia	SEV (C/I)	MOD (C/I)	MIL (C/I)		NORMAL				
Breathiness	SEV (C/I)	MOD (C/I)	MIL (C/I)		NORMAL				
Strain	SEV (C/I)	MOD (C/I)	MIL (C/I)		NORMAL				
Tremor	SEV (C/I)	MOD (C/I)	MIL (C/I)		NORMAL				
Nasality (+/-)	SEV (C/I)	MOD (C/I)	MIL (C/I)		NORMAL				
Prosody	S (C/I)	MOD (C/I)	MIL (C/I)		NORMAL				
Speech	SEV (C/I)	MOD (C/I)	MIL (C/I)		NORMAL				
Language	SEV (C/I)	MOD (C/I)	MIL (C/I)		NORMAL				
ACOUSTIC									
Fo ave (Hz)					185				
ST range (z)	-3.0	-2.0	-1.0		0		+1.0	+2.0	+3.0
I ave (dB 3')	50	55	60		65				
	80	75	70						
I range (dB)	10	20	30		40		50	60	70
PHYSIOL									
L-D rate (z)	-3.0	-2.0	-1.0		0		+1.0	+2.0	+3.0
L-D str	SEV weak	MOD weak	MIL weak		NORMAL				
	SEV tight	MOD tight	MIL tight						
L-D con	SEV	MOD	MIL		NORMAL				
S:Z (z)	+3.0	+2.0	+1.0		0				
	-3.0	-2.0	-1.0						
s-prolong (z)			+1.0		0				

Figure 9–6. Data summary (profile) sheet.

authors have expressed serious concerns about the consistency of auditory-perceptual measures in general (see, for example, Bassich & Ludlow, 1986), and, in the extreme, pessimism that a stable, common auditory-perceptual space *can* even exist across listeners

(Kreiman & Gerratt, 1996). One of the problems is that human listeners appear to shift internal criteria for ratings depending on a series of factors, including which voices they have just heard. Although most if not all of the work to this point has been conducted relative to voice quality as opposed to suprasegmentals, there is no reason to think that any auditory-perceptual judgments of voice are exempt from similar controversy. All told, there seems to be an unfortunate impasse. Virtually no clinician would conduct a voice assessment without listening to the voice and attempting to obtain information from it. Yet the outlook for obtaining reliable auditory-perceptual judgments appears controversial at best, and bleak at worst. Efforts are ongoing to solve the dilemma, but definitive solutions have not yet been forthcoming.

As clinicians, what shall we do in the face of such an impasse? I will propose a tentative tack in a few paragraphs. However, first a brief discussion is in order about what auditory-perceptual measures actually *are*. Virtually all auditory-perceptual measures involve a combination of *qualitative* and *quantitative* judgments. Relative to voice, the qualitative judgments involve the categorical description of voice, or labeling. Common terms partly familiar to the layperson include "hoarse," "breathy," "pressed," "harsh," "rough," "diplophonic" or two-toned voice, etc.[3] Relative to resonance, common terms are "hypernasal" ("talking through the nose") and "hyponasal" ("talking as if you have a cold"). Relative to prosody, common terms are "monotone" or "increased prosody" (increased pitch, loudness, and duration changes). For all types of auditory-perceptual judgments, quantitative judgments then involve severity ratings. Traditionally, ordinal scales are used (e.g., mild, moderate, and severe), although other scales are also possible that are beyond the scope of this discussion. For all auditory-perceptual judgments, the typical clinical procedure is simply to listen to the patient's voice, usually in conversational speech or reading, and to indicate qualitative and quantitative ratings of phonation, resonance, and prosody. If the patient is a singer or actor, or otherwise uses the voice in unusual ways, you should listen to the voice during other relevant activities as well.

In fact, given the concerns about the reliability of auditory-perceptual measures, there is every reason to suspect that the results of typical clinical practice are subject to instability (unreliability). Fortunately, there are some procedures that you can implement to enhance reliability in the clinical setting. The procedures are somewhat cumbersome, and, in some instances, not possible, but may be well worth the effort, particularly given the importance that most clinicians assign to auditory-perceptual measures. First, you should tape record your patient's voice during conversational speech or

---

[3]A written, verbal description of these terms is somewhat challenging because they refer to auditory concepts that are most easily demonstrated, not explained. For clarification, you can consult with an experienced clinician.

better, a standard reading passage. You should rate her voice on whichever parameters you consider important. For voice quality, you might consider the GRBAS scale, which stands for the parameters (overall) Grade, Roughness, Breathiness, Asthenia (weakness), and Strain (Hirano, 1981). I add Tremor and Nasality (distinguishing between hyper- or hyponasality) since these are relevant for some subsets of patients. Finally, depending on your practice, a gross indication of prosody and speech articulation is also warranted. For each parameter, you should indicate severity. A limited number of scalar judgments (normal, mild, moderate, severe) will yield more reliable measures than a large number (1–100). An example of a profile sheet to indicate the data is shown in Figure 9–6. For each abnormality noted, you should indicate if the abnormality is consistent or inconsistent. This parameter is important because some diagnoses are based on symptom consistency, for example, spasmodic dysphonia versus hyperfunction.

When you have completed your judgments, you should ask colleagues unfamiliar with the patient or her status in treatment (pre- or post) to independently rate the audiotaped sample, using the same scales. You should use as many independent judges as possible, so that the influence of any atypical judge is minimized. It is helpful to use judges who have been trained in your rating techniques, which are standardized across all clinicians for your clinic. For each parameter rated, the *median* response across all judges is probably the best estimate of the patient's true score (for description and calculation of median, see Chapter 1). Ideally, you should provide judges with audiotaped examples of similar age and gender patients, which serve as "anchors" for what you consider "normal" and "severely abnormal" (endpoint anchors) or "moderately abnormal" (midpoint anchor). Overall, whichever specific method you select to obtain auditory-perceptual judgments, you should use it consistently. Finally, you should be mindful of the potential limitations of auditory-perceptual measures when you interpret the data. Neither these nor any measures should be used as a sole basis for clinical conclusions, with rare exceptions.

Acoustic Index

Acoustic measures reflect the physical properties of sound. The most basic properties are fundamental frequency, intensity, spectral distribution, and duration. In the best cases, acoustic measures provide a physical window on what we hear, sometimes converging with what our ears tell us. As do many or most of the measures that we make in voice assessment, acoustic measures contribute to the establishment of baseline severity, and they may also provide information about possible etiologic and maintaining factors for a voice disorder.

A framework for acoustic observations can be erected around the four basic properties of sound: fundamental frequency, intensity, voice quality (timbre), and duration. We discuss each of these parameters and their relation to the voice assessment.

Fundamental Frequency Measures. Fundamental frequency (F_0) in speech directly reflects the number of vocal fold vibrations per second, in Hertz (Hz). F_0 and pitch are closely related, with the caveat that sometimes voice quality influences the perception of pitch. Although several F_0 measures are worth noting in a voice evaluation, only two are emphasized here. The most straightforward to obtain with limited instrumentation is average F_0 in speech. This variable sometimes reflects the *effect* of a laryngeal pathology; for example, accumulated fluid mass in Reinke's edema often causes a decrease in F_0, whereas stiffness from scarring may cause an increase in F_0 relative to norms. In other cases, F_0 abnormalities may indicate a *causal* factor for laryngeal pathology. The clearest case is for contact granuloma, in which low–F_0 vocal fold vibrations may result in arytenoid rocking and abrasion, ultimately generating ulceration and granulation. It is interesting that despite much speculation in the past about *pitch* abnormalities as a cause of laryngeal pathology, in fact the data do not support a role in most cases; most patients with laryngeal pathology demonstrate normal F_0 in speech.

A procedure for obtaining approximate average F_0 in speech, and for comparing the results to selected norms, is indicated in Appendix 9B. The reliability of F_0–extraction depends on the method and the clinician. If you use a pitch-matching method dependent on your own matching of the patient's pitch with your voice, your results will be reliable if you are good at pitch-matching. Otherwise, electronic equipment will be needed.

Other F_0 measures can be extremely valuable in some cases, as well. In particular, measures of F_0 variability may have value, including long-term F_0 changes in speech as an indication of prosody; F_0 variability during sustained vowel as an indicator of vocal tremor; cycle-to-cycle period stability, or "jitter," mentioned together with voice quality measures below; and F_0 breaks or shifts which may assist in the diagnosis of spasmodic dysphonia (Sapienza et al., 1998). If relevant, you should refer to other sources for more information (e.g., Colton & Casper, 1996; Titze & Verdolini, in preparation).

Finally, an F_0 variability measure that you can make with limited instrumentation is the total physiological F_0 range, often expressed as semitone pitch range. Many conditions including mass lesions and dysmotility disorders (paralysis) tend to yield restricted F_0 range. Procedures and norms are indicated in Appendix 9C.

Intensity Measures. As for F_0, there are several intensity measures that are clinically valuable; only two are described here. Intensity is roughly the acoustic correlate of loudness, at least for the midrange of intensities. At the least, you should obtain information about the patient's approximate average intensity during speech. As for the F_0, this measure may reflect causes or effects of a voice disorder. For example, a high intensity during speech probably implies large vocal fold oscillations which, if coupled with tight adduction, may produce large intercordal impact stresses, contributing to phonotrauma (nod-

Information from the history about vocal use in the workplace will be useful in making these estimates.

ules or polyps). In fact, high intensities are rarely observed in the clinical situation. This is probably because people tend to talk quietly in such settings. Low intensities might reflect poor laryngeal valving due to space-occupying lesions of the membranous folds, vocal fold bowing, or paralysis.

A procedure for establishing the average intensity during conversational speech, and approximate normative information, are indicated in Appendix 9D. Since the extraction of intensity depends on the use of a sound pressure level meter, the measure will be reliable and valid to the extent that the measurement device is properly functioning (with fully charged batteries), that you maintain a constant microphone-to-mouth distance (3 feet for the norms listed in Appendix 9D), and that your instructions are consistent across measurement times. A high-quality sound pressure level meter is preferable, such as the Bruel & Kjäer Sound Level Meter (approximately $5000); however, a less expensive model purchased at Radio Shack for about $35 can also yield clinically pertinent information, with some limitations.

As for F_0, measures of intensity variability may also be of value in clinical assessment. The measures include intensity variability during speech as a prosodic variable; intensity variability during sustained vowel production as an indicator of tremor; outright phonation breaks which may be useful in the differential diagnosis of spasmodic dysphonia (Sapienza et al., 1998); and cycle-to-cycle amplitude stability, or "shimmer," discussed under measures of voice quality. Other texts provide further information (Colton & Casper, 1996; Titze & Verdolini, in preparation).

Finally, it is helpful—and not expensive—to measure intensity range (in dB). Some conditions, such as mass lesions, tend to reduce the dynamic range on the quiet end (i.e., patients have difficulty producing sounds quietly). The same conditions and other ones may reduce dynamic range on the loud end (e.g., paralysis, in which patients have difficulty producing sounds loudly).

Spectral Measures and Other Possible Measures of Voice Quality. The sound spectrum is a plot of intensity over frequency for a given sound, at a given moment in time. A useful measure may be the ratio of intensity of the first harmonic (H1) relative to the intensity of the third formant (F3). This measure of "spectral tilt" is larger with poorly closing vocal folds than with well-closing folds (Hanson, 1997). A second spectral measure of potentially great clinical value is the signal-to-noise ratio (SNR), also called the harmonic-to-noise ratio. This measure indicates the amount of periodic sound in the voice in comparison to aperiodic sound or noise. As such, it should be an acoustic reflection of voice quality.

Although not spectral measures per se, other measures have also been proposed as possible indicators of the perceptual parameter that spectral measures are supposed to reflect: "voice quality." These are "perturbation measures," specifically jitter, which indicates the average cycle-to-cycle deviation in the acoustic period, and shimmer, which is the average cycle-to-cycle deviation in the acoustic amplitude.

Duration Measures. In the clinical voice assessment, duration is probably most relevant in relation to word duration, more simply expressed in words per minute. This measure can be obtained by simply audiotaping your patient's spontaneous speech or reading and counting the words produced in a minute or some fraction thereof.

Physiological Index

In this type of measure, we directly assess important aspects of laryngeal dynamics. Many aspects of laryngeal dynamics could be considered. If we want to restrict our observations to the most encompassing ones that are clinically relevant, we can ask: What types of abnormalities can affect the larynx, and what should be the physiological impact? The responses are relatively straightforward. Two basic types of abnormalities can affect laryngeal physiology: (1) structural abnormalities and (2) motility abnormalities. What should be the physiological impact of such deviations? Structurally, the most common laryngeal deviations are mass lesions of the vocal folds. This includes mass lesions of the membranous vocal folds, in predominance, such as edema, nodules, polyps, polypoid degeneration (Reinke's edema), cysts, papillomas, precancerous lesions, and cancer. Most of these lesions protrude from the free margins of the membranous vocal folds and, as such, preclude membranous vocal fold closure during vocal fold oscillation. Dynamically, the most common abnormalities involve paralyses and pareses of the recurrent laryngeal nerve or, more generally, arytenoid dysmotility. The fundamental physiological result is failure to achieve arytenoid approximation (closure) at phonation onset.

> In these measures, we attempt to describe physical aspects of the patient's voicing patterns.

From the foregoing observations, we can make predictions about the most common physiological abnormalities encountered clinically and the measures most likely to reflect them. Common structural abnormalities, likely to impede membranous vocal fold closure, are indicated by two primary measures: the S:Z ratio and minimum glottal flow. Dynamic or motility abnormalities, most likely to affect the recurrent laryngeal nerve (if not other laryngeal nerves as well) and thus arytenoid closure, are similarly reflected by the S:Z ratio and minimum glottal flow, but also by laryngeal diadochokinetic (L–DDK) performance and electromyography. Let us turn to a discussion of these measures next.

> For both of these measures, two or three trials may not be enough to yield a stable measure.

S:Z Ratio. The S:Z ratio is a dimensionless value that indirectly reflects membranous fold closure during phonation, described in Appendix 9E. It is computed by dividing maximum sustaining time for /s/ by maximum sustaining time on /z/. In the normative data that most clinicians use, the ratio is calculated from the best of two trials of both /s/ and /z/ (Appendix 9E). The rationale is that the primary difference between /s/ and /z/ is that voicing occurs during /z/, but not /s/. If the vocal folds are closing normally, airflow should be inhibited during the closed phase of each cycle during production of /z/, and /z/ should be longer than /s/, yielding a ratio less than 1.00. Conversely, if the vocal folds are closing poorly, airflow is not normally inhibited during voicing. In fact, for reasons that are not entirely clear, airflow through the glottis is actually *speeded up* in such cases during the voiced as compared with unvoiced sound, and the S:Z ratio becomes larger than 1. The S:Z ratio should indicate poor membranous vocal fold closure not only due to abnormalities of the membranous vocal folds themselves, but also due to incompletely adducting arytenoids. The S:Z ratio has been reported to be relatively reliable by Verdolini and Palmer (1997). One validity of the S:Z ratio in the detection of membranous vocal fold closure further appears much greater than for another measure often used to detect closure, maximum phonation time (MPT) on /a/ (92% vs. 65% "hit rates," respectively; Verdolini & Palmer, 1997).

Note that any measures requiring maximum sustaining should be interspersed with other measures, or recovery time should be provided between successive trials.

Minimum Glottal Airflow. Whereas the S:Z appears to be a grossly valid *indirect* indicator of membranous vocal fold closure during phonation, minimum glottal airflow more *directly* indicates closure. In short, minimum flow is the amount of air that passes through the larynx (in ml/s or cc/s) when the vocal folds are at maximum closure. Poor closure of the membranous folds and/or arytenoids should result in relatively large minimum flows. Good closure or tight closure should result in relatively small minimum flows. (Minimum flow is rarely zero, because some air does make it through the posterior commissure, behind the true vocal folds, in almost all cases.) You are referred to other texts for further information about this important measure (Baken, 1987; Colton & Casper, 1990; Titze & Verdolini, in preparation).

Laryngeal Diadochokinesis. Laryngeal diadochokinesis (L–DDK) refers to the rapid, repeated production of glottal plosives over a period of several seconds. For our purposes, there are three important parameters of L–DDK performance: (a) the rate of the productions (the number of glottal plosives per second), (b) the strength of the plosives, and (c) their consistency or steadiness across time. The procedure for L–DDK, and available normative data, are reported in Appendix 9F. L–DDK is presumed to indicate arytenoid closure capabilities. The reason is straightforward: glottal plosives are produced by tight approximation of the arytenoids, and sudden release. It stands to reason that, if the arytenoids cannot be tightly closed, and thus pressure cannot be built up below them to then release abruptly, L–DDK performance should be weak and/or slow. If the problem is caused by a peripheral disorder such as paralysis, or even ankylosis or arytenoid dislocation for that matter, performance should, however, be relatively consistent in time. On the other hand, if there is a problem in the central nervous system that affects arytenoid control, a primary problem might relate to the temporal aspect of the production, which is dysrhythmic. Available data indicate high reliability and validity, at least within a given clinic (Verdolini & Palmer, 1997).

The methodology for eliciting L–DDK measures, and the norms, are indicated in Appendix 9F.

Electromyography. As for minimum airflow, a thorough discussion of electromyography (EMG) is beyond the scope of this chapter. However, you should be aware of this measure because if the procedure is not available in your clinic, in some cases you may wish to request it at another clinic for special patients.

Briefly, EMG records electrical activity in muscle. There are two basic types of EMG. Surface EMG involves the placement of electrodes on the skin surface. Recordings then reflect muscle activity in the group of muscles below the electrodes. Deep EMG, on the other hand, involves the insertion of a needle electrode into the muscle of interest. In particular, deep EMG can confirm the presence of a paralysis or paresis of laryngeal, pharyngeal, or oral muscles and distinguish it from other conditions that may look like it, clinically. Deep EMG can also give information about how old a paralysis is and whether it is in a state of regeneration (improvement), degeneration, or stability.

Other Measures

In this chapter, we have focused on the simplest and most commonly used measures that you can make without expensive equipment. Of course, there are many other measures that you should be familiar with through your coursework in speech sciences and voice disorders and through your clinical practica. These include acoustic measures such as phonetograms (plots of a patient's intensity range across all frequencies); aerodynamic measures including AC flow, maximum flow, and subglottal pressure; respiratory measures such as vital capacity and other functional measures; electroglottographic and photoglottographic measures indicating closed and open quotient; and videostroboscopic measures. In particular, videostroboscopic measures are used in every major voice clinic and are derived from the direct inspection of the true vocal folds by videotape. For more information about these measures, see Baken (1987), Colton and Casper (1990), and Titze and Verdolini (personal communication, February 1999).

Impressions

After you have completed the case history and the voice measures, you should form cohesive impressions about the results. You should discuss your impressions with the patient and/or her family, and you should indicate the impressions in a specific section of the written report. In this section, include a description of the nature and severity of the disorder, at a general level ("The patient has a moderately weak speaking voice . . ."), the immediate underlying causes (". . . consistent with the otolaryngological diagnosis of a unilateral laryngeal paralysis . . ."), and factors that may have contributed to the onset and maintenance of the problem (". . . that may have originated from a viral infection about 2 years ago").

Eventually, we must put it all together!

Recommendations and Prognosis

Finally, you should make treatment recommendations and indicate what you think the prognosis is for improvement. Is voice therapy recommended? If so, how often, and how long will each session be? Over what period of time? What will be the focus of therapy? What is the likelihood of a partial or complete resolution of the problem with the treatment program recommended? Base your recommendations and prognostic statements on clinical experience and on reports available in the literature.

Section Summary

In this section on assessment, we discussed the important concepts behind a voice assessment in general and specific assessment approaches. The most important concepts, as we see them, are understandings of voice and voice disorders, of voice measures, of how voice measures are properly elicited, and of what their limitations are. With this information, and by applying careful analytic thinking to the results, we look for converging evidence across measures in answering critical clinical questions. In the next section, we give examples of the findings from a few different patients to illustrate some of these principles.

CASE EXAMPLES

In the case examples that follow typical findings from three classes of voice disorders are discussed: (a) those due to discrete mass lesions of the membranous vocal folds (Case 1), (b) those due to a movement disorder (Case 2), and (c) those due to a nonorganic condition (Case 3). In these case reports, we orient toward measures that can be made with a minimum of equipment. The findings are typical for the diagnostic categories discussed. However, you should not in any way take them as absolutes. Other outcomes are possible and, in fact, occur quite regularly.

Case 1: Vocal Fold Nodules

Relevant Case History

This patient is a 9-year-old boy who has moderate-sized, bilateral vocal fold nodules. According to his parents, he has been hoarse for about 2 years. Neither the parents nor the child recall any illnesses in conjunction with the onset of hoarseness. With the exception of common childhood illnesses (chicken pox, measles, and mumps), and vocal fold nodules, the general medical history is unremarkable, by the parents' report. The child concedes that he often screams on the playground at school. He describes a moderate effort level during speech. He also reports a moderate motivation level to improve his dysphonia.

Measures

The findings for this patient are shown in Table 9–1. The General Voice Index shows evidence of a voice disorder. As noted in the case history, the child reports some functional impairments. He also describes a high phonatory effort level during speech, and he has an overall moderate grade of dysphonia. Speech and language seem normal. The Acoustic Index indicates a normal F_0 and intensity in speech, but restricted semitone pitch and dynamic ranges. The Physiological Index reveals poor S:Z ratio, but normal L–DDK measures. Respiratory status, shown by prolonged /s/, appears borderline superior.

Tying It Together

This voice profile is quite typical for patients with discrete mass lesions of the membranous vocal folds. In addition to phonatory effort and hoarseness, which are generic findings, the distinctive pattern is an overall impairment in measures reflecting membranous vocal fold closure, but normal neural control (arytenoid closure) measures. Treatment was recommended to reduce the nodules and to improve hoarseness.

Case 2: Parkinson's Disease

Relevant Case History

This patient is a 73-year-old retired man with progressive onset of Parkinson's disease over the past several years. He is followed by a neurologist. Under her direction, he takes medication daily for treatment of Parkinson's symptoms. An otolaryngological evaluation revealed mild vocal fold bowing that did not persist during purposefully effortful phonation. The patient walks with characteristically

Table 9-1. Data summary (profile) sheet for Case 1.

VOICE/SPEECH PROFILE SHEET

Patient: Case 1

Date(s):

Referring diagnosis: Nodules

Clinician:

		POOR			NORMAL			SUPERIOR	
GENERAL									
VHI									
F	40	30	20	10	0				
P	40	30	20	10	0				
E	40	30	20	10	0				
Effort	x 4	x 3	x 2		x 1				
Voice									
Grade	SEV (C/I)	MOD (C/I)	MIL (C/I)		NORMAL				
Roughness	SEV (C/I)	MOD (C/I)	MIL (C/I)		NORMAL				
Asthenia	SEV (C/I)	MOD (C/I)	MIL (C/I)		NORMAL				
Breathiness	SEV (C/I)	MOD (C/I)	MIL (C/I)		NORMAL				
Strain	SEV (C/I)	MOD (C/I)	MIL (C/I)		NORMAL				
Tremor	S (C/I)	MOD (C/I)	MIL (C/I)		NORMAL				
Nasality (+/-)	SEV (C/I)	MOD (C/I)	MIL (C/I)		NORMAL				
Prosody	SEV (C/I)	MOD (C/I)	MIL (C/I)		NORMAL				
Speech	SEV (C/I)	MOD (C/I)	MIL (C/I)		NORMAL				
Language	SEV (C/I)	MOD (C/I)	MIL (C/I)		NORMAL				
ACOUSTIC									
Fo ave (Hz)					200				
ST range (z)	-3.0	-2.0	-1.0		0		+1.0	+2.0	+3.0
I ave (dB 3')	50	55	60		65				
	80	75	70						
I range (dB)	10	20	30		40		50	60	70
PHYSIOL									
L-D rate (z)	-3.0	-2.0	-1.0		0		+1.0	+2.0	+3.0
L-D str	SEV weak	MOD weak	MIL weak		NORMAL				
	SEV tight	MOD tight	MIL tight						
L-D con	SEV	MOD	MIL		NORMAL				
S:Z (z)	+3.0	+2.0	+1.0		0				
	-3.0	-2.0	-1.0						
s-prolong (z)			+1.0		0				

small movements. His wife, who has a hearing impairment, complains that she cannot understand her husband because he talks so quietly. The patient describes a comfortable level of effort during conversational speech, and he notes only marginal functional impairments related to voice. However, his wife reports a significant disruption in their communication because her husband talks quietly. Presently, the wife appears more motivated to seek an improvement in the situation than the patient himself.

Measures

Table 9–2 shows the findings for this patient. Again, the General Voice Index indicates a disorder. Although the patient's ratings of functional impairments and of phonatory effort do not reveal problems, the clinician's auditory-perceptual evaluation indicates weak voice, hypernasality, and monotone prosody (limited pitch and loudness variations during speech). Speech is slurred, but language appears grossly intact. The Acoustic Index confirms a somewhat high F_0 during speech, and a low intensity, both consistent with vocal fold bowing. Despite the vocal fold bowing noted, the physiological measures indicating membranous vocal fold closure during phonation (S:Z) is normal or even borderline low, indicating tight vocal fold approximation. Measures reflecting neural control of the larynx, L–DDK measures, show normal vocal fold adduction rate, but poor adduction strength and poor consistency.

Tying It Together

The profiles for patients with Parkinson's disease are variable, depending among other things on the stage of the disease and medication status. However, in our experience, the profile for this patient is quite typical of medicated patients with a moderate disease stage, without dementia. The most telltale findings are monotone speech prosody, weak voice, slurred speech, and impaired laryngeal neural control measures. Monotone prosody and weak voice reflect the limited range of motion in vocal fold elongation and vibration amplitude, characteristic of Parkinson's disease. The impaired neural control measures indicate a neurological problem. The marginally high fundamental frequency may reflect the vocal fold bowing noted by the otolaryngologist. Note that, despite the bowing, the membranous vocal fold closure measure (S:Z ratio) is normal. The reason is probably that the bowing does not persist for purposefully effortful tasks. For this patient the medical treatment recommendation was to continue with the current medication. The speech-language recommendation was to perform a more complete evaluation of communication status, including an evaluation of speech and language. On the basis of the combined results, speech-voice therapy was recommended.

Table 9–2. Data summary (profile) sheet for Case 2.

VOICE/SPEECH PROFILE SHEET

Patient: Case 2   **Date(s):**

Referring diagnosis: Parkinson's Disease   **Clinician:**

		POOR			NORMAL			SUPERIOR	
GENERAL									
VHI									
Functional	40	30	20	10	0				
Physical	40	30	20	10	0				
Emotional	40	30	20	10	0				
Effort	x 4	x 3	x 2		x 1				
Voice									
Grade	SEV (C/I)	MOD (C/I)	MIL (C/I)		NORMAL				
Roughness	SEV (C/I)	MOD (C/I)	MIL (C/I)		NORMAL				
Asthenia	SEV (C/I)	MOD (C/I)	MIL (C/I)		NORMAL				
Breathiness	SEV (C/I)	MOD (C/I)	MIL (C/I)		NORMAL				
Strain	SEV (C/I)	MOD (C/I)	MIL (C/I)		NORMAL				
Tremor	S (C/I)	MOD (C/I)	MIL (C/I)		NORMAL				
Nasality (+/-)	SEV (C/I)	MOD (C/I)	MIL (C/I)		NORMAL				
Prosody	SEV (C/I)	MOD (C/I)	MIL (C/I)		NORMAL				
Speech	SEV (C/I)	MOD (C/I)	MIL (C/I)		NORMAL				
Language	SEV (C/I)	MOD (C/I)	MIL (C/I)		NORMAL				
ACOUSTIC									
Fo ave (Hz)			165 Hz						
ST range (z)	-3.0	-2.0	-1.0		0		+1.0	+2.0	+3.0
I ave (dB 3')	50	55	60		65				
	80	75	70						
I range (dB)	10	20	30		40		50	60	70
PHYSIOL									
L-D rate (z)	-3.0	-2.0	-1.0		0		+1.0	+2.0	+3.0
L-D str	SEV weak	MOD weak	MIL weak		NORMAL				
	SEV tight	MOD tight	MIL tight						
L-D con	SEV	MOD	MIL		NORMAL				
S:Z (z)	+3.0	+2.0	+1.0		0				
	-3.0	-2.0	-1.0						
s-prolong (z)			+1.0		0				

Case 3: Nonorganically Based Voice Disorder

Relevant Case History

This patient is a 24-year-old elementary school music teacher, a woman, who complains of quick fatigue with voice use and occasional hoarseness. The otolaryngological examination failed to reveal notable findings. The patient is a nonsmoker and does not use alcohol or caffeine, with the exception of a small predilection toward chocolate. She reports loss of work days due to her voice problems and considerable distress over her problem. She also reports significant phonatory effort during speech and singing. She appears highly motivated to improve her condition.

Measures

Table 9–3 shows the results for this patient. The findings are largely within normal limits. Measures of functional impairment, phonatory effort, and auditory-perceptual status are the only abnormal ones. The remaining measures, including the measure indicating membranous vocal fold closure (S:Z ratio), neurological control measures, and acoustic measures, are all normal.

Tying It Together

This profile is quite typical for a patient with a nonorganically based voice complaint. The distinctive pattern is elevated phonatory effort, possibly some hoarseness, but otherwise normal (or nearly normal) functioning.

SOME SPECIAL CONSIDERATIONS

The discussions here have been general in order to provide principles and procedures that can be applied to any patient with a voice disorder as defined here. Obviously, these principles and procedures must be modified to fit a specific patient, and I have commented about that occasionally. Further comments about special patient populations follow.

Hoarseness and Throat Cancer

One example is our extreme concern that patients who are at risk for throat cancer be referred promptly for otolaryngologic examination. Adults, older than 50 who are hoarse or who have any change in voice for a period of 2 weeks or more that cannot be reasonably explained (a bad cold, the flu, hay fever), are clearly at risk and should be referred to an otolaryngologist immediately.[4] This is a rule of public health that should be familiar to every speech-language pathologist, regardless of the nature of her clinical practice.

Table 9–3. Data summary (profile) sheet for Case 2.

VOICE/SPEECH PROFILE SHEET

Patient: Case 3
Referring diagnosis: Non-organic

Date(s):
Clinician:

		POOR			NORMAL			SUPERIOR	
GENERAL									
VHI									
Functional	40	30	20	10	0				
Physical	40	30	20	10	0				
Emotional	40	30	20	10	0				
Effort	x 4	x 3	x 2		x 1				
Voice									
Grade	SEV (C/I)	MOD (C/I)	MIL (C/I)		NORMAL				
Roughness	SEV (C/I)	MOD (C/I)	MIL (C/I)		NORMAL				
Asthenia	SEV (C/I)	MOD (C/I)	MIL (C/I)		NORMAL				
Breathiness	SEV (C/I)	MOD (C/I)	MIL (C/I)		NORMAL				
Strain	SEV (C/I)	MOD (C/I)	MIL (C/I)		NORMAL				
Tremor	SEV (C/I)	MOD (C/I)	MIL (C/I)		NORMAL				
Nasality (+/-)	SEV (C/I)	MOD (C/I)	MIL (C/I)		NORMAL				
Prosody	SEV (C/I)	MOD (C/I)	MIL (C/I)		NORMAL				
Speech	SEV (C/I)	MOD (C/I)	MIL (C/I)		NORMAL				
Language	SEV (C/I)	MOD (C/I)	MIL (C/I)		NORMAL				
ACOUSTIC									
Fo ave (Hz)					220 Hz				
ST range (z)	-3.0	-2.0	-1.0		0		+1.0	+2.0	+3.0
I ave (dB 3')	50	55	60		65				
	80	75	70						
I range (dB)	10	20	30		40		50	60	70
PHYSIOL									
L-D rate (z)	-3.0	-2.0	-1.0		0		+1.0	+2.0	+3.0
L-D str	SEV weak	MOD weak	MIL weak		NORMAL				
	SEV tight	MOD tight	MIL tight						
L-D con	SEV	MOD	MIL		NORMAL				
S:Z (z)	+3.0	+2.0	+1.0		0				
	-3.0	-2.0	-1.0						
s-prolong (z)			+1.0		0				

When the Patient Is a Child

Another example that requires special consideration is the child with a voice disorder. I have defined a voice disorder as a condition in which voice functioning is unacceptable to the user. Young children, particularly those age 4 and younger, may not recognize that they are hoarse. Further, even children who do recognize that they are hoarse may not note any particular functional impairments because of it. These considerations pose some problems for a voice assessment and for voice therapy. When a child does not recognize that he is hoarse, and/or when he does not note any particular functional disruptions because of hoarseness, there is no "voice disorder" as we have defined it! Should you perform a voice assessment, or consider voice therapy at all? Regarding the assessment, this question is particularly relevant because voice norms are relatively less well established for children than they are for adults, and therefore the results may be tenuous. Further, hoarseness rarely signals a life-threatening condition in children, thankfully. Thus, health considerations rarely motivate an assessment of voice or voice therapy for children.

There are different opinions about how to proceed. You should be familiar with them and make your own decision. Some clinicians consider that hoarseness in children is maturational, in the sense that a large number of hoarse children develop clearer, normal voices as adults. This conclusion is implied by the relatively stable incidence of voice disorders across the life span (see Wilson, 1987). Further, there is concern that voice therapy may lead the child to be unusually self-critical of his abilities. Adding these to the considerations already mentioned, you might decide not to undertake voice therapy, and therefore you will not conduct a voice assessment. Or, if you do proceed, you will proceed in a guarded fashion.

Another view is that voice therapy and thus voice assessment may be valuable for many children. The child may not explicitly identify functional disruptions related to voice. However, disruptions may nonetheless exist, and therapy might improve them. For example, the child might suffer from low-grade, physical discomfort during voicing. He might not be aware of it, because he does not remember differently. Or, hoarseness may reflect problems with socialization patterns. A child may scream to get attention. Voice therapy might address these problems.

A complete discussion of such factors is beyond the scope of the present chapter. The point is that you will need to decide for yourself about the appropriateness of a voice assessment and voice therapy for children in general, and on a case-by-case basis. If you do proceed with an assessment and with therapy, you will need to adapt the

---

[4] Note that referral to an otolaryngologist is important for every patient that we see. I just emphasize the especially critical importance of a referral, and a prompt referral, for cases such as these.

usual procedures taking the child's age, overall cognitive abilities, and motivational status into account.

When the Patient Is an Older Adult

Complaints about the voice by the older adult have a double focus. One focus, quite naturally, is about the possibility that voice problems indicate serious disease or disorder. Obviously, such a concern is appropriate and leads to a very close working relationship with the otolaryngologist and, for this age group, the neurologist and perhaps the internist. As indicated earlier, sometimes our assessment findings are highly indicative of problems that require careful medical follow-up.

The other major focus, in my clinical experience, is on functional losses. Common complaints are that the patient is no longer able to sing or to be heard in a noisy room, or to call across the street to a neighbor, or to be heard easily by a hearing-impaired spouse or friend. These are very real problems, to be taken seriously. In the SLP assessment, you need to describe the nature and severity of the problem. In treatment, you need to assist the patient to accommodate as well as possible. Overall, the need is to be sensitive to the dimensions of the problem as it affects daily life.

Older patients, particularly those with apparent or diagnosed laryngeal disorders characterized by impaired motor or sensitivity function, often have voice and swallowing problems (dysphagia) in tandem. The patient with paralysis of a vocal fold (or the muscles regulating the arytenoid cartilage, to which the vocal fold is attached) in the open position probably has a breathy voice and, perhaps, aspiration during swallowing (leaking of some part of the bolus into the windpipe). Other patients, particularly older ones, report that the bolus "sticks" in the midthroat and "I can't get it down right." Issues about dysphagia are discussed in Chapter 15, but it is appropriate to remind ourselves of this relationship in this discussion of voice disorders as well.

What if the Patient Is a Professional Voice User?

For obvious reasons, there are many special considerations to be made when a patient uses her voice in her livelihood, and I have referred to them in many phases of the preceding discussion. Sometimes the questions are about competence ("I can't make myself heard as I need to, to do my job, in that noisy machine shop/factory/tavern/classroom/courtroom"). Sometimes, they are about durability ("I'm okay in the morning/when I begin my workday, but by noon, my voice gives out"). In the case of a singer or actor, the complaint may be about the "quality" of voice. If you work clinically with the latter groups (professional singers and actors), you may need special skills in assessment and treatment to be helpful. You should also work in close collaboration with the singing teacher or vocal coach. If your caseload involves a great number of such patients, you might consider some formal voice training yourself.

What About the Multicultural Perspective in Dealing With a Voice Disorder?

The need to be sensitive to differences among cultures in diagnosis in speech-language pathology is discussed in several sections of this book, and specifically in Chapter 2. This issue is also crucial in matters of voice disorders. It is directly relevant to our definition of a voice disorder that requires identification of the "disorder" by the individual in the context of her social group, and her social and work activities, that is to say, her culture. These are criteria against which her voice is measured that you must consider carefully in assessment and treatment.

CHAPTER SUMMARY

In this chapter, we discussed voice disorders and their assessment. To summarize, the following points are considered the important ones. First, the methodology that you use to assess the voice should be dictated by the clinical questions that you want to answer. Second, the most important tools for conducting a good voice assessment are a solid understanding of basic voice science and voice disorders, and good analytic skills. Sophisticated equipment does not guarantee a good assessment; your own abilities are much more important. Third, none of the available voice measures are without interpretative problems. You should be familiar with the rationale for each measure, and its limitations. Fourth, although no single measure is without problems, you can use a battery of measures together to generate an overall impression or, more formally, a voice profile that you can use to help answer your clinical questions. It should be emphasized that there is no cookbook approach to voice assessment, even with a profile approach. You need to interpret each profile based on the unique ensemble of information that each patient presents. Finally, in order for the individual measures that you make to be meaningful, you should obtain the measures using the same procedures that were used to develop the related norms, and you should compare the results to the norms.

I hope that these guidelines will provide you with a good start in the assessment of voice. I am confident that, with experience, you will develop more and/or other guidelines of your own. The important point is that your assessment procedure serve your patients well and that it contributes to the development of treatment recommendations that will enhance your patient's quality of life wherever possible.

REFERENCES

Baken, R. J. (1987). *Clinical measurement of speech and voice*. Boston, MA: College-Hill Press.

Bassich, C. J., & Ludlow, C. L. (1986). The use of perceptual methods by new clinicians for assessing voice quality. *Journal of Speech and Hearing Disorders, 51*, 125–133.

Colton, R. H., & Casper, J. K., (1990). *Understanding voice problems: A physiological perspective for diagnosis and treatment*. Baltimore, MD: Williams & Wilkins.

Hanson, H. (1997). Glottal characteristics of female speakers: Acoustic correlates. *Journal of the Acoustical Society of America, 101*, 466–481.

Hirano, M. (1981). *Clinical examination of voice*. New York: Springer-Verlag.

Hirano, M. (1989). Objective evaluation of the human voice: Clinical aspects. *Folia Phoniatrica, 41*, 89–144.

Jacobson, B. H., Johnson, A., Grywalski, C., Silbergleit, A., Jacobson, G., Benninger, M. S., & Newman, C. W. (1997). The Voice Handicap Index (VHI): Development and validation. *American Journal of Speech-Language Pathology, 6*(3), 66–70.

Kreiman, J., & Gerratt, B. R. (1996). The perceptual structure of pathologic voice quality. *Journal of the Acoustical Society of America, 100*, 1787–1795.

Ptacek, P. H., Sander, E. K., Maloney, W. H., & Jackson, C. R. (1966). Phonatory and related changes with advanced age. *Journal of Speech and Hearing Research, 9*, 353–360.

Sapienza, C. M., Murry, T., & Brown, W. S., Jr. (1998). Variations in adductor spasmodic dysphonia: Acoustic evidence. *Journal of Voice, 12*, 214–222.

Sederholm, E., McAllister, A., Sundberg, J., & Dalqvist, J. (1999). Perceptual analysis of child hoarseness using continuous scales. *Scandinavian Journal of Logopedics and Phoniatrics*. Submitted.

Smith, E., Kirchner, H. L., Taylor, M., Hoffman, H., & Lemke, J. H. (1998). Voice problems among teachers: Differences by gender and teaching characteristics. *Journal of Voice, 12*, 328–334.

Smith, E., Verdolini, K., Gray, S., Nichols, S., Lemke, J., Barkmeier, J., Dove, H., & Hoffman, H. (1996). Effect of voice disorders on quality of life. *Journal of Medical Speech-Language Pathology, 4*, 223–244.

Titze, I. R., Lemke, J., & Montequin, D. (1997). Populations in the U.S. workforce who rely on voice as a primary tool of trade: A preliminary report. *Journal of Voice, 11*, 254–259.

Verdolini, K. (1994). Voice disorders. In J. B. Tomblin, H. L. Morris, & D. C. Spriestersbach (Eds.), *Diagnosis in Speech-Language Pathology* (pp. 247–306). San Diego, CA: Singular Publishing Group.

Verdolini, K. (1999). Clinical analysis of common terminology in voice therapy: A position paper. *PHONOSCOPE, 1*, 1–8.

Verdolini, K., & Palmer, P. (1997). Assessment of a "profiles" approach to voice screening. *Journal of Medical Speech-Language Pathology, 5*, 217–232.

Wilson, D. K. (1987). *Voice problems of children* (3rd ed.). Baltimore, MD: Williams & Wilkins.

RECOMMENDED READINGS

Laryngeal Pathology

Colton, R. H., & Casper, J. K., (1996). *Understanding voice problems: A physiological perspective for diagnosis and treatment.* Baltimore, MD: Williams & Wilkins.

Movement Disorders Affecting Voice and Speech

Duffy, J. R. (1995). *Motor speech disorders: Substrates, differential diagnosis, and management.* Boston, MA: Mosby.

Voice Measurement

Baken, R. J. (1987). *Clinical measurement of speech and voice.* Boston, MA: College-Hill Press.

Kreiman, J., Gerratt, B. R., Kempster, G. B., Erman, A., & Berke, G. S. (1993). Perceptual evaluation of voice quality: Review, tutorial, and a framework for future research. *Journal of Speech and Hearing Research, 36,* 21–40.

Voice Therapy

Ramig, L. O., & Verdolini, K. (1998). Treatment efficacy: Voice disorders. *Journal of Speech, Language, and Hearing Research, 41,* S101–S116.

Verdolini, K., Ramig, L., & Jacobson, B. (1997). Outcomes measurement in voice disorders. In C. Frattali (Ed.), *Measuring outcomes in speech-language pathology* (pp. 354–386). New York: Thieme.

APPENDIX 9A
VOICE HANDICAP INDEX

Instructions: These are statements that many people have used to describe their voices and the effects of their voices on their lives. Circle the response that indicates how frequently you have the same experience.

F1. My voice makes it difficult for people to hear me.

P2. I run out of air when I talk.

F3. People have difficulty understanding me in a noisy room.

P4. The sound of my voice varies throughout the day.

F5. My family has difficulty hearing me when I call them throughout the house.

F6. I use the phone less often than I would like.

E7. I'm tense when talking with others because of my voice.

F8. I tend to avoid groups of people because of my voice.

E9. People seem irritated with my voice.

P10. People a   "What's wrong with your voice?"

F11. I speak with friends, neighbors, or relatives less often because of my voice.

F12. People ask me to repeat myself when speaking face-to-face.

P13. My voice sounds creaky and dry.

P14. I feel as though I have to strain to produce voice.

E15. I find other people don't understand my voice problem.

F16. My voice difficulties restrict my personal and social life.

P17. The clarity of my voice is unpredictable.

P18. I try to change my voice to sound different.

F19. I feel left out of conversations because of my voice.

P20. I use a great deal of effort to speak.

P21. My voice is worse in the evening.

F22. My voice problem causes me to lose income.

E23. My voice problem upsets me.

E24. I am less outgoing because of my voice problem.

E25. My voice makes me feel handicapped.

P26. My voice gives out" on me in the middle of speaking.

E27. I feel annoyed when people ask me to repeat.

E28. I feel embarrassed when people ask me to repeat.

E29. My voice makes me feel incompetent.

E30. I'm ashamed of my voice problem.

Note: The letter preceding each item number corresponds to the subscale (E = emotional subscale, F = functional subscale, P = physical subscale).

The patient is asked to indicate how often each symptom occurs. The words "never" and "always" are used as endpoint anchors, and scored as "4" and "0", respectively. Intermediate scores range between 1 and 3. The total scores are then computed for each subscale: Emotional, Functional, and Physical. [From The Voice Handicap Index (VHI): Development and Validation, by B. H. Jacobson, A. Johnson, C. Grywalski, A. Silbergleit, et al., 1997. *American Journal of Speech-Language Pathology, 6*(3), 66–70. Reprinted with permission.]

APPENDIX 9B
AVERAGE FUNDAMENTAL
FREQUENCY MEASUREMENT

Age/Sex	Norm	SD/Range	Authors[1]
7/F	294 Hz	–	Fairbanks, Wiley, &
7/M	281 Hz	–	Lassman (1949)
8/F	297 Hz	–	
8/M	288 Hz	–	
10 to 12/F	237.5 Hz	198 to 271 Hz	Horii (1983)
10 to 12/M	226.5 Hz	192 to 269 Hz	
17 to 25/F	217 Hz	1.7 semitones	Fitch & Holbrook (1970)
17 to 25/M	116.7 Hz	2.1 semitones	
20 to 29/F (nonsmoking)	224.3 Hz	192 to 275 Hz	Stoicheff (1981)
20 to 29/M	120 Hz	–	Hollien & Shipp (1972)
30 to 39/F (nonsmoking)	213.3	181 to 241 Hz	Stoicheff (1981)
30 to 40/F	196.3 Hz	171 to 222 Hz	Saxman & Burk (1967)
30 to 39/M	112 Hz	–	Hollien & Shipp (1972)
40 to 49/F (nonsmoking)	220.8 Hz	190 to 273 Hz	Stoicheff (1981)
40 to 50/F	188.6 Hz	168 to 206 Hz	Saxman & Burk (1967)
40 to 49/M	107 Hz	–	Hollien & Shipp (1972)
50 to 59/F (nonsmoking)	199.3 Hz	176 to 241 Hz	Stoicheff (1981)
50 to 59/M	112 Hz	–	Hollien & Shipp (1972)
60 to 69/F (nonsmoking)	199.7 Hz	143 to 235 Hz	Stoicheff (1981)
65 to 75/F	196.6 Hz	–	McGlone & Hollien (1963)
60 to 69/M	112 Hz	–	Hollien & Shipp (1972)
70+/F (nonsmoking)	202.2 Hz	170 to 249 Hz	Stoicheff (1981)
80 to 94/F	199.8 Hz	–	McGlone & Hollien (1963)
80 to 89/M	146 Hz	–	Hollien & Shipp (1972)

(continued)

[1]For all these normative studies, subjects read a passage and the average fundamental frequency was extracted using relatively expensive equipment. For clinical purposes, we have found that similar values are obtained using a simpler counting task and a portable keyboard or a pitch pipe. The procedure is as follows: Ask the patient to count out loud slowly from 1 to 5. Match the patient's pitch contour with your own voice. Sustain the vowel on the word "three" as the patient continues counting. (You may want to warn the patient that you will be counting along, but to ignore you.) Then match this pitch to a keyboard or a pitch pipe. (The reason for selecting a vowel in midutterance is that pitch tends to fall below average values at the ends of utterances and may be higher than the average at the beginning.) Convert the pitch to frequency (see page 276 [Appendix 9B, continued]). Use this as the average fundamental frequency in speech for that patient.

APPENDIX 9B *(continued)*
PITCH TO FREQUENCY

Pitch	Frequency (Hz)	Pitch	Frequency (Hz)
B1	61.7	C#4	277.2
C2	65.4	D4	293.7
C#2	69.3	D#4	311.1
D2	73.4	E4	329.6
D#2	77.8	F4	349.2
E2	82.4	F#4	370.0
F2	87.3	G4	392.0
F#2	92.5	G#4	415.3
G2	98.0	A4	440.0
G#2	103.8	A#4	466.2
A2	110.0	B4	493.2
A#2	116.5	C5	523.2
B2	123.5	C#5	544.4
C3	130.8	D5	587.3
C#3	138.6	D#5	622.3
D3	146.8	E5	659.3
D#3	155.6	F5	698.4
E3	164.8	F#5	740.0
F3	174.6	G5	784.0
F#3	186.0	G#5	830.6
G3	196.0	A5	880.0
G#3	207.7	A#5	932.3
A3	220.0	B5	987.8
A#3	233.1	C6	1046.5
B3	246.9	C#6	1108.7
C4	261.6	D6	1174.7

APPENDIX 9C
SEMITONE PITCH RANGE MEASUREMENT

Age/Sex	Norm	SD	Authors
18–38 yr, F	32.8	4.4	Ptacek et al., 1966
18–39 yr, M	34.5	5.2	Ptacek et al., 1966
66–93 yr, F	25.1	7.9	Ptacek et al., 1966
66–93 yr, M	26.5	6.3	Ptacek et al., 1966

To follow the normative procedure your patient should be sitting. Ask him to vocalize on a comfortable pitch, and to descend in pitch by semitones until the lowest pitch is produced. This is identified as the lower boundary of the pitch range. Then ask the subject to increase pitch by whole tones until the highest possible pitch is produced. This is identified as the high boundary of the pitch range. The lowest grunts and highest screeches are encouraged; i.e., the range is not "performable" but rather physiological range. The range is computed by counting the number of semitones from lowest to highest pitch (Appendix 9B). To compare the results to norms, subtract the normative semitone pitch range from the patient's range, and divide by the normative standard deviation. This will yield a z score which then is indicated on the Profile Sheet.

APPENDIX 9D
AVERAGE VOICE INTENSITY MEASUREMENT

NORM = 65 dB at 3 feet

This norm may be an overestimation of the values that we tend to encounter clinically. Nonetheless, the procedure is to position a dB meter with a microphone-to-mouth distance of about 3 feet. Use the A-weighting, and slow response mode. Ask the patient to converse about some appropriate topic ("Tell me about your favorite vacation"). Note the approximate dB value around which the meter indicator fluctuates.

APPENDIX 9E
S:Z RATIO MEASUREMENT

Age/Sex	Norm	SD	Authors
5/F	0.83	0.50–1.14	Tait, Michel, & Carpenter[1]
5/M	0.92	0.82–1.08	(1980)
7/F	0.78	0.51–1.10	
7/M	0.70	0.52–0.97	
9/F	0.91	0.75–1.26	
9/M	0.92	0.66–1.50	
8 to 88/F,M	0.99	0.36	Eckel & Boone[2] (1981)

[1]To compare your patient's values with those reported by Tait et al., use the following procedures. Tell the child, "Take a deep breath and say /s/ (or /z/) for as long as you can . . . Ready? . . . Begin." Repeat for each phoneme three times, with a rest between trials. Time each trial with a stopwatch. Vary the order of the phonemes within each child, and vary order across different children. Select the longest /s/ and the longest /z/ to compute the s:z ratio (dividing /s/ by /z/). Compare to the norm.

[2]To compare the results for your patient to those reported here, use the following procedure. Tell your patients to take a deep breath and to hold out /s/ (or /z/) as long as possible at a comfortable pitch and loudness. (Give the patient an example without sustaining it maximally.) Time the patient's performance with a stopwatch. Repeat for two trials each of /s/ and /z/. Vary the order of /s/ and /z/ randomly within and across patients. Use the longest /s/ and the longest /z/ to compare the s:z ratio (divide /s/ by /z/), and compare it to the norm.

Note: For both children and adults, it is valuable to separately indicate the best /s/ prolongation value as a gross reflection of respiratory sufficiency. The norms are based on the same studies as for the s:z ratio, and are as follows:

APPENDIX 9F
LARYNGEAL DIADOCHOKINETIC MEASUREMENT (PRODUCTIONS PER SECOND)

Age/Sex	Norm	SD	Authors
6/F, M	3.6	—	Based on Fletcher[1] (1972)
7/F, M	3.8	—	for /kʌ/
8/F, M	4.2	—	
9/F, M	4.4	—	
10/F, M	4.6	—	
11/F, M	5.0	—	
12/F, M	5.1	—	
14/F, M	5.4	—	
18 to 38/F	5.3	0.8	Ptacek et al.[2] (1996)
18 to 39/M	5.1	1.0	
66 to 93/F	3.9	1.3	
68 to 89/M	4.1	0.9	

[1]We have not found norms for children for laryngeal diadochokinesis. Rather than eliminating this test for children or not interpreting it, we use the norms from Fletcher (1972) for repeated /kʌ/. These values seem to most closely approximate those for /ʌ/. We use the same procedure as for adults, below.

[2]The procedure for these norms is as follows. Show your patient the sound "uh" graphically and tell her you will ask her to produce it as rapidly as possible. Demonstrate. (In the demonstration, we include an initial glottal stop. It is unclear whether Ptacek et al. did or not.) Then ask the patient to take a deep breath and make the sound as fast as possible until you say to stop (7 seconds). If the patient runs out of breath earlier, accept the trial if you think it is the best that can be done. In the absence of sophisticated counting devices, dot a pencil on paper for each production of "uh" for the duration of the trial (timed with a stopwatch). (Ptacek et al. used a more sophisticated system, but we find this approach an adequate approximation.)

In addition to counting the *number* of tokens produced over the trial period, you should also note the strength and consistency of the tokens. Strong glottal plosives produced with a highly consistent rate would be considered "normal" on both strength and consistency parameters. With some clinical experience, you will be able to confidently scale poorer performance as "mild, moderate, moderately severe, or severe" impairment for both strength and consistency.

SECTION III

Some Special Populations

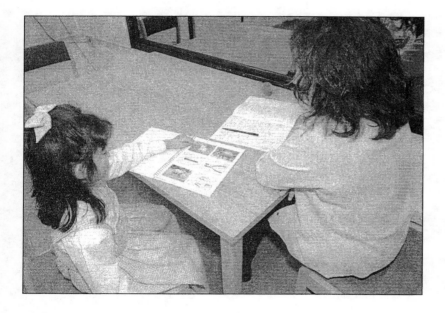

In this section, we have asked several master clinicians to write about specific disorders. We did this in an effort to help the student begin to apply the principles of diagnosis, described in the first two sections, to real-life problems. Admittedly, the list is not complete, but is intended to give examples. We join the authors in hoping that the discussions will further stimulate your interest in speech-language pathology.

10

Assessing Language in the Classroom and the Curriculum

Frank M. Cirrin, Ph.D.

INTRODUCTION

Language and Language-Learning Disorders in the Schools

Did you know that more than 50% of speech-language pathologists work in a school setting? Perhaps you remember a speech clinician in your school who helped students with articulation, voice, or fluency problems. Today, students who have *language-learning disorders* make up the majority of school speech-language pathologists' caseloads. Children with language-learning disorders are a heterogeneous group who have difficulty acquiring, comprehending, or expressing themselves with spoken or written language. The difficulties that these students have with language also place them at severe risk for academic and learning problems. That is not surprising given that language is the basis for virtually all learning, both in and out of school. Language is so embedded in school curricula that it is often difficult to separate learning the concepts of a subject from learning to use language to talk about these concepts. All aspects of the classroom environment are important to the learning process, but the most crucial ingredient is language.

A Rationale for Assessing Language Interactions in the Classroom

Gruenewald and Pollak (1990) suggest that there are three interacting language components in every learning or instructional task. There is a continuous interaction between the student's language, the teacher's language, and the language requirements and vocabulary in the curriculum or instructional materials. Many teachers assume that the causes of a student's learning problem lie in the language abilities and conceptual skills that the student brings to the task. A more accurate assumption is that the student's learning is also influenced by the other two language components that are always present in the classroom environment.

An example may help to clarify these language interactions. Jerry, a third grader, is typical of a student whose language-learning problems place him at risk for academic failure. In casual conversation, Jerry is spontaneously verbal, uses a mix of complete and incomplete sentences, and communicates messages effectively most of the time. However, in class he presents language and learning differences that affect his ability to participate in many learning activities. Jerry often engages in self-distracting behaviors, such as rocking in his chair or playing with pencils and paper clips. On these occasions Jerry needs repetition of directions that seem to be within his cognitive and language capabilities. He has difficulty following verbal and written directions for independent work sheets, and often turns in incomplete assignments. When he does not know what to do, he usually copies random sentences from the work sheet or the text. When participating in structured speaking tasks such as describing a sequence of directions, Jerry's verbalizations are short, incomplete, and difficult for a listener to follow. Although he often requires teacher repetition of directions and their sequence, Jerry has little difficulty remembering the gist of a story read to him, especially when the teacher uses a slow, conversational speaking style that includes periodic pauses for story-related comments from the class. In this task he can recall key vocabulary, characters, episodes, and other essential information. This suggests that when provided with a structure for remembering information (as in a story recall task) he has fewer problems retaining information, which in turn facilitates his understanding. Jerry's teacher was confused by the inconsistencies in his learning and was uncertain how to devise teaching strate-

> Do not assume that poor language abilities are the cause of a student's learning problem. Find out if the language used by the teacher and the language required by the lesson are contributing to the problem.

gies that would be more effective in helping him learn. The teacher needed to understand how Jerry's language abilities interacted with the classroom task (i.e., curriculum) and differences in teacher language and interactional style and how to help him within the context of the regular classroom.

The main goal of language intervention for students with language-learning disorders is to improve their functioning in real-life contexts, such as the classroom. This may seem obvious, but sometimes it is easy to lose sight of this basic fact. Speech-language pathologists must make sure that language interventions are relevant to the classroom, and that they will actually help students use language to communicate and learn in that context. To help students with language-learning disorders use language for learning, you (as a speech-language pathologist) must learn to observe and analyze the learning activities that students routinely encounter in school.

The need to assess the language interactions that occur in classrooms is also related to a major change in service delivery that has affected virtually all school speech-language pathologists. Recently, we have begun to provide services to many students with language-learning disorders *in their classrooms*. These classroom-based language services include team teaching with the regular classroom teacher, working with large and small groups of students in the regular classroom, and collaborating with teaching staff on creating classroom environments that foster language development, higher level thinking, and literacy. By working with students in the classroom, we are helping them use new skills and knowledge in the actual learning context. Speech-language pathologists and teachers need assessment information that can be used to connect language intervention to the day-to-day learning activities that the student encounters. This can only be accomplished by systematically observing and analyzing the language interactions between the student, teacher, and instructional materials in various classroom learning tasks.

The purpose of this chapter is to present specific assessment questions that a school speech-language pathologist needs to answer about classroom language interactions for students with language-learning disabilities. As we have seen, information should be gathered on at least three important language variables:

1. the student's ability to use language effectively in classroom speaking and listening tasks,

2. the teacher's language during teaching and other instruc-tional tasks, and

3. the language requirements, vocabulary and sentence structures that are found in the lessons and students' textbooks.

The process of assessing classroom language interactions is focused on understanding how each of these three variables may be

> Effective language assessment *and* intervention requires you to be *in the classroom.* The information you gather in the classroom is the most relevant to the real-life language and learning problems faced by your students.

contributing to the student's communication and academic difficulties. The teacher and the speech-language pathologist can then generate hypotheses about possible intervention strategies and modifications that can take place in the regular classroom to help the student.

Throughout this chapter we present a number of observational inventories that can help organize the classroom language information you collect and help you begin to answer these important assessment questions. We will also describe some strategies to make sure your classroom observations are efficient and go as smoothly as possible.

At this point you may be asking "what about students with articulation, voice, or fluency disorders? Isn't it important to observe these students communicating in the classroom?" The answer is "of course." Much of the information in this chapter can be applied to classroom-based assessments for students with other types of communication disabilities besides language-learning disorders. In fact, documentation of how a communication disability affects a student's classroom performance is a very good idea for all communication problems that children experience in the school setting.

Cautions When Observing Students From Diverse Cultural Backgrounds

As Westby pointed out in Chapter 2 on multicultural issues, current demographic trends make it important for all teachers, including school speech-language pathologists, to have a good understanding of cultural and linguistic diversity. For example, in my large urban school district almost 70% of the students are members of minority groups. Over 75 different cultures are represented by the students and their families. Classroom observation inventories, like the ones presented in this chapter, are excellent tools for collecting information on the communication needs of students from diverse cultural backgrounds. However, the possibility of harm exists if assessment information, including observational data, is interpreted without taking the appropriate cultural and linguistic variables into account. In Chapter 2, Westby describes a number of cultural differences that could affect a student's performance in classroom speaking and listening tasks, including telling or retelling stories as a monologue without assistance from the listeners.

Collaborating With Teachers

The first step in gathering relevant assessment data is to collaborate with those who know the child well. While this appropriately includes parents and peers, the focus of this chapter will be working with teachers. Speech-language pathologists need to collaborate with teachers to identify key classroom learning situations where communication and academic problems are evident, and to describe the language abilities of our students.

It is important that assessment of classroom language interaction be a collaborative venture between the teacher and the speech-language pathologist for at least two reasons. First, the teacher is the professional who has the primary responsibility for students' education. In this sense, the classroom is the teacher's "territory." An observation of a student, an examination of instructional materials, or an analysis of the teacher's language in that territory may be threatening. This is especially true if the teacher has not been an equal partner in identifying the problem, asking the assessment questions, and designing the assessment and observation plan.

Second, the teacher is usually very familiar with the student's language strengths and weaknesses as they affect that student's learning in the classroom. This is only natural because teachers spend the most time with students. In school settings, teachers are also the main referral source for students with language-learning disorders. They tend to be the first professionals who recognize that a student may be having difficulties with language and learning. Teachers will also have important information on students' academic performance, learning styles, social abilities, and other aspects of performance that must be integrated to obtain a picture of the "whole" child. Through collaboration, the teacher can add critical information to the analysis, and ultimately participate in seeking solutions to our students' language and learning problems.

Although a detailed discussion of collaborative classroom-based services is beyond the scope of this chapter, it is important to recognize that collaboration is a *voluntary* interaction between colleagues having a parity of knowledge and skills. This means that two (or more) professionals contribute their strengths and abilities to the assessment-intervention process. The intent of collaboration should be to solve identified student communication problems using the knowledge and skills of all professionals involved and to effect lasting changes in the student's behavior. Collaboration is also intended to increase the ability of teachers to handle similar student communication concerns that may arise in the future.

Because collaboration is based on the premise that individuals have entered into a voluntary, nonsupervisory relationship, it does not work to *require* teachers to engage in collaborative activities with speech-language pathologists, or vice versa. This caveat applies to the collection and analysis of assessment data on classroom language interactions. In this regard, speech-language pathologists may find interactions with teachers less problematic if they view their role as one of empowering teachers rather than one of simply giving advice. We need to recognize the teacher's strengths and needs in providing an atmosphere that is communicatively rich and language sensitive for students. There may be a tendency for a speech-language pathologist to view his or her role as language expert too narrowly. Identifying what teachers do not do "right" or often enough may justify to ourselves our role as "helper," but it does little to raise the awareness, competence, or acceptance of the teacher.

Speech-language pathologists and teachers must *share their professional knowledge* with each other in order for students to be successful with classroom language demands. It may take an entire school year to build a collaborative relationship with a teacher in your school, but it is well worth the effort.

ASSESSING STUDENT LANGUAGE USE IN THE CLASSROOM

For the remainder of this chapter we will follow the clinical problem-solving process that Tomblin proposed in Chapter 1. That is, we will (1) establish the clinical assessment question, (2) determine the information needed to answer the question, and (3) determine how to obtain this information. At the end of this chapter we will also discuss how the information that you collect can be used and interpreted.

Student language use is the first of the three interacting language variables we will address. Teachers expect students to be able to comprehend, produce, and use language competently in classroom speaking and listening tasks. Even though educators realize that learning is affected by both the teacher's language and the curricular materials themselves, students with language-learning disorders may not have all of the language skills that the learning task requires. In order to help a student who has been referred, you will need to examine the particular learning task that he or she is having problems with and determine if the student has the necessary speaking and listening skills. Several specific assessment questions must be asked about a student's use of language in the classroom.

Does the Student Have Sufficient Oral Language Skills to Do the Instructional Task?

Each instructional task requires the student to have knowledge of specific language forms (sentence structures) and language content (word and sentence meanings). To use language as a tool for learning and problem solving requires that students be able to produce a wide variety of simple sentences, compound sentences, and complex sentences, and to use age-appropriate vocabulary. Most students enter school with the ability to combine words into phrases, clauses, and sentences. Teachers are sometimes misled into assuming that, because a student uses language for social purposes (such as getting needs met or interacting with family and friends), he or she will be able to use language for the more formal types of verbal communication that are required in school. For example, a student with a language-learning disorder may not be able to use verb tense markers when asked to give an oral report on an activity that took place in the past, as the following monologue of a third grade student illustrates.

> Well, the kids get on the bus and we go to the mall and have some money to buy some stuff. Oh, and this man wants us to stop running in the store.

Retelling stories, another common classroom language task, requires students to use complex and compound sentences to talk about temporal and cause-effect relationships (*Well, the wolf tried to trick the sisters* because *he wanted to eat them*), and use pronouns as devices that help link the sentences of the story together (*The wolf climbed the tree to eat a nut. When* he *fell, the sisters escaped*). Many students with language-learning disorders do not have the expressive language abilities to perform adequately in this and other oral expression activities in the classroom.

Listening and language comprehension abilities are also required for academic success. Children with language-learning disorders often have difficulty drawing inferences about meanings that are not explicit. This will limit their comprehension of what they hear and read. The ability to go beyond the information given to make inferences or conclusions is expected at all elementary grade levels. An example is the following question from a fourth-grade workbook exercise:

Henry shook his dimes out onto	*Henry is_____.*
the bedspread.	*(a) in the store*
His expenses had been heavy.	*(b) in the house*
He wanted to buy Ribsy a new collar.	*(c) in his backyard*

In this exercise, students must not only understand the meanings of the printed words and sentences, but must go beyond these meanings to reach the appropriate conclusion.

These children also experience difficulties using grammatical rules to understand sentences produced by their teachers. They may try to rely on strategies that consist of identifying one or two key words and respond on that basis, rather than getting enough syntactic and semantic cues to understand the intent of the speaker or author. For example, the teacher's direction, "Before you go outside, make sure to finish your work packet," may be interpreted as the teacher giving permission to go outside and then come back to finish. This is because the student uses the order in which events are mentioned as the order in which they are to occur.

What Information Do You Need to Gather?

You need to gather information on the student's ability to communicate effectively meanings and ideas with sentence forms when *speaking*. Does the student use a variety of simple, compound, and complex sentences when speaking in the classroom? Information should be obtained on the student's use of appropriate verb tenses, plurals, prepositions, and other parts of sentences. You also need to find out if the student uses vocabulary appropriate for his or her age and grade level and uses words that have more than one meaning. Classroom language also requires the student to use humor (such as puns) and figurative language appropriately.

In addition to data on oral expression, information must be gathered on the student's ability to understand a variety of sentence forms and vocabulary when *listening* in the classroom. You need to obtain information on the student's general ability to attend to the teacher's explanations and instructions. It is important to know if the student can understand classroom directions and a variety of sentence structures. The student's ability to understand the concepts and main ideas presented in stories and lectures also needs to be assessed. Specific information that can be gathered on a student's classroom speaking and listening abilities is listed in Figures 10–1 and 10–2.

How Do You Gather the Information?

It is likely that some information on a student's expressive and receptive knowledge of language forms and content will be available from previously administered language tests and language samples. It is still necessary to find out, however, how the language-learning disordered student performs in actual classroom speaking and listening tasks.

Two assessment methods may be used to determine if a student has sufficient oral language skills to do a particular instructional task. First, checklists (see Figures 10–1 and 10–2) that contain the relevant behavior categories can be used to interview the student's teacher. As previously noted, the classroom teacher has the best opportunity to observe the student's comprehension and use of lan-

Teachers have information on student language in the classroom that *you need.* Approach them as a partner, *not   an expert,* and you will find that they are willing to collaborate.

Classroom Speaking Checklist	Yes	No	Sometimes
1. Uses correct grammar and sentence structure			
a. Formulates sentences correctly			
b. Uses verb tenses correctly			
c. Forms plurals correctly (regular and irregular)			
d. Uses pronouns correctly			
e. Uses prepositions correctly			
f. Uses negation correctly			
g. Forms compound sentences correctly (*with and, but, or*)			
h. Forms complex sentences correctly (with *when, if, because*)			
i. Asks grammatically well-formed questions			
2. Meaning			
a. Uses age-appropriate vocabulary			
b. Uses concepts of location, time, quantity, etc.			
c. Uses and understands multiple meaning words			
d. Uses humor, sarcasm, and figures of speech appropriately			
e. Produces complex sentences that contain:			
subordinate relationships			
relative clauses			

Figure 10–1. Student language checklist for speaking: Teacher interview and observation guide.

Classroom Speaking Checklist	Yes	No	Sometimes
A. Attention			
1. Attention span for oral presentations is adequate			
2. Attends to all or most of what is said in class			
3. Ignores auditory distractions			
4. Responds after first direction or presentation of information			
5. Asks for things to be repeated in class			
B. Comprehension			
1. Understands stories presented in class			
2. Understands material presented verbally (lecture) as well as those presented visually (written or drawn)			
3. Responds to questions within expected time period			
4. Follows a sequence of directions presented in class			
5. Understands concepts: temporal (before/after), position (above/below), quantity (more/several)			
6. Understands subtleties in word or sentence meanings (idioms, figurative language)			
7. Understands a variety of sentence structures			
8. Interprets meaning from tone of voice and other context cues			
9. Understands (verbally or nonverbally) the main idea of a verbal presentation			
10. Understands teacher's questions presented in class			
11. Understands words (vocabulary) used in class			

Figure 10–2. Student language checklist for listening: Teacher interview and observation guide.

guage in daily learning situations. By interviewing the teacher, or having the teacher fill out the checklist prior to your observation, you will obtain information on how he or she perceives the student's use of language in the classroom. Second, you need to observe the student using language during a specific instructional task. The same checklist that the teacher completed can guide your direct observation of the student. The main purpose of observing the student in one or more classroom speaking and listening tasks is to gain insights into how the student's language abilities interact with the language requirements of a specific learning situation.

Can the Student Use Language for a Variety of Academic Purposes?

Recently, we have become more aware of the language demands that are placed on children in school. It is not sufficient to be able to use language to communicate with others. In school, language must be used to regulate thinking; to plan, reflect, and evaluate; and to acquire knowledge about things that are not directly experienced.

The language demands of social conversation are comparatively simple, because people comment, request, state, and in other ways refer to events and activities *as they occur.*

The task demands in school are much different, extending to the literate end of what has been called the "oral-to-literate continuum" (Westby, 1985). The use of language in school is often *decontextualized,* relating to things not in the here-and-now. This requires that students use language that is more specific, less repetitive and redundant, more reflective on experiences, and more related to topics that the student may not have directly experienced. Students with language-learning disorders are likely to have difficulty using language to formulate ideas, compare and contrast, plan how to do a task, verbalize their experiences and feelings, and obtain information by asking questions. As teachers and speech-language pathologists, one of our most important jobs is to encourage students to use oral language for these purposes and to develop language as a tool for learning.

What Information Do You Need to Gather?

You need to determine how the student obtains information needed for school learning tasks and how effectively the student provides information to others. In addition, data should be gathered on how the student uses language to interact with teachers and classmates throughout the school day. For example, does the student use language to ask permission? Can the student use language to say what he or she wants to do, or to explain how he or she feels?

Information also needs to be collected on how the student uses language for academic purposes and learning. For example, it is important to know if the student can use language effectively to describe an object or event. Other lessons may require students to use language to make predictions and inferences, to make and defend judgments and opinions, and to compare and contrast. Figure 10–3 presents a language use inventory that can be used to record the student's use of language in a variety of structured and unstructured situations in the classroom.

How Do You Gather the Information?

Get into the classroom at least once per week for *all students on your caseload.* Watch how classrooms work and what it takes for a student to be successful. Don't feel guilty about doing lots of observation.

Because the classroom teacher has many opportunities to observe the student's use of language in learning situations, information can be obtained from the teacher using a checklist that contains the relevant behaviors (see Figure 10–3). The teacher can focus on the student's overall ability to use language as he or she has observed throughout the school year.

Information should also be gathered by direct observations. A language use inventory will help you record the student's use of language in specific instructional tasks. Because the use of language depends so much on the task, it usually makes sense to use this inventory to obtain information over several days or in a variety of learning situations.

I. How the Student Gives Information

1. Student gives information to others
   _____ usually on his or her own
   _____ sometimes on his or her own
   _____ only when asked

2. Student gives information
   _____ in classroom discussion
   _____ one-to-one conversation
   _____ play or free time with other students

3. When student gives information or explains something, people
   _____ usually understand
   _____ sometimes understand
   _____ have difficulty understanding

II. How the Student Gets Information

1. Student gets most of his or her information (learns best) through:
   _____ listening
   _____ seeing
   _____ reading
   _____ doing it on student's own
   _____ a combination of all of these

2. If student doesn't know something,
   _____ he or she usually asks
   _____ sometimes asks
   _____ rarely asks

III. How the Student Uses Language in the Classroom

A. Using Language for Basic School Communication

   1. Student uses language to ask permission.
   2. Student uses language to refuse to do something.
   3. Student uses language to criticize something/someone.
   4. Student uses language to praise something/someone.
   5. Student uses language to say what he or she believes.
   6. Student uses language to explain how he or she feels.
   7. Student uses language to say what he or she wants to do.

B. Using Language for Learning

   1. Student uses language to instruct, and provide sequential directions for how to do something.
   2. Student uses language to inquire, and gain information by asking questions.
   3. Student uses language to describe, or to tell about something; to give necessary information to identify.
   4. Student uses language to compare and contrast, or to show how things are similar and different.
   5. Student uses language to explain, or to tell why and provide specific examples.
   6. Student uses language to predict, or tell what might logically happen as a consequence.
   7. Student uses language to infer, or arrive at a conclusion from facts that are provided.
   8. Student uses language to evaluate, and judge the relative importance of an idea.

Figure 10–3. Student language use inventory: Teacher interview and observation guide. (Adapted from Gruenwald, L., & Pollak, S. [1990]. *Language interaction in curriculum and instruction* [2nd ed.]. Austin, TX: Pro-Ed.)

What Does the Student Know About the Classroom Rules, and the Various Routines or Scripts Followed in the Classroom?

Children's performance on many learning tasks is affected by what they know about how to act and interact in specific situations in the classroom. This knowledge is referred to as a script. Script knowledge includes information on the actors (who can participate), the props (what materials and tools are needed), the routine or required actions (what each actor is supposed to do and when to do it), and all of the possible variations.

Scripts can be used to describe virtually all classroom learning tasks. For example, the script for quiet in the classroom may include the teacher flicking the light and counting to 10. Students may be expected to know that they need to have the tops of their desks clear and be sitting quietly facing the front of the room by the time the teacher reaches the number 10. Other common classroom scripts include how teachers give directions for homework assignments and the rules for participating in class discussions, such as knowing when hands should be raised and when it is permissible to speak out.

Some classroom rules are stated by the classroom teacher. Other rules are implicit, and therefore never communicated directly to the student. Most children learn the stated and unstated classroom rules easily. Other children may have difficulty learning the rules given to the class as a whole, may be unable to generalize stated rules to new situations, or may not pick up on subtle verbal and nonverbal cues for learning the teacher's unstated rules.

Knowledge of the script enables the student to determine what is appropriate to do and say during the event or task. Some language-learning disabled students may have difficulty following classroom directions or participating verbally in classroom activities because they have not learned the appropriate scripts. The information that we gather during our assessment can be used to help students develop stronger school scripts.

What Information Do You Need to Gather?

To answer this question you need to obtain information on the scripts necessary for a variety of classroom instructional tasks and on the student's knowledge of various classroom scripts. It is important to determine if the student does not know the rules, perceives the rules and scripts differently from the teacher and classmates, or is not able to recognize subtle clues to identify the teacher's rules for various classroom tasks and the teacher's mood.

Figure 10–4 presents some questions that can help determine the behavior scripts for a particular classroom. Answering these questions will give you an idea of the explicit and implicit classroom rules that students are expected to follow.

A. Questions for determining the **behavior script** for a particular classroom
  1. When is talking allowed?
  2. When is it okay for the student to ask a question in class?
  3. What are students supposed to do when they need help? Is it permissible to get help from peers?
  4. When is it okay for the student to talk out without raising a hand?
  5. What is the first thing the student should do when class begins?
  6. When are students supposed to give a short, specific answer, and when is an elaborated answer expected?
  7. How important is it to use correct grammar and complete sentences when talking? Writing?

B. Questions for determining the **teacher's cues** for a classroom script
  1. How does teacher communicate satisfaction/dissatisfaction with student?
  2. What does the teacher say or do to indicate that something is really important?
  3. How does the student know when the teacher is joking or teasing?
  4. What does the teacher do when it is time for a lesson to begin?

C. Questions for determining the **child's awareness** of classroom scripts and teacher cues
  1. Does the student know when to be quiet?
  2. Does the student know when to ask a question?
  3. Does the student know when to raise his or her hand, and when it's okay to talk out?
  4. Does the student know when it's okay to answer in single words, and when to use complete sentences?
  5. Does the student know when the teacher is joking? Dissatisfied? About to say something important?

Figure 10–4. Classroom script inventory. (Adapted from Creaghead, N. (1992). Classroom interactional analysis/script analysis. In J. Damico [Ed.], *Best practices in school speech-language pathology: Descriptive/nonstandardized language assessment.* San Antonio, TX: The Psychological Corporation/Harcourt Brace Jovanovich.)

How Do You Gather That Information?

Information can be obtained on the teacher's perceptions of rules in his or her classroom by using the questions in Figure 10–4 as part of an interview. You can also gain insight into classroom scripts by making direct observations of various classroom routines. Select a specific lesson and attempt to answer the questions in Figure 10.4. Through observation, you are attempting to discover the classroom rules and scripts, both explicitly (stated by the teacher) and implicitly (not stated). It is important to talk with the teacher after the observation to verify the accuracy of what you saw, heard, and concluded about the script requirements of the classroom.

After determining the script requirements of a specific learning task, you should examine the teacher's cues for defining the script and alerting the children when a given script is to begin. It is helpful to compare the cues for scripts in which the child is successful and those in which he or she is not. This may allow you to identify specific teacher cues that facilitate the student's performance in the learning task.

Student problems with following directions may relate to their lack of script knowledge of what to do and how to participate in the classroom.

Finally, you need information on the child's awareness of the script and the teacher's cues. For example, does the student know when to be quiet? Does the student know when questions are allowed? Does the student know when it is okay to talk out without raising his or her hand? This information can usually be obtained by asking the student directly.

Section Summary

It is important to assess the student's language use in the classroom because it is one of the critical language components that interact in all learning activities. Three specific assessment questions need to be answered. Does the student have sufficient oral language skills to do the instructional task? Can the student use language for a variety of academic purposes? What does the student know about the various routines and scripts followed in the classroom? Formal tests of language can provide us with some information on student language abilities. Teacher interviews and direct observation, however, must be used to gather information on how the student uses language in real classroom contexts.

ASSESSING TEACHER AND INSTRUCTIONAL LANGUAGE

Teacher language is the second of the three interacting language variables we will address. The talk that students encounter in school can be quite different from the conversations they experience with family and friends outside of the classroom. School discourse places additional demands on the student's ability to understand language, which continues to become more context-free as age and grade level increase. Communication in the classroom relies heavily on the meaning expressed by the teacher's spoken words. In school there are fewer opportunities for the student and teacher to engage in communicative repair if a breakdown occurs in the child's comprehension. At home, parents may make revisions and repetitions as often as necessary, tailored to fit the child and the situation. In the classroom, however, teachers must try to accommodate the varying needs of all the listeners in their classrooms, and they often must do this with little prior knowledge of the individual student's experiences.

Other differences between school and home discourse are also apparent. The style of teacher talk can affect a student's ability to process incoming verbal information. Teachers often adopt an expository style that includes numerous directions, explanations, and a variety of questions, all centered around topics in the curriculum. Finally, the complexity of the sentence structures that teachers use, in addition to suprasegmental variables such as rate of speech, intonation, and stress, can either facilitate making the intended meaning of the message clear to the listener, or interfere with processing rather than aiding it.

The language used by the classroom teacher influences the responses of students in an instructional task. It is important to analyze the effect of teacher talk within an instructional task. This analysis provides clues about how a teacher's language interacts with the language abilities of a student who is having communication and academic problems. This information can help teachers become more aware of how their language affects the performance of students in their classroom, and allows them to tune in closely to the multiple verbal and nonverbal signs that individual children in their classrooms are comprehending or not. There are at least three specific questions that should be asked about teacher language.

What Are the Length and Rate of the Teacher's Verbal Instructions? How Much Talking Does the Teacher Do?

An excessive amount of teacher talk can create passive or confused listeners in students with language-learning problems. These students may have difficulty focusing on the important information if it is embedded in a lengthy discourse. Students may process academic information better if opportunities for student talk and questions are built into the lesson. Repeating or paraphrasing a direction may help some students who did not understand it the first time. While it may be beneficial to repeat instructions, lengthy or complicated repetitions may not positively affect student comprehension. It is important to determine whether the length of the direction is affecting the response of the student with a language-learning disorder. The rate of the teacher's speech also may affect the student's understanding of the message.

> When a student does not understand verbal directions, find out whether changes in teacher talk improve comprehension.

What Information Do You Need to Gather?

Information should be gathered on the rate and on the amount of teacher talk that occurs during a particular instructional task. First, identify the aspects of teacher talk that seem to match and support the student's comprehension in the task (strengths). Focusing on strengths of teacher talk is important for several reasons. Teacher talk behaviors that appear to facilitate student performance in one learning situation may be applied to other contexts and to other students with language-learning problems. In addition, discussing facilitative language behaviors with the teacher builds rapport and trust. This may make teachers receptive to examining their own language as it interacts with the language abilities of their students.

Teacher talk behaviors that do not appear to match the level of the student's comprehension (potential mismatches) should also be described. When potential mismatches are observed, they should be accompanied by a hypothesis of a modification that might foster a better match between teacher talk and student listening. For example, you might note that a teacher effectively used intonation to highlight important concepts or vocabulary words in a lesson (strength). This is an important strategy to use with students who have language-learning disorders. At some point in the lesson, the teacher might have asked three questions in a row without pauses for students to respond (potential mismatch). In this case, it would be appropriate to explore whether a strategy of pausing for several seconds between each question might facilitate the comprehension of the student with a language-learning disorder (hypothesis). The speech-language pathologist and the teacher might brainstorm about other possible hypotheses or strategies for increasing student comprehension and then systematically try them out in future lessons.

How Do You Gather That Information?

Information on teacher language can be gathered by observing an instructional task in the classroom and using the format in Figure 10–5 to take notes and write down examples in each category. To save time, try to limit your observations to classroom tasks that seem to be especially difficult for the student with language-learning problems. Consultation with the teacher prior to the observation can provide useful information about which task(s) to observe.

The Use of Tape Recording Equipment

Because it is difficult to write down everything that a teacher says during an observation, you may sometimes tape record the lesson for later analysis. If you and the teacher are in a collaborative relationship and he or she voluntarily agrees to participate, try to tape record a 5- or 10-minute segment of a lesson with an individual student who is experiencing difficulty in learning the task. The lesson should be an exchange between student and teacher. Initially, you can listen for examples in one or two teacher talk categories each time the tape is played. With practice, it is possible to chart several items during one listening session.

As a general rule, recording equipment should be considered when the communication is unfolding so quickly that it simply cannot be reliably heard and written down in real time. Recording equipment is also used when the language and communicative behaviors of interest are so complex that all aspects of language cannot be focused on simultaneously. The analyses of tape transcripts can provide insights that may not be available merely by listening to an exchange between a teacher and a student.

Cautions When Analyzing Teacher Language: Empower Rather Than Judge

It is important to keep in mind that one of our main goals is to help teachers become skilled in analyzing their own lessons to obtain insights into and control over the language of teaching. Increased knowledge can also allow teachers the opportunity to acknowledge

Teacher Language During Lesson	Strengths	Potential Mismatches	Hypothesis
1. Rate of teacher talk:			
Amount of teacher talk time:			
2. Teacher's instructional language			
a. Questions			
Number of questions asked:			
Pauses for students to answer:			
Types of questions			
Close-ended:			
Open-ended:			
b. Directions			
Number of directions given:			
Single concept directions:			
Multiple concept directions:			
c. Explanations			
Length of explanations:			
Clarity of explanations:			
3. Teacher's sentences			
a. Sentence Complexity			
Simple Sentences:			
Complex Sentences:			
b. Sentence Length			
Short Sentences:			
Long Sentences:			

Figure 10–5. Recording format for teacher's language. (Adapted from Gruenewald, L., & Pollack, S. (1990). *Language interaction in curriculum and instruction* [2nd ed.]. Austin, TX: Pro-Ed.)

their strengths or, if they think it necessary, to modify their instructional style as a tool for facilitating student learning. The overall purpose of analyzing teacher talk should not be viewed as judgmental.

There are several reasons why teachers might be reluctant to participate in this activity. Recording and analyzing language can be quite time-consuming. It also may make some persons uncomfortable or embarrassed to listen to their voices. In some cases it may be frustrating, disappointing, and threatening for a teacher to hear that what was intended to be conveyed was not. For these reasons, teacher participation must be voluntary.

How Syntactically Complex Are the Teacher's Messages in the Classroom?

The length and complexity of teachers' sentences may not match the language comprehension abilities of some students with language-learning disorders. When this occurs, these students may encounter difficulties when engaged in a specific instructional task. Sentence complexity refers to whether the teacher uses mostly simple, compound, or complex sentences. A simple sentence is defined as containing a subject, verb, and object; a compound sentence is composed of two or more simple sentences; a complex sentence includes dependent and independent clauses connected by conjunctions.

What Information Do You Need to Gather?

It is necessary to obtain information on the number of simple and complex sentences that are used by the teacher in a specific instructional task. You also want to know the approximate number of sentences that were short (for example, 7 words or less) and those that were long (for example, 8 words or more).

How Do You Gather That Information?

This information can be obtained by direct observation and/or a tape recording of a specific teacher–student interaction. The recording format presented in Figure 10–5 guides the observation.

What Instructional Style Does the Teacher Use, and How Varied Are the Teacher's Questions, Directions, and Explanations?

The expository style that most teachers use in the classroom contains many explanations, directions, and questions. Students with language disorders may not be able to process and remember directions and explanations that are lengthy or that contain multiple concepts. It is also difficult for some students to understand a rapid series of directions that are all given at one time.

Teachers spend a great deal of time asking questions during instructional activities. Students with language disorders may be overwhelmed by many questions unless there is sufficient pause time between questions. A pause time of at least 3 seconds gives students time to think and formulate an answer.

Questions may be close-ended or open-ended. Close-ended questions usually require "narrow thinking." This means that they often have a single answer that is correct. Teachers usually know the answers to close-ended questions that they give students. In most educational systems, these close-ended "knowledge" and "comprehension" questions allow students to demonstrate their knowledge verbally to teachers. This is a skill related to academic success, and something that students with language-learning disorders need to know how to do. Close-ended questions typically involve recalling facts, naming places, or yes or no responses. Open-ended questions focus on broader, higher level thinking skills such as making inferences and generalizations, predicting, or evaluating. Open-ended questions usually have many possible responses.

Both types of questions are appropriate, depending on the lesson, the teacher's goals for the lesson, and the language abilities of the students. Using majority of close-ended questions, however, does not assist students with language-learning problems in using language to develop the higher levels of thinking that are required in the upper grades. When teachers vary their questions, they allow students to practice using language to develop higher levels of thinking. Figure 10–6 presents examples of some close- and open-ended questions that might be used in the curricular areas of language arts, science, and social studies.

> The taxonomy of questions for "higher level thinking" (see Figure 10–6) makes an excellent tool to include in both classroom language assessment and intervention. Find out how your students answer these questions.

What Information Do You Need to Gather?

Information should be gathered on the instructional talk that teachers use in the classroom. You should analyze the types of questions that were asked in a given instructional task. Information should also be obtained on how the teacher gives directions or instructions, and if they appear to match student comprehension abilities. The approximate length and number of concepts expressed in teacher explanations should also be noted.

How Do You Gather That Information?

This assessment data can be obtained by direct observation and/or a tape recording of a specific teacher–student interaction. The recording format presented in Figure 10–5 guides the observation.

Teacher Language Example

The following example from Gruenewald and Pollak (1990, p. 11) illustrates how teacher language can interact with students' ability to solve a math story problem using subtraction.

> Teacher: I have a story problem I want you to do. I will do it, too. First, I want you to listen. Then, I will give you a copy of it and we will do it together and then we will do the figuring. The first thing we are going to do—I want to ask you to think whether or not you have to do addition or subtracting first. Think really hard. Just do the whole problem. Don't just write down plus or minus. Just do the whole problem whether you think it is adding or subtracting.

> *Yesterday Sue traveled 36 miles. Today Ed traveled 53 miles. How many more miles did Ed travel than Sue?*

Type	Definition	Language Arts	Science	Social Studies
Close-Ended/Narrow				
Knowledge	Memorizes and repeats information presented; answers simple questions.	What was the little girl's name in Charlottes Web? Where did Templeton the rat live?	What kind of rock is made of mud and clay pressed together?	Where did the Alaskan oil spill occur? What company owned the boat that caused the spill?
Comprehension	Demonstrates understanding by paraphrasing or stating information in another form.	What was the story about? Tell me the story you just heard.	Explain how metamorphic rock is produced.	Describe how the Alaskan oil spill occurred.
Open-Ended/Broad				
Application	Uses information or principles in new but similar situations.	Charlotte and Wilbur are friends. How can friends help each other?	(After discussion of the characteristics of granite) What could we use granite for?	What are some other ways that the wildlife could have been rescued?
Analysis	Identifies components, gives reasons, identifies problems.	How did Wilbur change over the course of the story?	How are limestone, shale, and sandstone alike?	What types of problems were caused by the spill?
Synthesis	Generalizes from previously learned knowledge to generate new solutions to problems.	What would have happened if Templeton hadn't found words for Charlotte to weave in her web?	How would the world be different if there were no volcanoes?	What kinds of problems would occur if there were a chemical spill in our town?
Evaluation	Compares alternatives, states opinions, justifies responses.	Which character do you like best in this story and why?	If you had to create a monument, what type of rock would you use and why?	Discuss who should be responsible for the clean-up and why they should be responsible.

Figure 10–6. Examples of open-ended (broad) and close-ended (narrow) questions in several curriculum areas. (Based on Bloom, B. [1956]. *Taxonomy of educational objectives: Cognitive domains.* New York: David McKay Co.; Westby, C. [1985]. Learning to talk—Talking to learn: Oral-literate language differences. In C. Simon [Ed.], *Communication skills and classroom success: Therapy methodologies for language-learning disabled students.* San Diego, CA: College-Hill Press; and Gruenewald, L., & Pollack, S. [1990]. *Language interaction in curriculum and instruction* [2nd ed.] Austin, TX: Pro-Ed.)

Teacher: Okay, let's see. Would you please put your sign down so I know exactly what you did? Okay, and let's see—David, you said you plussed 36 and 53, and Debbie, you said you plussed also. Okay what were the key words in that story?

Debbie: How many.

David: How many more.

Teacher: How many more. Does that tell you that you had to be adding?

Students: Yes.

Teacher: We want to know how many miles. Are we going to put them together or find a difference? Ed traveled more miles. Right? When we are finding more miles are we adding or subtracting?

Students: (no response)

Even though these students may have been able to perform the operation of subtraction when presented as a standard math problem (e.g., $53 - 36 = ?$), the language of the math story prevented them from solving the problem. The length and grammatical structure of the teacher's explanations did not appear to match the students' comprehension abilities. Also, the teacher asked a series of three questions without waiting for a response. A preliminary hypothesis might ask if opportunities for the students to use verbal language to solve the problem or ask questions would have aided student performance.

Section Summary

It is important for teachers to analyze the language they use during instruction because it interacts with student language and the curriculum in all learning tasks. Speech-language pathologists can help gather data on instructional language for teachers who choose to participate in these activities. There are three specific assessment questions that can be answered with regard to teacher talk. What is the length and rate of the teacher's verbal instructions? How syntactically complex are the teacher's messages in the classroom? How effective are the teacher's questions, directions, and explanations? In a collaborative environment, this information can help teachers become aware of how their language affects the comprehension of students with language-learning disorders.

ASSESSING LANGUAGE REQUIREMENTS OF THE CURRICULUM

The language of the curriculum is the third component that interacts with student language and teacher language in all learning tasks. What is the curriculum? As used in this chapter, the term "curriculum" refers to the lessons, textbooks, worksheets, and the scope and sequence of the actual content of what is being taught (and learned) in the classroom. For example, a third-grade class will have a curriculum for Math, Language Arts (including reading, writing and spelling), and Science. Nelson (1989) pointed out that there are other curricula in schools besides this "official" curriculum. She suggests that students must have knowledge of "school culture" curriculum (e.g., implicit and explicit classroom scripts) and "de facto" curriculum (e.g., lesson content determined by the "Teacher's Guide" to a particular textbook series), among others. The official curriculum will be the focus of this section.

To help students with language-learning disorders, speech-language pathologists and teachers must analyze the language of the lessons and textbooks that students are expected to use and understand. The language requirements of specific lessons and texts can be analyzed in at least three ways. First, we must examine both the prerequisite vocabulary and new vocabulary that will be needed to understand the information presented in the lesson. Second, we need to look at how the students will be expected to demonstrate their comprehension of the lesson and how they will be expected to express themselves orally and in written form. Third, we also want to look closely at the sentence structures that students encounter in the oral lessons and written materials. These three curriculum variables will affect the ability of students to learn and understand the lesson.

What Vocabulary and Concepts Do the Curriculum Materials Contain?

Effective assessment of the language of curriculum materials requires that you *read the books and worksheets that the student is expected to read.* School speech-language pathologists should attend the same district workshops on curriculum that regular education teachers attend.

In any given subject area, and in every instructional task and textbook, there is a set of *explicit vocabulary words* that is fundamental to the content or concepts that are being taught. When performing a curriculum analysis, it is critical to consider the prerequisite vocabulary a student is expected to know. Likewise, it is important to identify new vocabulary that will be presented in the lesson or text. For example, a fourth-grade science project might have many prerequisite vocabulary items that have been previously taught, including *grams, meter, width, height, length,* and *solid.* The new vocabulary that will be introduced in the lesson, and that will be the foundation for the new subject matter, might include the terms *kilometer, centimeter, liquid, volume, mass* and *density.*

In addition to the vocabulary, each instructional task requires the student to have knowledge of some underlying concepts. These concepts are just as important to learning as the explicit vocabulary words, but may not be as obvious to the student or the teacher. For example, the concept knowledge required for performing a science experiment on measurement includes *conservation* (as expressed by the vocabulary items *more, less*) and *seriation* (as expressed by the vocabulary items *big, bigger, biggest*).

In this chapter it is not feasible to cover all of the possible concepts and vocabulary that are taught in the various curricula in the schools. However, there are several basic concepts that you can describe and analyze in a variety of curricular materials in the classroom.

Classification

Classification operations are strategies for organizing and grouping objects, symbols, and events. Each classification task has its own specific vocabulary. For example, classifying objects by their perceptual attributes requires the use of words to describe their color, shape, size, texture, and form. Classifying objects by their function requires vocabulary words to talk about the uses of objects and how they function. If objects are grouped into categories, the relevant vocabulary words include the names of classes of objects (e.g., fruits, animals, words that start with the letter A).

Classification skills are embedded in many academic areas including Math (formation of sets, story problems), Social Studies (outlining, historical concepts, geography), Reading Comprehension (main ideas, part/whole relationships), and Science (classes of plants and animals).

Conservation

Conservation is defined as the ability to realize that certain attributes of an object are constant, even though that object may change in appearance. For example, pouring liquid from a short, fat glass into a tall, thin glass may change the appearance but not the volume. The ability to conserve is basic to the understanding of number, measurement, and space.

The vocabulary items associated with conservation concepts differ depending on the nature of the instructional task. For example, the vocabulary for Number includes the terms *more, less, the same as, all, half, whole, few, before,* and *after*. The vocabulary for Size includes the terms *tall, short, thin, fat, wide, narrow, high,* and *low*. The explicit vocabulary for Length includes the terms *taller than, shorter than,* and the *same length*.

Time

Time, or temporal concepts, can be expressed in two ways: temporal order (sequence) and duration (the time interval between two events). Vocabulary words used to express temporal order include *first, second, before, during, after, next, last, earlier,* and *later*. Vocabulary words used to express duration or time include *morning, afternoon, old, young, long time, today, tomorrow, yesterday, hour,* and *day*. Time concepts are found in the academic areas of Social Studies (dates, times), Language Arts (order of events in a story), Math (measurement), and Science (seasons, changes over time).

Seriation

The concept of seriation involves the ability to learn the relationships between objects and put them in order. Vocabulary associated with seriation includes number (*first, second, third,* etc.), size (*big, bigger, biggest*), length (*long, longer, longest*), height (*tall, taller, tallest*), space/time (*in front of, behind, before, after*), and amount (*least, most*).

Space

Spatial concepts are required to locate the position of objects in relation to one another. This requires the ability to view an object from different points of view. Vocabulary used to talk about the location of an object in space includes *over, under, above, below, in front of, in back of, behind, next to, right and left, in, out, on, off, inside, outside, top,* and *bottom*.

What Information Do You Need to Gather?

Information should be obtained on the prerequisite vocabulary and concepts that students are expected to know, and the new vocabulary that will be presented in the lesson and instructional materials and text.

How Do You Gather That Information?

The only way to gather information on vocabulary and concepts in curriculum materials is for you to read the books, materials, and worksheets that the students will be exposed to. It is important to confer with the teacher and decide which specific curriculum materials should be examined. If finding a time for meeting with the teacher is difficult, the speech-language pathologist can request to see the curriculum objectives and the text pages or materials the teacher will use over the next few weeks. To analyze these materials, simply list the important prerequisite vocabulary and concepts and the new vocabulary presented in the materials, and check these with the teacher at a later time. Examples of the vocabulary and conceptual content of lessons can be recorded on an analysis guide like the one in Figure 10–7.

What Are the Language Comprehension and Expression Requirements of the Lesson?

What Information Do You Need to Gather?

When reviewing the language requirements of specific curriculum lessons and materials, Prelock et al. (1993) suggested that an analysis should be performed of the three major ways that students are expected to demonstrate mastery of the subject material. The fol-

A. Vocabulary Review of Curriculum

    1. Identify **prerequisite** vocabulary necessary for achieving lesson objectives:

    2. List **new** vocabulary to be introduced:

B. Concepts Necessary for Achieving Lesson Objectives

    Check appropriate line for underlying concepts required in the instructional task:

    _____ Conservation (number, size, length, amount)

    _____ Time (temporal order, duration)

    _____ Spatial

    _____ Causality (cause/effect)

    _____ Classification (sorting, inclusion/exclusion, regrouping)

    _____ Order/seriation (number, length, height, space/time, amount)

C. Language Requirements Review

    1. Comprehension: Student must demonstrate comprehension by (check all that apply):

_____ pointing/showing	_____ circling, drawing
_____ sequencing pictures/words/sentences/numbers	_____ manipulating objects
_____ role playing	_____ answering questions
_____ following oral directions	_____ following written directions
_____ demonstrating or restating directions	
_____ other (please specify):	

    2. Oral Expression: Student must express self verbally by (check all that apply):

_____ defining vocabulary	_____ storytelling or retelling
_____ talking in complete sentences	_____ reciting known information
_____ answering and asking questions	_____ oral reading
_____ explaining answers	_____ clarifying responses
_____ other (Please specify):	

    3. Written Expression: Student must express self in writing by (check all that apply):

_____ writing numbers/letters	_____ copying numbers/letters/words
_____ spelling words	_____ filling in sentences
_____ making outlines	_____ writing complete sentences
_____ writing stories	_____ writing book reports
_____ writing explanations	_____ creating word problems
_____ writing equations/formulas	
_____ other (please specify):	

Figure 10–7. Format for recording vocabulary, concepts, and language requirements in curriculum Materials. (Adapted from Gruenewald, & Pollack, [1990], and Prelock, Miller, & Reed [1993]).

lowing assessment questions can be asked. First, how will students demonstrate comprehension of the lesson? For example, will they be asked to follow oral directions, manipulate objects, or answer questions? Second, how will students be expected to express themselves orally? Will they need to define vocabulary words, explain their answers, or talk in complete sentences? Last, how will students be expected to express themselves in written form? For example, will they need to write complete sentences, make outlines, or fill in sentences?

How Do You Gather That Information?

Information on the comprehension, oral expression, and written expression skills required by the curricular materials, texts, or lessons can be gathered by observing an instructional task in the classroom and using the analysis format in Figure 10–7. Consultation with the teacher prior to the observation can provide useful information about which task(s) to observe. Try to limit your observations to classroom tasks that seem to be especially difficult for the student with language-learning problems. This practice can save you time.

What Sentence Structures Do the Curriculum Materials Contain?

The language in a reading assignment or in the instructions on a worksheet may include sentence structures that do not match the comprehension abilities of students with language-learning disorders. Complex sentence forms that the student can understand in spoken social communication may be incomprehensible when encountered in written form. Thus, it is important to analyze the sentence structures and grammatical forms embedded in curriculum materials.

What Information Do You Need to Gather?

To answer this question, you need to obtain information on the major sentence structures and the constituent parts of sentences that are contained in the curriculum materials. Constituent parts of a sentence include verb tenses, comparatives, prepositions, conjunctions, negatives, questions, and modifiers.

There are two ways to analyze this information. First, you should determine what sentence forms the task requires the student to *produce*. For example, is the student expected to write the answers to reading comprehension questions in complete, syntactically correct sentences? If so, does the student need to use simple, compound, or complex sentences? Second, you should determine what sentence structures the materials require the student to *understand*. For example, does the student need to understand prepositional phrases and comparatives? Are the instructions written in simple sentences, or are they complex? Figure 10–8 presents a list of major sentence types and constituent parts of sentences that guide the analysis of curriculum materials.

How Do You Gather That Information?

The only way to determine the conceptual content and the sentence structures in curriculum materials is to analyze carefully the materials themselves. Examples of the major sentence structures and sentence parts required by the curricular materials, texts, or lessons can be listed on an analysis guide like the one presented in Figure

	Production (Speaking and Writing)	Comprehension (Listening and Reading)
A. Major sentence structures required by the task		
1. Simple sentences		
2. Compound sentences (*and, but, or*)		
3. Complex sentences (*when, if, because*)		
B. Constituent parts of sentences		
1. Morphological endings		
Plurals: regular (*-s, -es*)		
irregular (*man/men*)		
Tenses: regular (*-ed, -t*)		
irregular (*went, run*)		
Possessives:		
Comparatives (*-er, -est*):		
2. Other sentence parts		
Prepositions		
Conjunctions		
Negation		
Questions (*what, where, who, when, how, which, why*)		
Modifiers (adjectives, adverbs)		

Figure 10–8. Guide for analyzing sentence structure in curriculum materials. (Adapted from Gruenewald, L., & Pollack, S. [1990]. *Language interaction in curriculum and instruction* [2nd ed.]. Austin, TX: Pro-Ed.)

10–8. The classroom teacher can help select the curricular materials that seem most difficult for the student. These may come from a wide variety of learning tasks, such as written instructions on a worksheet, an assignment in a textbook, or even sample class tests and quizzes.

Curricular Concepts Example

The following example from Gruenewald and Pollak (1990, p. 26) illustrates concepts and sentence forms embedded in a fourth-grade math lesson.

> *A turkey is to be cooked 20 minutes for each pound. If a turkey weighing 10 pounds is to be done at 5 P.M., what time should it be put in the oven to cook?*

The explicit vocabulary representing the temporal concepts in this example are *5 P.M.* and *20 minutes*. The underlying temporal concepts and operations (implicit) include duration of time (length of cooking time is 20 minutes × 10), number of minutes to the hour (200 minutes/60 = 3⅓ hours), and reversibility (working backward from 5 P.M. to 1:40 P.M.). Syntax requirements include complex sentences with *if—what then* constructions.

There are several possible reasons why a fourth-grade student with a language-learning disorder might have difficulty with this problem. One reason is that the student may not understand that the concepts of *a.m.* and *p.m.* are equivalent to morning, afternoon, and evening (e.g., the concept of a day). It is also possible that the student may not have the concept of *duration* as being equivalent to the interval between two points. Another possibility is that the student might not understand complex sentences with *if-then* constructions.

This type of analysis allows teachers and speech-language pathologists to hypothesize whether aspects of the language in curriculum materials match the level that our students can process. From these hypotheses, we can systematically implement one or more interventions that might result in a better match between the materials and the student's cognitive and language level. For example, instructions for an assignment could be rewritten or rephrased using different syntactic constructions. The teacher might try having a peer read instructions to the student. The student could be asked to paraphrase the instructions and ask clarification questions if parts were not understood. The speech-language pathologist might try preteaching the required concepts or vocabulary to the student.

Section Summary

The language embedded in texts, lessons, and other instructional materials in the curriculum must be carefully examined. These language forms and content will interact with student language and teacher language, and affect the ability of students to learn. There are at least three specific assessment questions that can be asked. What vocabulary and concepts do the curriculum materials contain, both explicitly and implicitly? How must students demonstrate comprehension of the lesson, and how must they express themselves orally and in writing? What sentence structures do the curriculum materials contain? Answers to these questions can lead the speech-language pathologist and the teacher to generate hypotheses about possible interventions to help students with language-learning disorders.

USING AND INTERPRETING CLASSROOM LANGUAGE INFORMATION

The information you gather on a student's classroom speaking and listening skills, teacher and instructional language, and the language and vocabulary requirements of the curriculum can be used in several important ways. To illustrate how this information can be used we will refer back to the diagnostic questions presented by Tomblin in Chapter 1. First, classroom language information can be used to *help determine the existence of a communication disorder.* In addition to the student's performance on norm-referenced tests of language, it is best practice to include classroom observation data in any assessment process designed to determine if a student has a language-learning disorder and is in need of (and eligible for) special education services. In fact many states and local school districts *require* that a classroom observation be performed for all initial assessments for special education eligibility. Second, classroom language information can help *determine factors causing or exacerbating the student's language problem.* As we have seen, the main purpose of classroom language assessment is to determine how student language, teacher language, and the language of the curriculum interact to help explain a student's language-learning problem. It is quite possible that a student's performance will be affected by teacher language or the language of instructional materials and lessons. Finally, and perhaps most importantly, the classroom and curriculum language information that you gather is appropriately used to *determine treatment alternatives* for a student who has a language-learning disability. Specifically, classroom observational assessment data can help a team determine IEP objectives that are valid, functional, and based on the curriculum that the student is expected to know. With good data from a classroom language assessment, the team can attempt modifications in the presentation of the curriculum material to meet the language and vocabulary requirement needs of our students. Speech-language pathologists and teachers can brainstorm about instructional strategies and develop teaching methods to assist student learning. Teaching methods such as appropriate teacher models and prompts, and visual organizers and aids, can be tried to improve student performance in classroom speaking and listening tasks.

PREPARING TO GATHER INFORMATION IN THE CLASSROOM

Speech-language pathologists need to collaborate with teachers and observe in the classroom to answer specific assessment questions about classroom language interactions. This section describes some strategies that can make the assessment of language interactions more effective.

1. Prior to the observation, set up a 15-minute block to interview the teacher using one or more of the checklists presented in this chapter, in the recommended supplemental readings, or one that you and the teacher have designed. If it is difficult to find a time to meet, it may be easier to leave the checklist and have the teacher return it to you in a day or two. Once the teacher returns the checklist, it is important to meet briefly to plan the observation.

   The teacher and you should agree on which classroom activities will be observed, when the observation(s) will take place, and the length of observation. For example, it may be possible to obtain the necessary information by observing one session, or it may be necessary to observe different sessions over several weeks. The instructional tasks that you select to observe should be those in which the student is having difficulties.

2. You may want to visit the classroom as a helper one or two times prior to your observation. This will allow you to become familiar with the general layout of the classroom and allow the children to become familiar with you. An observer's presence in the classroom is soon forgotten by the children. There should be close coordination with the teacher so that classroom disruption is kept to a minimum.

3. Record information such as the child's name, and contextual features that may be important for interpreting the assessment data at a later time. The following contextual information should be noted: time of day; information about the instructional activity; a sketch or map of the classroom including the student's, teacher's, and peer's place/position; the types of instructional materials used; and other information that will allow you to analyze the physical, temporal, and social organization of the activity, including its communication requirements.

4. Check with the teacher the morning of the observation to confirm that the student is present, and that the learning activity will go on at the scheduled time as planned.

   How long should the observation be? The amount of time per observation should be kept within reason. Start with 10- or 15-minute observation periods. By limiting the observation to a student's specific problem in an instructional task, it does not have to be an enormous task requiring extensive time.

5. It is necessary to compare notes with the teacher sometime shortly after your classroom observation. This allows you to integrate the viewpoint of the teacher and confirm the accuracy of your own observations. Discrepancies in the viewpoint of the teacher about the accuracy of these written records should be discussed.

If the teacher has previously volunteered to collaborate and analyze a tape recording of a lesson, schedule a time when this activity can take place. The teacher's role is to stop the tape when the child (or the teacher) is engaged in behaviors that are related either to the reason for a potential referral or to the initial problem. The tape should also be stopped when a contrast is noted between the target child's behaviors and those of other children in the activity, or when something occurs that the teacher would like to comment on.

CONCLUSION

Formal or standardized language tests can not provide you with all of the information you need to help students with language-learning disorders succeed in school. Spending time in classrooms and becoming familiar with the language requirements of instructional activities allows you to gather relevant assessment data. Current classroom-based service delivery models emphasize the need for collaboration with regular classroom teachers, both to plan and carry out valid assessments and to design intervention strategies and classroom modifications.

Assessing language interactions takes time, effort, and training. Given the time constraints that affect all teachers and speech-language pathologists who work in schools, it is sometimes tempting to limit language assessment to an initial assessment battery that focuses primarily on student strengths and weaknesses. Classroom-based language assessment is well worth the time and effort. The information you gather in the classroom is the most relevant to the real life language and learning problems the student faces. Language interventions that are based on relevant classroom assessment data have the best chance of making a real difference for students with language-learning disorders.

REFERENCES

Bloom, B. (1956). *Taxonomy of educational objectives: Cognitive domains.* New York: David McKay Co.

Creaghead, N. (1992). Classroom interactional analysis/script analysis. In J. Damico (Ed.), *Best practices in school speech-language pathol-*

ogy: Descriptive/nonstandardized language assessment. San Antonio, TX: The Psychological Corporation/Harcourt Brace Jovanovich.

Gruenewald, L., & Pollak, S. (1990). *Language interaction in curriculum and instruction* (2nd. Ed.). Austin, TX: Pro-Ed.

Nelson, N. (1989). Curriculum-based language assessment and intervention. *Language, Speech, and Hearing Services in Schools, 20*(2), 170–184.

Prelock, P., Miller, B., & Reed, N. (1993). *Working with the classroom curriculum. A guide for analysis and use in speech therapy.* San Antonio, TX: Communication Skill Builders.

Westby, C. (1985). Learning to talk—Talking to learn: Oral-literate language differences. In C. Simon (Ed.), *Communication skills and classroom success: Therapy methodologies for language-learning disabled students.* San Diego, CA: College-Hill Press.

ADDITIONAL REFERENCES

Silliman, E., & Cherry Wilkinson, L. (1991). *Communicating for learning: Classroom observation and collaboration.* Gaithersburg, MD: Aspen Publications.

Simon, C. (Ed.). (1985). *Communication skills and classroom success: Assessment of language-learning disabled students.* San Diego, CA: College-Hill Press.

CHAPTER

11

Aphasia and Related Disorders

Julie A. G. Stierwalt, Ph.D.
Heather M. Clark, Ph.D. and
Donald A. Robin, Ph.D.

"Yes, yes," says Mrs. Fraizer, nodding vigorously from her hospital bed as you introduce yourself as the speech-language pathologist, "I have it. It's all here, but I can't talk it" (Jordan, 1994).

In a university speech-language and hearing clinic, Jim, a tall, lanky 15-year-old describes a lawnmower, "Push back on it like this, pull into like that and just pull around like this all the time."

The preceding are examples of an acquired language impairment, or aphasia. To "break it down," as one would any medical term, the prefix (a-) means without or lacking, and the root (-phasia) means speech (Stevens & Adler, 1992). The purpose of this chapter is to introduce you to the concepts related to this medical diagnosis and to the principles involved in the assessment of aphasia and related disorders.

We begin our discussion with two important ideas. The first is that, in helping the patient with aphasia, we work as members of a rehabilitation team of several professionals. The second is that mem-

Mrs. Frazier's friends and relatives who have visited her in the hospital report that she is talking, but she is not making sense.

Jim tries hard to communicate, but can not seem to find the right words and must rely on gesture and description.

bers of the team address problems such as aphasia on several levels, namely, impairment, disability, and handicap (World Health Organization, 1980).

Impairment is a disruption of, a loss of, or a change in the physiological structure of function. The impairment is identified by the name of the disease state. For example, "hemorrhage," "blood clot," "vision loss," or "hypertension" label possible impairments for individuals (Jordan, 1994). The goal of treatment for an impairment is prevention of future impairments (Frey, 1984) or avoiding exacerbation of the present impairment. While for some communication disorders, identifying the impairment is straightforward (e.g., an impairment in some types of dysarthria is muscle weakness), the impairment in aphasia and other language disorders is not well understood. That is, a term like "brain weakness" is not very useful, since it does not differentiate the specific impairments that are affecting language performance. The same is true for the terms that describe the etiology of the impairment, such as "stroke," "tumor," or "swelling," since these etiologies result in many other impairments in addition to language disturbance. Nonetheless, because the underlying impairment in aphasia is not well understood, direct treatment of the impairment is a focus primarily of physicians, who treat the disease process causing the impairment. As speech-language pathologists, we should understand the disease process, and try to facilitate the patient and family's understanding of the implications for communication.

> Family and friends need a great deal of education regarding the nature of impairment in aphasia.

Disability is defined as the functional consequence of an impairment (Frattali, 1998). Assessment of disability requires exploration of the patient's ability to perform certain tasks. In the case of aphasia, a speech-language pathologist might examine the patient's ability to think of names, follow directions, read printed material, or write checks (Jordan, 1994). Disability is an area of focus for the entire rehabilitation team. As speech-language pathologists, we strive to provide treatment to enhance the patient's ability to compensate for impairment and maximize the use of residual skills. In addition, it is important to provide continuing education for the individual and their family regarding changes in communication ability and the impact on their lifestyle.

> Aphasia can lead to disability in almost every communication context.

Finally, each member of the "team" will deal with the handicap which results from the impairment. The *handicap* is defined as the social consequence or disadvantage resulting from the impairment or disability, which limits or prevents an individual from fulfilling a role that is normal. In the case of aphasia, an individual who relied on verbal communication a great deal in his vocation prior to the neurologic trauma might demonstrate a greater handicap than someone who had little need for such interaction in her vocation. Our role as members of the treatment team will include educating others about the nature of aphasia as an impairment, disability, and/or handicap. This education should extend from the patients and their families to service providers, policy makers, and the voting and taxpaying public (Jordan, 1994).

> Communicative disability can result in withdrawal from social situations.

Now we return to the task of defining aphasia. While on the surface, the medical definition explains the disorder as a disruption in verbal expression, it does little to inform us about the nature and complexity of aphasia. Moreover, a simple definition of the medical term does not differentiate aphasia as an impairment in language from an impairment of the motor speech system.

To better understand aphasia as an impairment of language, we need to revisit the model of language introduced by Weiss and colleagues in Chapter 6. Weiss, Tomblin, and Robin provided a model (Figure 6–1) that depicts the complex relationship between communication and the many components that contribute to expressing and understanding language (pragmatics, syntax, morphology, semantics, phonology). Each of these parts plays an important role in successful communication, through expression or comprehension. This illustration of the complexity of language warrants a more comprehensive definition of aphasia.

Such a definition comes from the work of McNeil (1982). He wrote that,

> Aphasia is a multimodality physiological inefficiency with greater than loss of verbal symbolic manipulations (e.g., association, storage, retrieval, and rule implementation). In isolated form it is caused by focal damage to cortical and/or subcortical structures of the hemisphere(s) dominant for such symbolic manipulations. It is affected by and affects other physiological information processing and cognitive processes to the degree that they support, interact with, or are supported by the symbolic deficits. (p. 693)

From the definition proposed by McNeil, we can better understand the complexities present in the language processing of an individual who has aphasia. Based on this account, it is apparent that evaluation will include a comprehensive assessment of each of the components of the model that contribute to linguistic processing.

DETERMINATION OF THE COMPLAINT

Our knowledge of the impairment of aphasia provides us with insight on how to approach the evaluation process. Even so, evaluating the complex linguistic functions that comprise language can seem an overwhelming task. Given the model of language and the definition of aphasia, it may seem difficult to know just where to begin. Fortunately, there are basic principles of evaluation that guide us in our task. In Chapter 1, Tomblin provided us with perspectives for the assessment of communication disorders. A first step in the assessment sequence is to determine the nature of the complaint, which can be examined by obtaining a comprehensive patient history. When collecting a case history there is information that is standard to any case, regardless of etiology. However, in the case of neurogenic communi-

Inefficiency with language may be more frustrating for the patient than if language abilities were totally lost.

"I was sitting in my chair watching television, when I began to feel funny. When I tried to get up, my right leg wouldn't support me. I tried to call out but the words wouldn't come."

cation disorders there are features to review that relate specifically to neurologic function (Johnson, George, & Hinckley, 1998).

Such information would include the following:

Details of the current complaint

Neurologic symptoms

Time postonset

Nature of the onset (i.e., slow or sudden)

Course of performance

Results from neuroimaging

CT

MRI

Family history of neurologic or communication disorders

Episodic disorders

Seizures

Fluctuations in consciousness

Headaches

Fluctuations in communication abilities

This information can help to illuminate the current problem that has resulted in aphasia. Obtaining such details will guide us in our evaluation and treatment procedures.

To further define the nature of the complaint, and because aphasia is an acquired impairment secondary to brain damage, we must examine the patient's history to determine the nature of the neurologic insult. The importance of isolating the type of injury lies in the fact that variation in etiology might result in varied neurophysiologic consequences, manifestations of aphasia (or other language disturbances), and a different course of the disorder, thus leading to different prognoses for recovery of function. Etiologies that result in aphasia or related language disorders are typically related to vascular, traumatic, inflammatory, neoplasm, and/or progressive diseases.

Aphasia secondary to vascular disease typically means that the individual has suffered from a cerebral vascular accident (CVA) or stroke. A stroke may be a case of "not enough blood supplying the brain." This scenario indicates that there is a blockage somewhere in the vascular system of the brain. A CVA might also be a result of "too much blood within the brain." This type of stroke is a hemorrhagic stroke and is typically secondary to a rupture or tear within the vascular system from an abnormality such as an aneurysm, an arteriovenous malformation (AVM), or a traumatically induced dissection.

A cutoff or reduction in blood supply to the brain is called an ischemic stroke.

Because vascular malformations or abnormalities can be congenital, hemorrhagic strokes can be seen in all ages.

When there is a rupture or tear of the vascular system, there is bleeding within the brain, which results in increased pressure within the cranium.

The typical onset of stroke is sudden with a dramatic manifestation of symptoms within minutes/hours. It is anticipated that following the stroke, depending on the severity and barring complications, the symptoms will begin to resolve. Presenting symptoms will continue to evolve and improve, with the most dramatic change in the weeks/months postonset.

Another etiology that might result in a language disturbance is traumatic injury. Traumatic brain injury (TBI) is defined as an injury from a blow to the head. Although the onset is sudden, like that of a CVA, the resultant sequelae are different from an individual who has suffered from a stroke. The difference can be explained by examining the pathophysiology of injury. Injury sustained as a result of stroke is considered focal and confined to the area of blockage or hemorrhage and surrounding tissues. Neuropathology from TBI is likely more diffuse in nature. In a traumatic event, individuals probably sustain damage not only at the site of impact, but throughout the brain from shearing and rotational forces. More detail about recovery patterns for TBI patients is presented later.

> Posttraumatic amnesia is a confusional state in which individuals are disoriented to person, place, and time.

Inflammatory processes that might result in disruptions in language function include those that impact the brain (e.g. encephalitis, vasculitis, meningitis). These processes may be bacterial or viral in origin and result in inflammation within the vascular system of the brain or the coverings of the brain. With proper medical treatment, such conditions are curable; therefore, the resultant language symptoms may be transient in nature and the prognosis good.

> One form of encephalitis (herpes encephalitis) does result in long-term memory impairments that are quite severe.

The next two etiologies for consideration tend to manifest language difficulty from a more gradual onset than those previously discussed. Cancer (neoplasm) is an insidious disease that may be present in a subclinical state for some time prior to the onset of symptoms. Aphasia symptoms, in the case of a brain tumor, arise from a growth or "mass" that may be located in or adjacent to crucial language areas. The tumor applies increasing pressure as it increases in size, which can disrupt the function of these critical areas. Because of the diverse nature of brain tumors, the prognosis for aphasia secondary to brain tumors varies considerably with tumor type and stage of the disease.

> Aphasia symptoms secondary to slow growing tumors may be very subtle and slow to develop. As a result, others may write it off to

A slow onset of language disturbance can also be seen in individuals with progressive conditions such as dementia. Advances in healthcare have resulted in longer life; thus illnesses associated with aging such as this are more prevalent. Roughly 15% of individuals over the age of 85 present with some form of dementia (Davis, 1993). Although there is some debate whether the language disturbance seen in dementia is "aphasia," speech-language pathologists are frequently called upon to evaluate language and set up programs to facilitate communication interaction for individuals that fit into this diagnostic category.

Additional information regarding the nature of the complaint should also include any results from instrumental evaluation. Neuroimaging techniques have contributed greatly to our understanding of the basis for neurogenic communication disorders. Until 25–30 years ago, our knowledge of language following brain damage was comprised of results from behavioral study of individuals following neurologic trauma and when possible, postmortem examination of their brains. The advent of computerized axial-tomography (CAT) and magnetic resonance imaging (MRI) has markedly increased our understanding of the neurological bases of language (George, Vikingstad, & YueCao, 1998). These techniques have allowed us to identify specific sites of lesion and conduct more in-depth study and correlation analyses on brain-behavior relations. Additional advances in neuroimaging techniques such as positron emission tomography (PET), single photon emission computed tomography (SPECT), and functional magnetic resonance imaging (fMRI) give us the opportunity to see the brain "in action" during the performance of various tasks.

Testing for Aphasia

After gathering available information about the nature of the complaint, the next question is whether the presenting symptoms are indeed aphasia. To answer this question, we must compare the patient's current level of performance with premorbid skills, especially in mild cases. In most instances, we must make estimates based on premorbid education and occupation. If there is a reduction from expected abilities in the comprehension and/or expression of language or in any of the components that contribute to language, then a diagnosis of aphasia is warranted.

As reviewed previously, language is comprised of many components. Most often, we measure each by use of a standardized test that was designed with the specific purpose of diagnosing aphasia. There are at least two benefits of standardized tests, certainly applicable to tests of aphasia. One is that norms are available, for most tests, for comparison of the performance of this patient with other patients and sometimes normal subjects. Another is that information is usually available about test reliability and validity, two concepts described in detail by Tomblin in Chapter 1. However, there are cautions to be taken. Primarily they are related to variability of performance of the individual patient (he may do well on Tuesday but not on Wednesday) and the important issue of distinguishing in performance between memory and aphasia. For example, test items should be chosen with a careful eye toward items with which he is familiar.

Four test batteries have been widely used in the United States to assess aphasia (Davis, 1993). Details of those tests are provided in Table 11–1. Although there are differences among these tests, there is a common thread. This commonality lies in the communicative

Table 11–1. Most widely used test batteries for evaluating aphasia.

Test Name	Administration Time	Number of Subtests	Standardization
Minnesota Test for the Differential Diagnosis of Aphasia	2–6 hours with an average of 3 hours. It is recommended to divide the test across two sessions.	46	157 patients with aphasia for the majority of the test
Porch Index of Communicative Ability	1 hour for a well–trained clinician	18	130 normal adults.
Boston Diagnostic Aphasia Examination	1–3 hours	27	242 patients with aphasia
Western Aphasia Battery	2–6 hours. It is recommended to divide the test into shorter segments	8 (?)	Several groups with and without aphasia or neurologic compromise

Source: Adapted from *A survey of adult aphasia and related language disorders*, by G.A. Davis, 1993. Englewood Cliffs, NJ: Prentice-Hall.

modalities tested. If you remember our discussion about the definition of aphasia, you will remember that there are many components that make the expression and comprehension of language successful. Consequently, each of the tests that evaluate aphasia examine performance on tasks that represent various components of language. Although there are many individual subtests, there are four main themes: auditory comprehension, control of the oral motor system, verbal expression, and writing and reading.

Auditory Comprehension

Evaluating auditory comprehension involves exploring the individual's ability to understand messages that are presented through the auditory modality. A look at subtests in aphasia batteries (Table 11–2) illuminates the range of tasks evaluated under this heading. In order to fully understand where a breakdown in comprehension exists, tasks range from simplistic to complex in forms of both content and length. One method for evaluating comprehension abilities is to ask questions that are unexpected. Individuals with aphasia may become quite proficient at masking comprehension deficits because they learn the responses to the routine questions that are asked of them. If the questions are novel or unexpected, however, you might find that the individual is not fully comprehending day-to-day interaction. We also want to examine factors that facilitate comprehension, such as a slow rate, a repeat of the question or stimulus, or a reduction in the complexity of the language presented. Such techniques should be included in our evaluation of aphasia.

Sometimes comprehension abilities can be maximized through manipulating the environment. For example reducing speed and complexity of delivery may facilitate comprehension.

"My husband nods and smiles during our conversations, even when we are discussing something sad."

Table 11–2. Some common tasks utilized to evaluate auditory comprehension.

Test Battery	Subtest	Tasks
Minnesota Test for Differential Diagnosis of Aphasia	Section A (Auditory Disturbances)	Recognizing common words, discriminating between paired words, following directions, repetition
Porch Index of Communicative Ability	Six subtests	Demonstrate object function, point to object when given function, matching picture to object, point to an object given the name, matching duplicate objects
Boston Diagnostic Aphasia Examination	II. Auditory Comprehension Subtests A–D	Word discrimination, body part identification, commands, complex ideational materials
Western Aphasia Battery	II. Comprehension (Subset of WAB)	Yes/no questions, auditory word recognition, sequential commands

Verbal Expression

Verbal expression is another area to examine when evaluating aphasia. Is the output fluent without disruption in the overall flow, or is it nonfluent with hesitations, groping, and false starts? In addition, when errors are present in the verbal output, what is the nature of those errors? A variety of error types (paraphasias) might be present in the verbal output of an individual with aphasia. The most frequently occurring consist of three types: semantic paraphasias, phonemic paraphasias, and neologisms.

An aphasic patient with semantic paraphasia might substitute a word that is semantically similar to the intended or target word. For example, a man might tell his wife that he is going to the freezer for "fish" when he meant to say "steak." The word substitution is related in that it is in the same semantic class, "meat," but it was not the intended word.

A phonemic paraphasia differs from a semantic paraphasia. It is not a whole word substitution; rather, the phonemes in the target word might be omitted or scrambled, or others might be added. Examples of phonemic paraphasias might be "knipe" for "knife" or "bellyjean" for "jellybean."

Finally, there may be utterances that are similar to words in their arrangement of consonants and vowels, but unlike any words in the language of the speaker. An example might be calling a comb a "planker." These errors are known as neologisms. When neologisms are present in the speech of an individual their verbal output can seem nonsensical or like jargon, even though once uttered, the patient may look to you expectantly for a response.

You may find paraphasic errors even in the speech of individuals who are not aphasic.

Once error types are noted, we want to examine the individual's level of awareness and/or frustration after she makes the error. We may notice that some automatic speech tasks are easily elicited with relatively few errors, but others are very difficult for the individual. Such contextual influences are important to note in your evaluation of verbal expression. Table 11–3 illustrates typical tasks used to test verbal expression from our standardized tests.

Control of the Oral Motor System

Although aphasia is defined as an impairment in language, there are sometimes concomitant difficulties with the planning of motor activity for speech. It is for this reason that we must look at the individual's control of the oral motor system (Chapter 12). The fact that dysfunction of the motor speech system often coincides with aphasia and will be evaluated as a part of the aphasia diagnostic battery is worth mention here, however.

> Behaviors that characterize apraxia of speech often coincide with aphasia.

Reading

Another modality of communication that is important to assess in evaluating aphasia is reading ability. It is imperative to examine this skill in depth, for in addition to being able to "read," individuals

> The act of reading and comprehension of what has been read are separate abilities and may be differentially affected in aphasia.

Table 11–3. Some common tasks utilized to evaluate verbal expression.

Test Battery	Subtest	Tasks
Minnesota Test for Differential Diagnosis of Aphasia	Section C (Speech and Language Disturbances)	Repetition of words and phrases, automatic speech, sentence completion, naming, answering questions, expression of ideas, describing pictures
Porch Index of Communicative Ability	I IV IX XII	Describing function, naming objects, sentence completion, imitation
Boston Diagnostic Aphasia Examination	I. Conversational and Expository Speech	Conversation, response to questions, picture description, automatized sequences
	III. Oral Expression	Recitation, word/phrase repetition, naming, verbal fluency
Western Aphasia Battery	I. Spontaneous Speech	Spontaneous speech, responsive speech
	III. Repetition	Repetition
	IV. Naming	Naming, verbal fluency, sentence completion

must understand what they are reading. One might assume that these two functions represent the same ability. But sometimes they do not.

For example, Mr. Johns is being tested for the presence of aphasia. Subtest VII of the Porch Index of Communicative Ability asks that Mr. Johns read a card and complete the action printed there. Mr. Johns picks up the card and accurately reads aloud, "Put this card to the right of the comb." He pauses, then repeats the direction several times under his breath while looking at the objects spread out on the table before him. Mr. Johns then shakes his head and looks at you in bewilderment. Although he was able to read the card, he had no idea what it said or how to carry out the direction. Now imagine that you had tested his reading ability and made the assumption that, because he could read directions, that ability implied that he understood and could follow written directions. Given that scenario, would you want Mr. Johns to return home and be independent in reading and following the directions on the labels of the myriad of new prescription medications? As an astute clinician, you would never make such an assumption. This rather extreme example illustrates that reading ability is a highly routinized activity that might be preserved after stroke, but the comprehension of what is read might be impaired. Such a caveat points to the importance of testing all parameters of reading when evaluating aphasia (Table 11–4).

Writing

The final communicative modality to be examined in our assessment protocol is writing. Like the other modalities, writing should be ex-

Table 11–4. Common tasks used to evaluate reading ability.

Test Battery	Subtest	Tasks
Minnesota Test for Differential Diagnosis of Aphasia	Section B Visual and Reading Disturbances	Matching letters, matching words, oral presentation, visual presentation, reading comprehension, sentences, paragraphs
Porch Index of Communicative Ability	V, VII	Following written directions
Boston Diagnostic Aphasia Examination	IV. Understanding Written Language	Symbol/word discrimination, word recognition, written, orally spelled, word-picture matching, reading sentences and paragraphs
Western Aphasia Battery	V. Reading, Writing and Nonverbal tests	Comprehension of sentences, matching word to picture, matching word to object, letter discrimination, spelling

amined through a variety of tasks so that the level of breakdown in ability can be determined (see Table 11–5 for examples). Writing is a form of expression and, like its verbal counterpart, requires the ability to formulate thoughts into a form that is recognized by others. Because both of these abilities (written and verbal expression) are similar, you may see parallels between them. For example, the same types of errors may be observed in both (semantic paraphasias, phonemic paraphasias, or neologisms).

> Individuals with aphasia may not be able to write with their preferred hand. This makes writing tasks even more difficult for them.

Screening Testing

Although comprehensive evaluation of aphasia is necessary, a look at Table 11–1 reminds us that the time required to administer some of these total test batteries is extensive. Given the current situation of shrinking medical resources, efficient time management is often foremost in the minds of clinicians. It may be necessary to forego extensive testing, with all its benefits, in favor of screening tools. Table 11–6 provides several examples of these tools.

In-depth Testing

Additional diagnostic tools have been designed to specifically explore one or more of the modalities tested in traditional protocols reviewed above. For example, let's reconsider Mr. Johns and his read-

Table 11–5. Some common tasks utilized to evaluate writing ability.

Test Battery	Subtest	Tasks
Minnesota Test for Differential Diagnosis of Aphasia	Section D: Visuomotor and Writing Disturbances	Writing numbers, copying letters, writing letters to dictation, spelling, writing sentences, writing paragraphs
Porch Index of Communicative Ability	Graphic Subtests: A–F	Writing the function of objects, written naming, oral presentation, visual presentation, spelling, copying, words, shapes
Boston Diagnostic Aphasia Examination	V. Writing	Writing mechanics; writing sequences; alphabet; numbers; writing letters, numbers, and words; copying; written picture description
Western Aphasia Battery	V. Reading, Writing, and Nonverbal tests	Personal information, picture description, written sentence, written words/letters, oral presentation, visual presentation, copying

Table 11–6. Screening batteries administered to evaluate aphasia.

Test Name	Administration Time	Description
Aphasia Language Performance Scales (ALPS)	20–30 minutes	Uses common objects in the patient's room to test comprehension and expression
Bedside Evaluation Screening Test (2nd Ed.) (BEST–2)	20 minutes or less	Assesses conversation, comprehension, reading, repetition and naming using common objects
Acute Aphasia Screening Protocol (AASP)	10 minutes	Uses objects easily found in the patient's room. Examines orientation, attention, comprehension, and expression

ing ability. Based on formal evaluation, it was apparent that reading had been impaired. Prior to discharge from the hospital, the medical team must consider the patient's abilities before making placement decisions. If Mr. Johns were to return home it would be necessary for him to be independent/alone for a large portion of the day while his wife works. To determine if Mr. Johns is capable of this, it may be necessary to assess his reading ability in greater depth to determine if he could follow simple written directions from his wife relating to, for instance, meal preparation and medications. The *Reading Comprehension Battery for Aphasia* (RCBA–2; LaPointe & Horner, 1998) might be a tool that you would consider for such a purpose. Table 11–7 lists other modality specific tests that allow us to measure specific communicative abilities.

Functional Communication Abilities

There is a recent trend in health care that emphasizes the importance of evaluating the impact of impairment on functional performance. This trend is not isolated to speech pathology but is growing in every discipline that works for the benefit of individuals with disabilities. Research has focused on elements in connected discourse and the pragmatics or rules of language displayed in the communication of individuals with aphasia. These analyses of language provide a more "functional" index of performance. Frattali (1992) defined functional communication as "the ability to receive a message or convey a message, regardless of the mode, to communicate effectively and independently in a given environment" (p. 64). She and her colleagues later reported on an assessment instrument (Frattali, Thompson, Holland, Whol, & Ferketic, 1995), designed to provide a short, sensitive, reliable, and valid tool for examining functional communication. This tool looks specifically at disability rather than handicap

Table 11–7. Several examples of assessment batteries that provide an in-depth examination of various components of aphasia.

Test Name	Modality	Description
Reading Comprehension Battery for Aphasia (2nd ed.) (RCBA–2)	Reading comprehension	Assesses reading comprehension for words, sentences, paragraphs, and functional reading tasks (i.e., prescription labels)
Revised Token Test (RTT)	Auditory comprehension	Assesses comprehension of commands from simple to complex. The commands require the manipulation of tokens of various colors and sizes.
Boston Naming Test (BNT)	Naming or word finding ability	Assesses naming ability and response to cues
Test of Adolescent/Adult Word Finding (TAAWF)		Also assesses naming or word finding ability, but in a variety of contexts (nouns, verbs, categories, sentence completion, and description)
Boston Assessment of Severe Aphasia	All modalities	This tool evaluates all aspects of aphasia, but is designed specifically for individuals with severe aphasia who may not be able to complete other standardized tests.

(Holland & Thompson, 1998). The assessment is comprised of rating the individual on a number of functional communication tasks. Based on these ratings, a profile is determined that reflects level of communication independence and the qualitative dimensions of communication. The tool is completed by a speech-language pathologist or through an interview with someone who is familiar with the individual in question.

Patient and Family Reactions and Attitudes to the Disorder

One of the most important roles we have as speech-language pathologists is to provide ongoing education about the impairment and resultant disabilities secondary to aphasia. The typical lay person has little if any experience interacting with individuals who have aphasia. You may remember your grandparents referring to one of their friends/relatives who "talked out of their head" following their stroke. Such a characterization makes it appear that the individuals

Including friends and loved ones in evaluation and treatment not only motivates the patient, but also provides much needed education regarding how to facilitate communication.

who have suffered strokes have little awareness of their surroundings or are "crazy." With only a little background on aphasia, even the beginning clinician knows that this is not the case.

We can only imagine the pain and frustration encountered by individuals who have survived a life-threatening event, only to realize that basic communication abilities have been disrupted so that even simple interaction is difficult, if not impossible. One method for easing the distress for individuals and their families is to provide them with pertinent information/education about their disability. In many instances, you can provide suggestions that optimize or even facilitate communication interaction.

Patient and family reactions/attitudes regarding the communication disability can influence prognosis for success in treatment. Those who resign themselves to a lifetime of devastating handicap will mostly likely become a self-fulfilling prophecy. On the other hand, patients and their families who tackle aphasia and make every attempt to maximize their skills will likely make great gains in treatment. Through patient education and training, we must make every attempt to prevent the former situation from occurring.

Identifying Concomitant Problems

Conditions that result in aphasia do not affect speech-language in isolation. Frequently there are concomitant problems to be considered that impact the individual's interaction with his or her environment. Some examples are hemiplegia or paresis (weakness on one side of the body); cognitive impairments (attention, memory, problem solving); psychological factors such as depression; and increased fatigability.

> Aphasia symptoms can become much worse when an individual is depressed or fatigued.

Related Language Disorders

This chapter has been devoted to introducing the beginning speech-language pathologist to concepts related to the assessment of aphasia and related disorders. Some brief discussion of other acquired disorders classified as "language disorders," but whose symptoms are not entirely consistent with the definition of aphasia, is needed. These disorders are also related to a neural event and should be reviewed here as an integral part of differential diagnosis for the speech-language pathologist.

Traumatic Brain Injury

As previously described, traumatic brain injury results from neural damage sustained from an external blow to the head. The impact of the injury results in diffuse brain damage. This kind of brain damage can result in disordered language, but is quite different from that found in the aphasias. The language characteristics of TBI were initially described as subclinical aphasia, that is, language deficits that are apparent in conversation but are not revealed on standard aphasia test batteries (Sarno, 1980). There may be anomia and impaired auditory comprehension, but expression is not clearly aphasiclike (Coehlo, 1997).

The potential for focal and diffuse injury to numerous areas of the brain, depending on the location and nature of impact, results in a wide range of linguistic and cognitive behaviors. Consequently, there are few standardized batteries that encompass the range of performance that must be addressed. In fact, many diagnosticians have continued to rely on aphasia batteries that do not accurately assess the abilities of TBI patients. It is the cognitive deficits that set individuals with TBI apart from those with aphasia. It is likely that these cognitive disturbances interact with language performance to result in disordered processing of language.

One disturbance frequently seen immediately following TBI injury is amnesia. The patient may have difficulty recalling personal, temporal, and geographical orientation because there is no continuous memory. If information cannot be stored from moment to moment, the individual's language might seem confused or disjointed. Formalized testing is not indicated because the findings do not provide a representative sample of true capabilities in such a state of confusion. Usually the amnesia resolves, orientation improves, and testing of other cognitive/linguistic areas can begin such as attention, memory, and so-called executive functions. Both attention and memory can be tested according to various components (Parente & Herman, 1996; Sohlberg & Mateer, 1989).

Executive functions are those high level cognitive skills that integrate information from all brain centers in order to plan, implement, and evaluate goal-directed behavior. These abilities appear to reside in the frontal lobes, which are highly susceptible to damage from TBI. Skills such as judgment, problem solving, and social skills are all included under the heading of executive functions. Disturbances in these areas, combined with potential orientation, attention, and memory impairments can have a deleterious effect on every aspect of language performance from naming objects to connected discourse.

Right Hemisphere Communication Disorders

Another group of individuals that demonstrates acquired language deficiency is the group that has sustained right hemisphere damage (RHD). Although the left hemisphere has long been regarded as the dominant hemisphere for language, recent investigation has revealed that the right hemisphere also contributes to successful communication. A patient with this sort of damage might show deficits in extralinguistic features, such as generating and maintaining topics of conversation and making inferences. There may also be disruption in the ability to appreciate or understand abstraction in language. This might be demonstrated in a decreased ability to appreciate humor or

> Attentional abilities are important to formulating, expressing, and understanding language.

> Conversations often rely on recalling bits of information from short-term and/or long-term memory.

> Disinhibition may lead to poor social skills in communication tasks. Such behavior might lead to imposed isolation because no one wants to be confronted with such potentially embarrassing situations.

> Individuals with RHD might talk and talk, giving little warning before changing topics and paying no heed to social cues that the listener might be sending.

to recognize figurative language. The patient often interprets language at a very concrete level. For example, during an RHD evaluation, Janie was asked to complete a visual scanning sheet. This sheet consisted of a matrix of randomly occurring letters. The directions included underlining the letter M every time it occurred, circling the letter R in blue ink each time it occurred, and crossing out the letter T in red ink each time it occurred. At the onset of the task these instructions were reviewed and colored pens were provided. Janie studied the paper for several moments, then looked up and reported that she could not complete the task because there were no Rs in blue ink or Ts in red ink. This situation demonstrates how literal interpretation can lead to miscommunication and/or a misunderstanding.

Like most acquired language disorders, RHD also results in a fairly specific set of cognitive deficits, the most notable of which is so-called visual left neglect. It is an attentional problem in which the patient ignores the left side of her world. She will eat only the items on the right side of her tray. She will not react to her environment on the left, frequently bumping into things. She may even neglect clothing the left half of her body. The amount of space or degree of neglect varies, but you can imagine the impact on communication. For instance, she may not even interact with others in conversation who are sitting on her left! Reading ability can also be disturbed, with only the right half of words on the right side of the page in view.

Among the other problems experienced by individuals following RHD are difficulty in interpreting and/or conveying emotion, reduced prosody, anosagnosia (an inability to recognize their disability), and visual/spatial impairments. All of these skills are important for successful communication and thus have the potential to cause communication problems if disrupted. In particular, the disruption of prosody (Robin, Klouda, & Hug, 1991) results in difficulty understanding speech that changes meaning based on subtle changes in intonation or produces changes in meaning that are driven by intonation patterns. For instance, persons with RHD may have difficulty producing a characteristic rise in pitch at the end of sentences to signal a question.

Dementia

The final diagnosis for consideration under related language disorders is dementia. As reviewed earlier, dementia is present in a large portion of the population who are 85 years and older. Dementia is an acquired syndrome characterized by persistent intellectual decline, secondary to neurologic changes (Shekim, 1997). Dementia can be seen as a component contributing to a variety of neurologic conditions: Parkinson's disease, Huntington's disease, or following multiple infarcts. The most common form of dementia, however, is dementia of the Alzheimer's type.

Although the initial symptom of dementia is memory impairment, language performance parallels that of the overall intellectual decline. Because of that parallel, researchers have recommended that linguistic decline be included in the clinical definition of dementia (Murdoch, Chenery, Wilks, & Boyle, 1987). Language performance in dementia is classified according to severity of presenting deficits. Although the progression of dementia of the Alzheimer's type is continuous, some have attempted to divide the disease into three distinct stages (Davis, 1993). These stages are arbitrary but allow the beginning clinician to understand better how the disease changes over time. The patient in Stage I may be forgetful and demonstrate carelessness in daily routines but follows those routines well. Language performance in Stage I is marked by good comprehension, word-finding errors, and vague terminology. In Stage II, deficits become more pronounced with a marked reduction in working (short–term) memory. The language of an individual in Stage II reflects a reduction in auditory comprehension, paraphasias in expression, verbose, sometimes irrelevant speech, and a decreased awareness of language dysfunction. The final stage of this kind of dementia is characterized by minimal ability to store or recall events or people; the patient may be unresponsive to the environment and essentially mute.

An examination of the language of individuals with dementia reveals similar types of language performance to that produced by individuals with aphasia. However, the unremitting, progressive course of dementia makes this diagnosis very dissimilar to individuals with nonprogressive aphasia. Our task in evaluating individuals with dementia is to determine the current level of language and how we as professionals might structure the environment or communication tasks to facilitate successful interaction.

Determining the Course of the Problem (Prognosis)

Throughout this chapter, we have discussed factors that influence a patient's prognosis for a variety of disorders. First, we discussed the nature of the neurologic insult. If aphasia symptoms are related to a slow-growing benign tumor then, following surgical excision, prognosis is good. However, if the symptoms are related to a large left-hemisphere CVA, the prognosis may be less favorable. Other factors that influence prognosis are patient and family attitudes.

Factors that we have not discussed but may have an impact on prognosis, are characteristics of the individual. One such factor is the patient's age. Age has been found to influence an individual's ability to benefit from rehabilitation (Katz & Alexander, 1994). Namely, individuals in the age range from 20 to 40 years fared better than those in the age range of 40 to 60 years, and 60 years and beyond.

Another factor that might influence prognosis is premorbid language abilities. In an earlier edition of this text, Jordan (1994) provided an example of the influence of premorbid language abilities. Individuals with aphasia may be called upon to recognize the need to produce and accept alternative responses as a result of their disabili-

Many factors play into the prognosis for an individual with aphasia or a related language disorder.

Highly motivated individuals with severe disability may have a better functional outcome than an individual with mild disability who suffers from depression.

ty. Premorbid skills that were based on rich and varied language experiences might provide the individual with more strategies with which to deal with communication breakdown. It is important then to consider a multitude of variables (personal as well as injury) when providing a prognosis, not just the type and severity of injury.

The Evaluation Report

Now that you have completed the evaluation, you must generate a report of your findings. Most clinical reports follow a standard format that may vary slightly from facility to facility but contain the same elements. While generating a report, it is imperative to remember those elements that third-party payers (private insurance, Medicare/Medicaid) are looking for. Appendix 11A provides an example of an evaluation format with details on elements to include.

Treatment Factors

Congratulations, you have completed the process of evaluation, carefully weighing all factors, and generated the evaluation report. This is a big hurdle, but you have only just begun the journey. After you have determined the presence of aphasia, you begin the task of sifting through your diagnostic findings for potential treatment directions. It is tempting to look at the results of testing with the desire to remediate those areas determined to be the weakest. However, this would not provide the greatest benefit for the patient. Instead, the focus should be on communicative strengths that you might optimize through treatment. These strengths can then be used to compensate for weaknesses in communication abilities. Examine the results of your testing with one question in mind: What skill can we work on that will make the greatest functional impact on this individual's communication abilities? Treatment focused on these areas will result in more immediate gains and patients and their families will likely maintain their motivation for ongoing treatment.

SUMMARY

The purpose of this chapter was to introduce you to concepts related to the evaluation of aphasia and related disorders. Assessment of patients with these disorders includes not only the determination of specific disabilities related to the impairment, but also the level of handicap, which is determined by their functional abilities. Your assessment battery can include standardized tests, screening tools, and tests of overall functional abilities, as well as tests devoted to specific areas of communication function. With all of these diagnostic tools available, you have the flexibility to pattern your assessment to the needs of the individual. When the evaluation is complete and the report has been generated, the treatment journey begins. The direction of treatment is one that should be determined by the information that you have obtained in your assessment as well as the wants and needs of your patient. But that journey is another tale.

REFERENCES

Coehlo, C. A. (1997). Cognitive-communicative disorders following traumatic brain injury. In C. T. Ferrand & R. L. Bloom (Eds.), *Introduction to organic and neurogenic disorders of communication: Current scope of practice* (pp. 110–138). Boston, MA: Allyn and Bacon.

Davis, G. A. (1993). *A survey of adult aphasia and related language disorders.* Englewood Cliffs, NJ: Prentice-Hall.

Frattali, C. M. (1992). Functional assessment of communication: Merging public policy with clinical views. *Aphasiology, 6,* 63–83.

Frattali, C. M. (1998). *Measuring outcomes in speech-language pathology.* New York: Thieme.

Frattali, C. M., Thompson, C. K., Holland, A. L., Whol, C. B., & Ferketic, M. M. (1995). *Functional assessment of communication skills for adults (ASHA FACS).* Rockville, MD: ASHA.

Frey, W. D. (1984). Functional assessment of communication: Merging public policy with clinical views. *Aphasiology, 6,* 63–83.

George, K. P., Vikingstad, E. M., & YueCao (1998). Brain imaging in neurocommunicative disorders. In A. F. Johnson & B. H. Jacobson (Eds.), *Medical speech-language pathology: A practitioner's guide* (pp. 285–336). New York: Thieme.

Holland, A. L., & Thompson, C. K. (1998). Outcomes measurement in aphasia. In C. M. Frattali (Ed.), *Measuring outcomes in speech-language pathology* (pp. 245–266). New York: Thieme.

Johnson, A. F., George, K. P., & Hinckley, J. (1998). Assessment and diagnosis in neurogenic communication disorders. In A. F. Johnson & B. H. Jacobson (Eds.), *Medical speech-language pathology: A practitioner's guide* (pp. 337–554). New York: Thieme.

Jordan, L. (1994). Aphasia. In J. B. Tomblin, H. L. Morris, & D. C. Spriestersbach (Eds.), *Diagnosis in speech language pathology* (pp. 165–177). San Diego, CA: Singular Publishing Group.

Katz, D. I., & Alexander, M. P. (1994). Traumatic brain injury. Predicting course of recovery and outcome for patients admitted to rehabilitation. *Archives of Neurology, 51,* 661–670.

LaPointe, L., & Horner, J. (1998). *Reading comprehension battery for Aphasia* (2nd ed.). Austin, TX: Pro-Ed.

McNeil, M. R. (1982). The nature of aphasia in adults. In N. J. Lass, L. V. McReynolds, J. L. Northern, & D. E. Yoder (Eds.), *Speech language, and hearing: Vol. III. Pathologies of speech and language* (pp. 692–740). Philadelphia: W. B. Saunders.

Murdoch, B. E., Chenery, H. J., Wilks, V., & Boyle, R. S. (1987). Language disorders in dementia of the Alzheimer type. *Brain and Language, 31,* 122–137.

Parente, R., & Herrmann, D. (1996). *Retraining cognition: Techniques and applications.* Austin, TX: Aspen Publishers.

Porch, B. E. (1971). *The Porch Index of Communicative Ability.* Palo Alto, CA: Consulting Psychologists Press.

Robin, D. A., Klouda, G., & Hug, L. N. (1991). Neurogenic disorders of prosody. In D. Vogel & M. P. Cannito (Eds.), *Treating disordered motor speech control: For clinicians by clinicians* (pp. 241–274). Austin, TX: Pro-Ed.

Sarno, M. T. (1980). The nature of verbal impairment after closed head injury. *Journal of Nervous and Mental Disease, 168,* 685–692.

Shekim, L. O. (1997). Dementia. In L. LaPointe (Ed.), *Aphasia and related disorders* (2nd ed., pp. 238–249). New York: Thieme.

Sohlberg, M. M., & Mateer, C. A. (1989). *Introduction to cognitive rehabilitation theory and practice.* New York: Guilford Press.

Stevens, N., & Adler, J. (1992). *Introduction to medical terminology.* Springhouse, PA: Springhouse Corporation.

World Health Organization. (1980). *International classification of impairments, disabilities, and handicaps.* Geneva: Author.

RECOMMENDED READINGS

German, D. J. (1990). *Test of Adolescent/Adult Word Finding.* Austin, TX: Pro-Ed.

Goodglass, H., & Kaplan, E. (1983a). *Boston Diagnostic Aphasia Exam.* Philadelphia: Lea & Febiger.

Goodglass, H., & Kaplan, E. (1983b). *Boston Naming Test.* Philadelphia: Lea & Febiger.

Helm-Estabrooks, N., Ramsberger, G., Morgan, A.R., & Nicholas, M. (1989). *Boston Assessment of Severe Aphasia.* Austin, TX: Pro-Ed.

Kertez, A. (1982). *The Western Aphasia Battery.* New York: Grune & Stratton.

McNeil, M. R., & Prescott, T. A. (1978). *Revised Token Test.* Austin, TX: Pro-Ed.

Schuell, H. (1965). *The Minnesota Test for Differential Diagnosis of Aphasia.* Minneapolis, MN: University of Minnesota Press.

APPENDIX 11A.
SAMPLE REPORTING SHEET

Speech-Language Hearing Center
Diagnostic Clinic
Speech/Language Evaluation Report

Name:

MR#:

DOB:

SSN:

Admit Date:

Date of Injury:

Referring Physician/Agency:

Attendance

State the number of units spent evaluating the patient

Background and History

Reason for referral

Date of onset

Significant PMH

Premorbid status

Speech/Language Evaluation

State the type of evaluation conducted and some comment on pt. behavior/performance throughout testing:

Patient performance on assessment tasks indicated the following:

Auditory Comprehension

The first statement should be a statement that refers to auditory acuity ("Hearing sensitivity was not formally assessed but _____ responded to speech presented at a conversational level" or "Hearing screening indicated _____ . ") The rest of this section should address all testing which assessed auditory comprehension. Use quantification of results as much as is possible.

Verbal Expression

This section should discuss syntax, semantic and word-finding problems. Consideration should be given to the ease/difficulty with which verbalization is elicited. If probed with various cues, those that were most facilitative should be discussed.

Control of the Oral Motor Mechanism (Speech)
This section should include comments on intelligibility, fluency, and prosody. Discuss the examination of the speech mechanism for speech and nonspeech movements.

Written Expression
Comment first on whether the patient is using the preferred hand for writing. Follow with results from assessment.

Reading Expression
Include any information from the chart regarding visual acuity, disturbance, etc. Follow with results from assessment.

Cognition
Include any assessment results from:
Attention
Memory
Visual disturbance/neglect
Pragmatics
Problem solving
Judgment

If warrante additional sections may be added such as:
Augmentative/Alternative Communication
Gestural Communication

Impressions and Prognosis
Speech/Language
Speech/Language Diagnosis
Prognosis
Expectation for recovery

Recommendations
Treatment recommendations may include the following:
Mr/s. _____ is being transferred to _____ .
Mr/s. _____ is being discharged to his/her home where he/she will be seen on an outpatient basis by _____ .
Continued remediation is recommended (at what schedule) to address the following long-term goals:
      Long-term goals

Or if being discharged fully:
Mr/s. _____ has made satisfactory progress as evidenced by
1.
2.
3.

As a result of the progress made to date, continued remediation is not warranted at this time.

12

Motor Speech Disorders

Heather M. Clark, Ph.D.
Julie A. G. Stierwalt, Ph.D., and
Donald A. Robin, Ph.D.

INTRODUCTION

The purpose of this chapter is to introduce the beginning speech-language pathologist to the assessment of acquired motor speech disorders, specifically dysarthria and apraxia of speech (AOS). Motor speech disorders are speech production deficits that result from impairments in the neuromuscular and/or motor control system. Motor speech disorders are distinct from language disorders, such as aphasia. Recall from Chapter 11 that aphasia affects the understanding and formulation of linguistic messages. In motor speech disorders, the nervous system signals that control speech musculature are affected, thereby altering the speech signal.

The two primary diagnoses that fall under the category of motor speech disorders are dysarthria and apraxia of speech. *Dysarthria* is defined by Darley, Aronson, and Brown (1969) as "a group of speech disorders resulting from disturbances in muscular control" (p. 246). Dysarthria may impact the ability to use the voice effectively, or to move the muscles of the respiratory system, the soft palate, or the ar-

Two primary motor speech disorders are dysarthria and apraxia.

ticulators quickly or accurately. These impairments may result in speech that sounds slurred, uneven, harsh or quiet, or slow.

Apraxia of speech (AOS), on the other hand, is thought to reflect a disruption of motor planning and programming. It is manifest, not by disrupted neuromuscular function or by deficits in sensory or language processing, but by a reduced ability to program the articulators for speech movements (McNeil, Robin, & Schmidt, 1997). In essence, patients with AOS have difficulty "telling the muscles what to do." The speech of patients with AOS may sound slow, effortful, and uneven and might include sound distortions. In both AOS and dysarthria, you may hear substitutions, additions, and/or omissions.

The pathophysiology of dysarthria and AOS in adults is typically related to acquired neurologic injury or disease. However, dysarthria may also be a component in congenital conditions. For example, individuals with cerebral palsy are frequently born with neuromuscular deficits that result in dysarthria.

Strokes are the most common cause of AOS and are a common cause of dysarthria as well (Duffy, 1995). Dysarthria and AOS may also result from traumatic brain injury or tumors. The implications of stroke, tumors, and traumatic brain injury are discussed in detail in Chapter 11. In addition to these etiologies, several progressive diseases frequently result in dysarthria. What follows is a description of common disease processes that present with some form of dysarthria.

Amyotrophic lateral sclerosis (ALS) is a rapidly progressing disease that affects both the upper and lower motor neurons. Parkinson's disease, which results from basal ganglia dysfunction, is characterized by rigidity and tremor and may ultimately result in dementia as well. Basal ganglia dysfunction may also result in Huntington's disease, which is characterized by involuntary movements and dementia. Multiple sclerosis (MS) is caused by a stripping away of myelin and the formation of scar tissue on axons in the central nervous system. The most common form of MS exhibits a relapsing and remitting pattern and may be characterized by sensory, motor, and/or cognitive deficits (Yorkston, Miller, & Strand, 1995).

Each of the above diseases presents different underlying impairments and thus different speech characteristics. Each disease has a different progression of symptoms and prognosis. Some diseases may be treated medically; others are considered medically untreatable. Because of the variety of issues associated with degenerative diseases, it is important to become familiar with the implications of specific diagnoses. A useful resource is *Management of Speech and Swallowing in Degenerative Diseases* (Yorkston et al., 1995), which provides detailed information about the degenerative diseases listed above.

When considering the assessment of motor speech disorders, it is critical for you to consider the various levels and methods of measurement available. As also discussed in Chapter 11 (Stierwalt, Clark, & Robin), the World Health Organization describes different levels of disorder, including impairment, disability, and handicap (WHO, 1980). *Impairment* is defined as the underlying physiologic condition

Causes of motor speech disorders include stroke, tumors, TBI, and degenerative diseases.

that impairs performance. *Disability* refers to the actual behavioral/ performance deficits resulting from the impairment. The effect of a disability on an individual's quality of life is defined as *handicap*. While it seems as though clinicians should be able to predict disability from impairment, and handicap from impairment and disability, several examples will illustrate how this is not always the case.

Imagine two people who have similar *impairments* of muscle weakness and reduced range of motion. One individual, who is a theater performer, is able to produce speech that is reasonably intelligible, because she has had practice producing carefully and clearly articulated words. Thus, she would have only a mild disability. The second individual, who is not practiced in compensatory strategies, may produce speech that is barely intelligible, resulting in a severe disability. We see, then, that impairment does not necessarily predict disability.

It is critical to assess impairment, disability, and handicap.

To continue the example, imagine that the second individual is an artist who lives alone, communicating with friends primarily through correspondence. Even though he has a severe disability, the inability to speak may not disrupt his ability to work or communicate with family and friends. Thus, the artist with a severe disability may experience only a mild handicap. In contrast, the performer who has a relatively mild speech disability may no longer be able to work in the theater, thus experiencing significant handicap. These examples indicate that it is very difficult to predict handicap from disability.

A final point is that the diagnostician must determine the underlying impairment that leads to the speech disorder. For example, unintelligible speech (disability) can result from a variety of impairments, including muscle weakness, muscle incoordination, or disrupted motor planning. Additionally, depending on the impairment, there may be an expectation of recovery or the expectation may be that the symptoms will worsen in their severity. In order to determine the best therapeutic approach, it is necessary for you to identify the underlying impairment contributing to the observable disability. Therefore, the rest of this chapter will be devoted to a detailed overview of assessment relating to identifying impairments, disabilities, and handicaps.

Determination of the Complaint

Medical History

The first step in the assessment process is obtaining previous medical history. At the impairment level, this most often involves a review of medical records to provide information about the medical conditions that caused the impairment or are contributing to it. We gain access to medical records in two ways. If we are an employee of the agency holding the medical records, we have access to them. If not, we must submit a request to the appropriate agency (or agencies), with a release of information signed by the patient. For

Impairment information may be obtained from the medical history.

some patients, it will be necessary to request information from several agencies, including acute care hospitals, rehabilitation facilities, and outpatient clinics.

Table 12–1 identifies the type of information that we need to obtain from medical records of these patients, and where within the medical record this information is most often found.

Patient and Family Interview

Disability and handicap information may be obtained partially through the diagnostic interview.

A comprehensive case history from the patient and family, including the onset and progression of symptoms, as well as current functioning, is needed to describe the disability and handicap. Table 12–2 provides examples of questions that will be helpful to obtain the needed information. It is important to remember that the patient and the family may not share the same perceptions about the severity or impact of the speech disorder, so it is good to interview both the patient and members of the family. Sometimes we conduct separate interviews. Frequently, we must modify interview methods to accommodate to the level of communication skills of which the patient is capable. For example, some of these patients may have difficulty understanding interview questions; that is, they may also have cognitive or language impairments; or they may have difficulty expressing themselves or making themselves understood. If that is the case, we must simplify our language, or simplify the questions so that only single-word responses are sufficient.

Table 12–1. Information to be obtained from medical records.

Information to Obtain	Area of the Medical Chart Information Is Typically Found	Specific Findings
Reason for admission	Admission note, History and Physical	Date of admission, circumstances surrounding admission, admitting diagnosis
Pertinent medical history (PMH)	Admission note	Neurological history (history of stroke, dementia, brain injury, seizures, disease), ENT history (head and neck cancer, laryngeal pathology). Medications
Prior level of functioning	Admission note, Social Worker's note	Level of independence, family support
Current medical and mental status	Physician's progress notes, Nurses notes	Level of alertness, medical frailty
Site of lesion	Imaging reports	CT scan, MRI, PET results.
Therapy history	Therapists' notes (OT, PT, SLP)	Ability to participate in treatment, progress made to date, physical limitations

Table 12–2. Interview questions.

Disability

Onset and Course
Do you have any difficulty with your speech? Do others think you have difficulty with your speech?
How long have you had this problem? Did it occur suddenly or develop gradually?
Did any other difficulties occur at the same time as the speech problem began?
Is your speech getting any better or worse over time?

Associated Deficits
Do you have any difficulty with chewing or swallowing? (If yes, complete clinical swallowing assessment.)
Do you drool?
Do you have any difficulty expressing your emotions?

Perception of Deficit
Describe your speech problem and how it has changed over time. How does it sound? How does it feel?
How do others describe your speech?

Management
Does anyone have difficulty understanding you? What do you do when this happens?
What things have you tried to compensate for your speech difficulties? Have you ever had speech therapy?
How important is it to you to improve your speech now?

Awareness of Diagnosis and Prognosis
Do you know the cause of your speech problems? If so, what is going to happen?

Handicap

Professional
How well are you able to perform your job duties?

Social
Do you do the things you used to do for enjoyment with friends and family?

Communicative
Are you able to understand what people say, and can others understand you?

Physical
Do you feel tired or ill?

Emotional
Do you feel strong emotions—sadness, anger, frustration—because of your impairments?

Sources: Adapted from Duffy, 1995, and Verdolini, 1994.

Determining the Existence of a Motor Speech Disorder

After the history and information about the nature of the complaint have been reviewed, we examine the symptoms to determine if the diagnosis of motor speech disorder is warranted. Many types of measurement methods and assessment tools are now clinically available, each providing different types of information. In general, assessment tools can be categorized as being perceptual, acoustic,

Measurement systems may be perceptual, acoustic, or physiologic.

or physiologic. Most observations made by speech-language clinicians are perceptual in nature, meaning that little instrumentation, such as computers, transducers, or other electronic devices, is required. Perceptual observations are particularly critical in the assessment of motor speech disorders, since the types of motor speech disorders are differentiated on the basis of perceptual characteristics. That is, how a person with a motor speech disorder "sounds" will play a primary role in helping to determine what, if any, motor speech disorder is present.

There are several measurement systems that do not rely on perceptual observations. Acoustic observations utilize transduction of the speech signal into visually or digitally represented signals. Such observations provide specific information about the acoustic signal that is not always discernable to the auditory perceptual system. With the advent and growing availability of the desktop computer, acoustic analysis systems are increasingly available in clinical settings and may be a valuable tool for the assessment process.

Physiologic observations allow observation of specific physiological functions. Typically, these are observations not readily visible or audible, such as muscle activity or airflow. Physiologic observations require instrumentation and skilled interpretation and thus are not available in many clinical settings. However, they can provide valuable information to the diagnostician. For example, the *Iowa Oral Performance Instrument* (Robin & Luschei, 1992) is a device that measures tongue strength and endurance. By obtaining an objective measure of tongue strength, the clinician can determine whether muscle weakness is contributing to reduced articulatory precision. Based on this information, the clinician may choose to include tongue-strengthening exercises in the patient's treatment plan. Table 12–3 includes examples of commonly used perceptual, acoustic, and physiologic measurements.

Assessment of the Impairment

Because neuromuscular impairments can differentially affect various parts of the body, it is necessary to evaluate the integrity of

Table 12–3. Examples of perceptual, acoustic, and physiologic observations.

Perceptual	Acoustic	Physiologic
Slurred speech, monoloudness, slow rate, reduced intelligibility	Voice onset time, format transitions, fundamental frequency, intensity	EMG, kinematic measures (displacement, velocity, acceleration of articulators), vital capacity, air flow rate

each of the speech subsystems individually (Table 12–4). However, during speech, the subsystems interact, with individual subsystems affecting the performance of other subsystems. For example, a patient with poor respiratory support (respiratory subsystem) may compensate by using excessive glottal closure to sustain voicing (phonatory subsystem). These interactions may mask the contribution of specific impairments or may lead us to erroneously conclude that a particular subsystem is impaired. In the above example, we may think that the patient has poor phonatory control (since it seems like the voice is the primary problem) when, in fact, it is the respiratory subsystem that is impaired.

Because of the difficulty in measuring "true" interactions during speech, it is necessary to use nonspeech tasks to assess impairments of the subsystems.

Nonspeech tasks are valuable for a variety of reasons (Robin Klouda, & Hug, 1991). Nonspeech tasks allow the clinician to examine subsystems individually. Additionally, nonspeech tasks remove the influence of language from the task. That is, during speech, the speaker is using linguistic processes to formulate a message and motor processes to produce the actual speech movements. Nonspeech tasks permit us to observe motor performance without the influence of linguistic processes. Removing linguistic influences can be particularly important during the assessment of motor speech disorders, since many of these patients also exhibit language impairments. Therefore, nonspeech tasks can help the clinician determine which speech behaviors are related to language impairments and which are related to motor impairments.

Several examples of nonspeech tasks are included in Table 12–4. Some of the tasks are speechlike (e.g., diadochokinetic tasks) and/or require the interaction of more than one subsystem (e.g., maximum phonation time involves the respiratory and phonatory systems). These "maximum performance tasks" are included as nonspeech tasks because, even though they are speechlike, performance on these tasks may not predict speech performance. For example, a patient may be able to sustain phonation for only 10 seconds (which would indicate an impairment), but demonstrate the ability to use her respiratory and phonatory subsystems effectively during connected speech (no disability).

Assessment of Disability

Description of the disability is critical in the assessment of motor speech disorders, since at this level, we can identify how speech production is affected by underlying impairments. As was true with impairments, it is important to assess the performance of each of the subsystems during tasks that address disability. Because, during speech, each of the subsystems interacts, it may not be possible to perfectly differentiate the contribution of specific subsystems to performance (e.g., both the respiratory and phonatory subsystems affect maximum phonation time); however, the careful observer will be

> The speech subsystems interact during speech production

> Nonspeech tasks facilitate assessment at the impairment level.

Table 12–4. Observations of subsystems made at the impairment level.

Subsystem	Method	Task/Observation*	Standard of Performance
Respiratory	Perceptual	Take a deep breath and let it out as audibly and slowly as possible*	At least 5 seconds
		Observation of resting breathing*	Observe rapid (> 25 cycles per minute) or shallow respiration
		Sniff, pant	At least 1 per second
		Blow bubbles through straw into water	Sustain bubbles for 5 seconds in 5 cm of water
	Physiologic	Vital capacity	Refer to standards provided by manufacturer
		Pressure and flow during resting breathing or maximum performance respiratory tasks	Kent (1994)
Phonatory	Perceptual	Maximum phonation time*	15–20 seconds
		Raise and lower pitch during sustained /a/*	Range of at least 6 notes
		Raise and lower volume during series of /a/*	Noticeable change in loudness
		s/z ratio*	[.7 – 1.3]
	Acoustic	Fundamental frequency range during sustained /a/*	At least one octave
		Intensity range during sustained /a/*	Range of 25–50 dB
	Physiologic	Laryngeal function, including adduction and vibratory pattern	Karnell (1994)
		EMG during sustained /a/	
Resonatory	Perceptual	Observation of velum at rest*	Observe symmetry, structural integrity
		Observe velar elevation during /a/*	Observe symmetry, excursion
		Note nasal flow with nasal mirror during sustained /a/	Mirror should not fog
	Physiologic	Nasendoscopy during sustained /a/	Closure of velar port
Articulatory	Perceptual	Oral mechanism exam assessing symmetry, strength, range of motion, coordination during nonspeech tasks*	Dworkin & Culatta (1996)
		Diadochokinetic tasks*	/pʌ/, /tʌ/, /kʌ/: 4 per second /pʌtʌkʌ/: 3 per second
		Praxis during nonspeech oral tasks (blowing, whistling, licking lips, etc.)*	Observe groping or effort
	Physiologic	Tongue strength and endurance	Robin & Luschei (1992)
		EMG during nonspeech tasks	

*Many of these tasks are the same or similar to ones described by Dabul (1979), Robertson (1987), Enderby (1983), and Drummond (1993).

able to gain valuable information from speech tasks. Table 12–5 provides examples of tasks that allow us to assess performance of the speech subsystems at the disability level. Tables 12–4 and 12–5 illustrate how perceptual, acoustic, and physiologic observations can be used to identify both impairment and disabilit.

Table 12–5. Observations of subsystems made at the disability level.

Subsystem	Method	Task/Observation*	Standard of Performance
Respiratory	Perceptual	Count to 20 on one breath* Observe breathing during conversation or reading* Words per exhalation during reading and counting*	Observe depth, rate, speaking on exhalation, inhalation, stridor Reading: 5 WPE Counting: 10 WPE
	Physiologic	Shape during speech Pressure and flow during speech	Solomon & Hixon (1993) Kent (1994)
Phonatory	Perceptual	Quality during connected speech* Ability to vary pitch and loudness during speech*	Note breathiness, harshness, wetness, strain Noticeable change in pitch and loudness
	Acoustic	Fundamental frequency range during connected speech* Intensity range during speech*	Men: 110–150 Hz Women: 175–210 Hz Range of 25–50 dB
	Physiologic	Laryngeal function, including adduction and vibratory pattern during speech tasks EMG during speech	Karnell (1994)
Resonatory	Perceptual	Note nasal resonance during speech* Note nasal flow with nasal mirror during speech*	Note hypernasality, nasal emission, or hyponasality Mirror should fog during nasal consonants and surrounding vowels (dialectical variations)
	Physiologic	Nasendoscopy during connected speech	Adequacy and efficiency of velar port closure
Articulatory	Perceptual	Articulatory accuracy during single words, reading, and connected speech* Repeated productions of multiple syllable words* Repeat words of increasing complexity* Automatic speech tasks (counting, days of week)*	Note distortions, omissions, additions, trial and error groping Observe consistency of errors Observe increased errors with increased complexity Observe decreased errors with decreased volitionality
	Acoustic	Segment durations, format frequencies, format transitions, consonant spectra	Forrest & Weismer (1995)
	Physiologic	EMG during speech tasks	

*Many of these tasks are the same or similar to ones described by Dabul (1979), Robertson (1987), Enderby (1983), and Drummond (1993).

Measurement of intelligibility is critical to the assessment of disability.

An important perceptual measure of disability is *intelligibility*. While assessing the integrity of individual subsystems is important, it is essential to examine how the subsystems interact to produce understandable speech.

Intelligibility (defined as how well a person is understood) can be measured in many different ways. One of the most common is to compute the percentage of words accurately identified by the listener. Such a rating is often used as the foremost indicator of disability. However, the assessment of intelligibility is complex, because intelligibility ratings are influenced by a variety of factors, some of which have little to do with the speaker's speech abilities. Variables that might influence intelligibility ratings are included in Table 12–6.

Measures of intelligibility should control for these variables as much as possible, and reported ratings of intelligibility should describe specifically how intelligibility was defined and measured. Several different methods of obtaining intelligibility ratings are commonly used and are included in Table 12–7. One standardized instrument designed specifically for use with dysarthric speakers is *Assessment of Intelligibility of Dysarthric Speech* (Yorkston & Beukelman, 1984), which assesses intelligibility of single words and sentences of increasing length. Because stimuli are randomly selected from a large sample, it may be administered to the same patient many times. Thus, it is a useful tool for measuring changes in intelligibility, thus changes in disability.

Two other perceptual measures of disability are *prosody* and *speech naturalness*. It is possible for a patient with a motor speech

Table 12–6. Factors affecting intelligibility.

Speaker variables	Speech sample (single words, connected speech, commonly used words, etc.)
	Speech rate
	Speaker appearance
	Compensatory strategies
	Motivation
	Cognitive and language status
Listener variables	Manner of response (transcription, multiple choice, etc.)
	Familiarity with dysarthria
	Familiarity with speaker
	Motivation
	Sensory status and processing capacity
Environmental variables	Contextual cues (phonologic, syntactic, semantic)
	Signal-to-noise ratio
	Presence of distractors (visual, auditory, tactile)
	Natural versus clinic setting, familiar versus unfamiliar setting

Table 12-7. Tasks to assess intelligibility.

Types of Stimuli*	Elicitation Techniques	Judgment Mode
Single words* Sentences of varying length* Reading of paragraph* Connected speech*	Repetition Reading	Listener blind to versus aware of stimuli Word-by-word transcription Multiple choice Subjective judgement of comprehensibility (on-line judgements of connected speech)

* Many of these tasks are the same or similar to ones described by Dabul (1979), Robertson (1987), Enderby (1983), Drummond (1993), and Yorkston and Beukelman (1984).

disorder to be quite intelligible (that is, listeners can understand what was said), but still sound "funny." She may speak with unnatural rhythm or melody. These are characteristics that contribute to an aspect of speech termed "prosody." Terms commonly associated with prosody are tempo, intonation, stress, and rhythm. Prosodic variation is accomplished primarily through adjustments in pitch, loudness, duration, and pause, and can be used to signal differences in meaning or to convey emotion (Hargrove & McGarr, 1994). We need to assess prosody and speech naturalness in a variety of situations (Table 12-8). As noted in Table 12-8, prosody can also be assessed acoustically.

Assessment of Handicap

Handicap is perhaps the most difficult area to assess but still important, particularly to the patient. In many evaluation settings, assessment of the handicap will consist entirely of self-report by the patient. Specifically, we ask the patient to describe the effect of the motor speech disorder on various aspects of his life. Table 12-2 includes several interview questions adopted from Verdolini (1994), which address issues of handicap.

Handicap may be reported or observed.

Ideally, we also want to directly observe the effects of the motor speech disorder on the patient's life as part of the assessment process. For example, the patient's interactions with family members are often easily observed, although, unless these observations are made in the home, they may not be fully representative of these interactions during daily activities.

Observations of the patient at work or in social situations also provide valuable information about the impact of the motor speech disorder. These observations are more easily obtained in some settings (e.g., vocational rehabilitation centers) than in others. Sometimes observation is simply not possible. If that is the case, we can ask the patient or any other available informant about performance in those situations. Reports from others are important in comparing them to the patient's perceptions.

Table 12–8. Tasks for assessing prosody.

Method	Task/Observation*	Standard of Performance
Perceptual	Speech rate and judgments of prosodic adequacy during connected speech and reading*	140–200 wpm Perceptual judgment of adequacy
	Ability to imitate stress variations and speech rates during sentences*	Perceptual judgment of adequacy
Acoustic	Average sentence duration and average sentence F_0 range*	< 2.0 seconds per sentence >50 Hz range

* Many of these tasks are the same or similar to ones described by Dabul (1979), Robertson (1987), Enderby (1983), and Drummond (1993).

Differential Diagnosis

Speech-language
pathologists diagnose
motor speech disorders
not the und(' ing
medical conuiuon causing
the speech disorder.

After collecting information about the impairment, disability, and handicap, the next step in the diagnostic process is to interpret the findings to develop a diagnosis. With regard to motor speech disorders, the diagnosis will include identification of the type of dysarthria, the presence or absence of apraxia of speech, and a severity rating. While a detailed discussion of differential diagnosis of motor speech disorders is beyond the scope of this chapter, Table 12–9 identifies those features identified at the impairment and disability levels which are most commonly associated with the various types of dysarthria and apraxia of speech. It is important to remember that we, as speech-language pathologists, provide a speech diagnosis, not a medical diagnosis. Thus, while we may diagnose dysarthria and provide the physician with information that contributes to the medical diagnosis, we do not diagnose the medical etiology, such as Parkinson's disease or stroke.

Determining the Prognosis

Developing a prognosis
involves understanding
common disease
processes.

We also want to determine a prognosis, describing the potential for improvement in speech, either with or without intervention. Many factors influence the prognosis for motor speech disorders, including the patient's medical diagnosis and current health status. If a patient has a degenerative disease such as Parkinson's disease or ALS, recovery may not be expected. For such cases, the predicted outcomes might be use of compensatory strategies or use of an augmentative communication device.

For patients in the acute stages after a stroke, it may be necessary to defer a statement of prognosis until the patient is alert and medically stable enough to participate in a complete evaluation. Other prognostic factors to consider include the patient's age, speech, and language abilities prior to the onset of the motor speech disorder, motivation and ability to participate in therapy, and the presence (and role) of family and other social support systems.

Table 12–9. Differential diagnosis.

	Flaccid Dysarthria	Spastic Dysarthria	Ataxic Dysarthria	Hypokinetic Dysarthria	Hyperkinetic Dysarthria	Unilateral UMN Dysarthria	Apraxia of Speech
Impairment	weakness, atrophy, hypotonicity	hypertonicity, weakness	incoordination, dysmetria, tremor	bradykinesia, rigidity, tremor	variable tone, involuntary movements	unilateral lower facial or tongue weakness	
Respiratory Subsystem	reduced respiratory support for speech	reduced respiratory support, control	irregular respiratory patterns	shallow breaths, reduced breath support	sudden, irregular respiratory patterns	typically normal	typically normal
Phonatory Subsystem	breathiness, monoloudness monopitch	strained-strangled, reduced pitch and loudness variation	hoarse or breathy, irregular pitch, loudness changes	reduced loudness	sudden changes in pitch, loudness, quality	harshness, reduced loudness	rare, irregular changes in pitch or loudness
Resonatory Subsystem	hypernasality	hypernasality	typically normal	typically normal	typically normal	typically normal	typically normal
Articulatory Subsystem	reduced articulatory precision	reduced articulatory precision	reduced and irregular articulatory precision	reduced articulatory precision, often with reduced range of motion	sudden, irregular breakdowns in articulatory precision	reduced articulatory precision, irregular alternate motion rates	sound distortions, substitutions, omissions, and additions groping of the articulators
Prosody	short phrases	excess and equal stress, short phrases	irregular pitch and loudness changes, irregular speech rhythm	rapid bursts of speech, long pauses	rapid bursts of speech, inappropriate phrasing	typically normal	slow rate, irregular pauses and prolongations

Sources: Adapted from Duffy (1995), and Dworkin (1991).

Determining Treatment Alternatives

Closely related to determining prognosis is providing treatment recommendations. Patients with motor speech disorders often have additional clinical findings. They may be medical, as in the case of a stroke, or physical, such as paralysis or tremor; or communicative, such as aphasia. Usually, then, treatment recommendations are determined by a rehabilitation team, including physicians, physical and occupational therapists, speech-language pathologists, and the patient and his/her family. The objective is to meet all of the patient's needs systematically.

One of the first decisions the team will make is the setting in which the patient will receive the recommended services. Options might include an intensive rehabilitation center, a skilled nursing or long term care facility, or an outpatient therapy setting. For each of these settings, the team will estimate the length of time the patient will be expected to receive therapy, as well as the frequency of therapy. The team will also determine the anticipated outcomes, or goals.

CONCLUSIONS

This chapter provided an overview of the assessment process for motor speech disorders. It is important to remember that patients with motor speech disorders often have related impairments in language, cognition, and/or swallowing. The speech-language pathologist will assess these areas as well; Chapters 11 and 15 will provide direction for these concomitant disorders.

REFERENCES

Dabul, B. (1979). *Apraxia battery for adults.* Tigard, OR: C. C. Publications.

Darley, F. L., Aronson, A. E., & Brown, J. R. (1969). Clusters of deviant speech dimension in the dysarthrias. *Journal of Speech and Hearing Research, 12,* 462–496.

Drummond, S. S. (1993). *Dysarthria examination battery.* Tucson, AZ: Psychological Corporation.

Duffy, J. R. (1995). *Motor speech disorders.* St. Louis, MO: Mosby.

Dworkin, J. P. (1991). *Motor speech disorders: A treatment guide.* St. Louis, MO: Mosby.

Dworkin, J. P., & Culatta, R. A. (1996). *Dworkin-Culatta oral mechanism examination and treatment system (D-COME-T).* Farmington Hills, MI: Edgewood Press.

Enderby, P. M. (1983). *Frenchay dysarthria assessment.* Austin, TX: Pro-Ed.

Forrest, K., & Weismer, G. (1995). Acoustic analysis of dysarthric speech. In M. R. McNeil (Ed.), *Clinical management of sensorimotor speech disorders.* New York: Thieme.

Hargrove, P. M., & McGarr, N. S. (1994). *Prosody management of communication disorders*. San Diego, CA: Singular Publishing Group.

Karnell, M. P. (1994). *Videoendoscopy: From velopharynx to larynx*. San Diego, CA: Singular Publishing Group.

Kent, R. D. (1994). *Reference manual for communicative sciences and disorders*. Austin, TX: Pro-Ed.

McNeil, M. R., Robin, D. A., & Schmidt, R. A. (1997). Apraxia of speech: Definition, differentiation, and treatment. In M. R. McNeil (Ed.), *Clinical management of sensorimotor speech disorders* (pp. 311–344). New York: Thieme.

Robertson, S. J. (1987). *Dysarthria profile*. Tuscon, AZ: Psychological Corporation.

Robin, D. A., Klouda, G. V., & Hug, L. N. (1991). Neurogenic disorders of prosody. In J. Vogel & M. P. Cannito (Eds.), *Treating disordered speech motor control* (pp. 241–274). Austin, TX: Pro-Ed.

Robin, D. A., & Luschei, E. S. (1992). *IOPI Normative database, linear regression model*. Iowa City, IA. Laboratory of Speech and Language Neuroscience, University of Iowa.

Robin, D. A., Solomon, N. P., Moon, J. B., & Folkins, J. W. (1997). Nonspeech assessment of the speech production mechanism. In M. R. McNeal (Ed.), *Clinical management of sensorimotor speech disorders* (pp. 49–61). New York: Thieme.

Solomon, N. P., & Hixon, T. J. (1993). Speech breathing in Parkinson's disease. *Journal of Speech and Hearing Research, 36*, 294–310.

Verdolini, K. (1994). Voice disorders. In J. B. Tomblin, H. L. Morris, & D. C. Spriestersbach (Eds.), *Diagnosis in speech language pathology*. San Diego, CA: Singular Publishing Group.

World Health Organization. (1980). *International classification of impairments, disabilities, and handicaps*. Geneva: Author.

Yorkston, K. M., & Beukelman, D. R. (1984). *Assessment of intelligibility of dysarthric speech*. Austin, TX: Pro-Ed.

Yorkston, K. M., Miller, R. M., & Strand, E. A. (1995). *Management of speech and swallowing in degenerative diseases*. Tuscon, AZ: Communication Skill Builders.

13

Head and Neck Cancer

Shirley J. Salmon, Ph.D.

Head and neck cancer is diagnosed in a laboratory from analysis of a tissue biopsy. Most often, the findings are interpreted to the patient and significant others by the physician. As you can imagine, learning the diagnosis of cancer is devastating. Most individuals react with shock and, often, denial. When they do acknowledge the diagnosis, patients usually agree to the recommended treatment and rehabilitation procedures. Because more men than women have cancer of the oral tract and/or larynx, I use male pronouns to refer to patients and female pronouns to refer to speech pathologists or significant others.

The cancer may be dealt with medically by surgery, irradiation therapy, chemotherapy, or a combination thereof. These treatments may cause speech, voice, resonance, and/or swallowing problems. When such problems are anticipated, a speech pathologist will be asked by the surgeon to see the patient and significant others for pre-treatment counseling.

The speech pathologist is an important member of the treatment team for these patients.

Following treatment, a speech pathologist will be involved with appraisal and diagnosis of the communication and/or swallowing disorders, counseling, and follow-up therapy. Since oral communication is such an integral part of an individual's personality, you, as a speech pathologist, must consider your patient's lifestyle, occupation, availability of family support, and other pertinent factors when carrying out these responsibilities. Also, you must thoroughly understand the related anatomy and physiology, the ramifications of various cancer treatment procedures, and the psychosocial implications of head and neck cancer. The intent of this chapter is (a) to acquaint you with some of the issues involved in the appraisal of speech and/or voice that is impaired or lost because of cancer and (b) to sensitize you to the emotional reactions of those involved with such losses or impairments.

These emotional reactions are never to be minimized!

MULTIDISCIPLINARY INTERACTIONS

After head and neck cancer is diagnosed, the physician will recommend that it be treated by surgery, radiation, chemotherapy, or any combination of these. Treatment may differ from one person or place to another depending on various factors such as site and size of lesion, general health and age of the patient, physician preference, equipment availability, support personnel's expertise, and patient input. Regardless of the treatment selected, a number of changes may result, which could be temporary, fluctuating, or permanent. Many of the changes are predictable, but some are not. Consequently, you must be knowledgeable about the most common types of aftereffects and be flexible enough to deal with those that are unexpected.

In larger facilities, a team of professionals will meet in pretreatment planning conferences to discuss the selection of treatment, a rehabilitation strategy, and the emotional state of the patient (Logemann, 1989). Generally, the team is headed by a surgeon and includes representatives from dentistry, dietetics, nursing, oncology, pharmacy, physical medicine, psychology, radiology, social work, and speech pathology. In smaller facilities, formal pretreatment planning conferences may not be held. Nevertheless, depending on the complexity and severity of the case, the surgeon will consult with the professionals whom he expects to be involved in the rehabilitative process. It is essential that each professional understand and respect the unique contributions made by the others.

Treatment of the whole person can only be accomplished with a team effort.

Factors associated with the voice and speech problems that generally require speech pathologists' involvement will be discussed in the remaining pages of this chapter. Those associated with swallowing disorders (dysphagia) will be discussed in Chapter 15.

ORAL CANCERS

It was estimated that there would be 30,300 new cases of oral cavity and pharynx cancer in 1998 (Landis, Murray, Bolden, & Wingo, 1998). This number represents about 2.5% of all cancers in that year.

Conventional methods of treatment for oral cancers are surgery, radiation therapy, or both. With selected cases, chemotherapy is used in combination with radiotherapy and/or surgery. Depending on the location, size, and treatment of the cancer, the patient will be faced with cosmetic alterations, dental modifications, swelling or hardening of tissue, drooling or pooling of saliva, dysphagia, resonance changes, and impaired speech production. If swallowing, speech, or voice is impaired, the patient will be referred to the speech pathologist.

Pretreatment Counseling

Surgical reconstruction and/or prosthetic management of the oral structures or oral and nasal cavities usually will affect resonance, swallowing, and speech production. Of particular concern is the possibility of partial (under 75%) or total (75% or more) glossectomy (surgical excision of the tongue). The tongue is vital for speech and swallowing, and it cannot be replaced by a prosthesis. When these problems are anticipated, the surgeon will request the speech pathologist to provide pretreatment counseling. It is essential that you review the medical chart and determine the treatment plans before you meet with the patient and significant others.

> Demonstrating familiarity with the patient's history will increase your credibility with him and his family.

Your goals will be to help the patient understand the treatment plan, so that he is cognizant of the major ramifications of treatment, is aware of the services that will be provided by speech pathology, and is prepared for posttreatment rehabilitation.

After a few social exchanges with the patient, I try to determine how well he understands the planned treatment procedure. Depending on his response, I reiterate, clarify, or expand on his knowledge and correct any misunderstandings. Concurrently, I include family members in the conversation and correct any of their misconceptions. I make a real effort to use lay terms, imagining that I am talking to my father or the neighbor down the street. If I use diagrams, I draw simple lines to illustrate basic structures and function. Often, we laugh about my ineptness and lack of artistic talent; momentarily, it lightens the somberness of the situation. I avoid predicting specific problems. I acknowledge that the patient will experience difficulties with speech and swallowing, but point out that individual differences and variations of treatment determine the extent of deficits and, also, whether they will be transitory or permanent. In other words, I encourage a wait-and-see attitude.

> A friendly, gentle, clinical manner is important in this situation

At this point, I usually mention that, because speech will be affected, we need to consider a temporary alternative means of communication. Writing is the more commonly used method unless either the patient or caregiver is illiterate. In such cases a picture board should be provided. If writing is to be used, I always obtain a sample of the patient's writing or printing to determine legibility.

> **Warning:** Some patients are reluctant to admit that they have limited literacy skills.

I do not rush these sessions and, typically, plan for them to last 60–90 minutes. Always, I listen for comments that may reveal attitudes about the patient's willingness to comply and to participate in the rehabilitation process, and the various family members' perception of their own involvement. When a spouse uses the pronoun "we" in place of the pronoun "he," I am always encouraged.

Posttreatment Counseling

The posttreatment counseling and assessment sessions blend together in terms of professional goals and interactions with the patients. Those who have undergone recent surgery, radiation, or both, often present with asymmetry of facial or oral structures, swelling of the affected area(s), loss of teeth, and swallowing problems that cause pooling of secretions and drooling of saliva. They often carry a cup into which they can expectorate, and a large number of tissues with which to wipe excess saliva. Many patients are not able to produce intelligible speech because of this pooling, dental problems, or restricted movements of the articulatory structures, and so they communicate by writing and gesturing. Usually patients are accompanied by a significant other who is eager to help by providing, or at least supplementing, the medical/surgical history. These friends or family members often seem more desperate than do the patients to receive information about the short- and long-term plans for speech rehabilitation. I think this is particularly so if they know they will be the primary caregiver and must somehow achieve clear communication with the patient.

In the case of patients who have undergone glossectomy (partial or total removal of the tongue), the speech pathologist's goal is to determine whether intelligible speech likely can be developed. When the soft palate or pharynx is involved, one must determine whether velopharyngeal closure can be attained with or without a palatal prosthesis. Because normal swallowing is dependent on coordinated movements of tongue, pharynx, larynx, and esophagus, swallowing function also must be assessed.

Because the tongue is the primary structure used to achieve vowel and consonant articulation, it is amazing that any intelligible speech can be produced following glossectomy. However, some patients demonstrate that it can be accomplished, presumably by compensatory strategies using any remaining tongue structure and other pharyngeal and oral structures. It remains a mystery as to how some individuals are able to compensate and overcome severe deficits in ways that might never have been predicted. In your rehabilitation planning, you should never discount the potential resources or resiliency of some human beings.

When the wound is sufficiently healed and pain has subsided, I conduct a careful evaluation of function. The results will help me formulate plans for speech and swallowing therapy. I begin from the outside and work inward. First, I observe facial structures, noting symmetry, muscle tone, ability to maintain closure of the mouth, flaring of the nares, or drooling. Asymmetry, or drooping of one side of the face, might result in poor coordination and precision during articulation. Drooling or inability to maintain closure of the mouth might indicate swallowing problems, and flaring of the nares may be an indication of inadequate velopharyngeal closure.

We must be careful, before surgery, about predicting the postsurgical range of ability.

During these examinations, we're trying our best to determine *what* the patient is capable of doing.

Next, I perform an oral mechanism examination that begins with an assessment of lip mobility, range of motion, and strength. I then check the presence of teeth and note the extent of mouth opening. I do this because I know that compensatory lip movements against teeth, the alveolar ridge, or a dental plate are frequently used by some patients to produce consonants formerly made with the tongue tip. Obviously, teeth and jaw movements also contribute to precise articulation. Providing a mirror and demonstration when necessary, I next instruct the patient to puff out his cheeks so I can assess the buccal musculature, the strength and completeness of the lip seal, and the ability to attain intraoral pressure, all of which contribute to intelligible articulation.

Simultaneously, I watch to see whether intraoral pressure can be maintained and listen for nasal emission. Air leakage through the nose may indicate velopharyngeal incompetence. Because resection of some portion of the velopharynx is relatively common with oral cancer patients, velopharyngeal competency must always be evaluated. Such competency is vital for swallowing, intelligible speech production, and normal vocal resonance. Specific techniques related to diagnosis and appraisal of velopharyngeal insufficiency are discussed in Chapter 15, so I will not discuss them further here.

When I examine the residual tongue, I first observe how it rests on the floor of the mouth and note asymmetries in structure. Then I assess movement, focusing more on mobility and strength than on mass (Imai & Michi, 1992). I instruct the patient to look at my modeling and then into the mirror to observe his attempts to imitate. First, I appraise the vertical and anteroposterior range of motion. Then, using a tongue blade to provide resistance, I note the strength of the tongue remnant during lateralization and elevation. I want to determine areas that the tongue cannot reach or contact. Recent findings indicate that patients with anterior tongue involvement tend to have more difficulty producing intelligible consonants and that those with posterior tongue involvement experience more difficulty producing intelligible vowels. These findings also indicate that patients who undergo mandibulectomy (excision of the mandible) that crosses the midline, or who are edentulous (without teeth), exhibit a high risk of speech impairment (Leonard, Goodrich, McMenamin, & Donald, 1992).

At this point, I may instruct the patient to produce a few selected vowels and consonants in isolation. However, because speed and coordination of the articulators are better taxed during the act of speaking, I continue my appraisal by administering an articulation test. I believe that the pictures used in articulation tests to elicit single word responses are too juvenile for use with adults. Consequently, I ask the patient to read sentences from the *Fisher-Logemann Test of Articulation Competence* (1971) or the *Sentences for Phonetic Inventory* (Fairbanks, 1960). In addition, I make an audiotape recording of the patient reading a standard passage, "The Rainbow Passage," from the *Voice and Articulation Drillbook* (Fairbanks, 1960). If the patient cannot read, I ask him to repeat sentences from one of the tests mentioned and audio record his responses during a conversational interview. We all must remember that these tests are not easy for the patient to endure, physically or emotionally. Consequently, we must frequently reward the patient's efforts and reassure him that we need this information to determine speech rehabilitative treatment plans.

When scoring these assessment tools I am, of course, interested in the sounds produced correctly; but, for treatment plans, I focus more on those that are omitted or distorted. Depending on the structures involved, possible compensatory articulation mechanisms include pharyngeal widening or narrowing and exaggerated tongue, lip, jaw, epiglottis, or larynx movements (Weber, Ohlms, Bowman, Jacob, & Goepfert, 1991). The distortions may help me decide what exercises to recommend so that compensatory movements may become more accurate. The omissions may indicate compensatory movements toward the articulatory target that are imperceptible and need to be strengthened, or articulatory positions that the patient cannot achieve. For example, if tongue mobility is significantly reduced vertically or laterally, the contact between the tongue and palate may be incomplete. In such cases, I may want to recommend that a palate-lowering or augmentation prosthesis be constructed soon after surgery. If you are interested in a detailed description of how such a device is constructed and utilized, I suggest you refer to Logemann (1989).

Finally, in my assessment, I evaluate the patient's ability to modify rate, pitch, and loudness. Patients who have undergone glossectomy sometimes speak too rapidly; use a low, monotonous pitch; and an inappropriate loudness level for conversation (Skelly, Donaldson, Fust, & Townsend, 1972). The adverse impact glossectomy often has on swallowing is profound. The consequences must not be neglected and are discussed in Chapter 15. You should address all of the parameters mentioned in this section when developing your treatment plan.

> This information will be helpful when we begin to plan treatment.

Further Considerations

In addition to treating the speech, resonance, and dysphagia problems commonly associated with oral/pharyngeal cancers, there are other aspects to consider such as prosthetic management, nutritional education, financial alternatives, and psychological counseling regarding the cosmetic, anatomical, and physiological ramifications of such diseases. Because of the diversity of such factors, it is imperative that these patients be managed, both pre- and postoperatively, by a team of professionals experienced with these types of complications. Myers, Barofsky, and Yates (as cited by Casper & Colton, 1998) underscored the benefits derived from a team of experts. They stated that a team approach will "provide the best means of avoiding many of the pitfalls that threaten patients who are managed by a single physician and exposed sequentially to other disciplines only when problems develop" (p. 189). Even though patients have been treated by a team of experts, they may still require follow up for speech, voice, and swallowing therapy after discharge from the major care center. So, if you have acquired additional training and achieved appropriate expertise, you may find yourself working with a specialty team and planning pre- and immediate postoperative rehabilitation treatment. Conversely, you may be practicing in the home community of a patient many miles from a major cancer treatment center. The patient may be scheduled for routine follow-up appointments with team members at the center but would not be receiving therapy. In this case, he might seek therapy from you, the local speech pathologist. If so, I encourage you to consult with the appropriate speech pathologist at the cancer center to help you determine realistic treatment goals.

Section Summary

In this section, I have attempted to acquaint you with issues involved in the appraisal of speech and/or voice impairment due to oral cancer. I have suggested ways to approach the patient and to evaluate his deficiencies as well as his remaining abilities. Always, the goal is to determine the potential for compensatory articulation movements and to recommend treatment procedures that will facilitate viable communication.

CANCER OF THE LARYNX

It was estimated that there would be 11,100 new cases of laryngeal cancer in 1998 (Landis et al., 1998). This number represents about 1% of all cancers expected to be diagnosed in that year. Even considering the 50,000 laryngectomized individuals in the current United States population, this is not a large number of people. The average age at time of laryngectomy is 62.5 years, so usually these people are employed. Although they represent a small part of any caseload, their rehabilitation needs are so conspicuous that they are given primary consideration by most speech pathologists to whom they are referred.

To enhance your appreciation of the communication skills achieved by many laryngectomized persons, I recommend a visit to a New Voice or Lost Cord Club meeting. There are approximately 300 such clubs throughout the world. All are affiliated with the International Association of Laryngectomees (IAL). Most are associated with their local cancer society. Their primary purpose is to serve as support groups for laryngectomized individuals and their significant others. The individual clubs and the IAL are valuable resources for both professionals and patients. I use the literature and videotapes they provide extensively in my practice.

The address:
International Association of Laryngectomees, 7440 N. Shadeland Avenue., Suite 100, Indianapolis, IN 46250.

Surgical Procedures

Small, less invasive cancers of the larynx commonly are treated by irradiation therapy; patients with such cancers usually are not referred for speech appraisal. Generally, more advanced cancers of the larynx are treated with surgery preceded or followed by radiotherapy. In these instances, the surgery is considered a life-saving procedure.

Surgeons are acutely aware of the traumatic consequences associated with loss of voice due to total removal of the larynx. Consequently, they are diligent about developing better or newer surgical techniques that permit salvaging whatever part of the larynx is free from cancer so that some type of laryngeal voice can be achieved, and oral feeding can be maintained without chronic aspiration. Thus, depending on site and extent of the lesion, a surgeon may perform a total laryngectomy or a partial laryngectomy. Total laryngectomy is excision of the entire larynx. Partial laryngectomies include (a) hemilaryngectomy, (b) supraglottic laryngectomy, (c) subtotal laryngectomy, and (d) near total laryngectomy. Therefore, it is important for you to know which surgical procedure is planned since your counseling, assessments, and rehabilitation plans will vary accordingly.

Preoperative Counseling

Let's begin this discussion with a general precaution. Because the patient and family are likely coming to grips with the reality of cancer, the prospect of surgery and the changes it will bring, and fears of pain and death, they may or may not show much interest in what you need to discuss with them. Nevertheless, the surgeon has referred them to us knowing there is much information they should have and so we proceed, in as much or as little detail as we judge they can follow. For example, my explanation of the various methods of speech following laryngeal surgery is fairly brief, unless they ask for more detailed information.

Before meeting with the patient and significant others, I review the medical chart to determine the specific surgical procedure planned. If a partial laryngectomy is proposed, you must be sure that the patient and family members understand that his voice will be different; swallowing may be more difficult; and he may breathe, permanently or temporarily, through a hole in his neck. If a total laryngectomy is anticipated, you should determine whether radical neck surgery will be included and whether a tracheoesophageal fistula (TEF) (see section on *tracheoesophageal fistula speech*) is planned as a primary procedure in conjunction with the laryngectomy or as a secondary procedure after total laryngectomy is performed. Unilateral or bilateral radical neck surgery will cause the patient discomfort with arm raising and neck turning immediately following surgery; a referral to physical therapy is appropriate. Neck surgery also may influence the choice of an artificial larynx. If a TEF is planned as a primary procedure, you should provide much more information about this method of laryngeal speech preoperatively (refer to the final paragraphs of this section).

Obviously, a close working relationship with the surgeon is required if this preoperative counseling is to be maximally helpful to the patient and family

The patient's general health also should be considered. Previous cancer or irradiation treatments, hiatal hernia, ulcer, or respiratory difficulties may have adverse effects on some types of speech after laryngeal surgery.

When you meet with the patient and family members, try to gain some insight about the patient such as personality, motivation, coping strategies, and inquisitiveness. Does he express an interest in voice and speech rehabilitation? Is he attentive? Do his questions or responses reflect an orientation to reality? Does he appear shy or outgoing? Do the spouse and he share in their communication or does she seem to do all the talking for him? Laryngectomized individuals who receive emotional support from peers and family tend to move more rapidly through the rehabilitative process, so try to glean some information about family relationships. Do family members show or express concern for each other and talk about their plans to help the patient after surgery?

Other areas to probe are the patient's vocation and avocations. To what extent does he rely on speech for his job, home life, and social activities? Does he plan to return to his current job, request a transfer to a different position that is less demanding of oral communication skills, or to retire? Would he be interested in discussing these issues with an appropriate counselor?

Finally, you will want to assess his speech and language behaviors. Typically, this is carried out in a fairly informal way. After all, you have been conversing with him throughout the interview and so already should have reached some conclusions. The patient's voice quality may be impaired because of the cancer, but what about resonance? Does velopharyngeal closure seem adequate? Is his speech rate within normal limits? Is he missing teeth or does he wear dentures? Are his articulation skills proficient? What percent of his conversational speech would you judge to be intelligible? Does he use gestures and facial expressions? Does he exhibit manual dexterity and coordination? Also, ask about his and his spouse's hearing. Consider a referral of one or both for an audiological evaluation.

Before discussing anything about the surgery or its ramifications, determine the patient's perception of what he already has been told. He may not understand that, when he wakes up in the recovery room, he will be breathing through an opening in his neck (tracheostoma) and mouthing words without a voice. At the very least, it is imperative that he understand these two basic consequences of laryngectomy. Ask the patient, "What have you been told about the planned surgery?" Or say, "Well, it sounds as if you are scheduled for some pretty serious surgery. Tell me about it." Listen carefully to his response. Reinforce or elaborate on his accurate information; correct any misconceptions.

Typically, I explain that, when all or a portion of the larynx is removed, a tracheostomy must be performed to protect the lungs from being filled with food or liquid. I estimate that the tracheostoma will range in size from a dime to a quarter. Finally, I mention that in

The emphasis here is on what he understands, not on what we assume that he's been told!

the future, if the tracheostoma will be permanent, the patient will wear homemade or commercially available stoma covers for both aesthetic and hygienic reasons.

My explanation of the various methods of speech following partial laryngectomies is fairly brief and includes mention of possible swallowing problems. If total laryngectomy is planned, I first explain why an alternative source for voice is required following removal of the larynx. I do this by drawing a simple, line sketch of the involved structures (nose, mouth, tongue, pharynx, area from where larynx was excised, trachea, lungs, esophagus, and stomach). To lighten the moment, I personalize the drawing with curly hair, a pug nose, or a long, thin neck (Figure 13–1). At this point, I am ready to provide a simple explanation of the relevant anatomy and physiology. My goal is to increase the patient's understanding, so I use laymen's terminology in both my discussion and on the diagram. I explain that food or liquid moves from the mouth, into the back of the throat (pharynx), through a ring of muscles at the top of the esophagus (pharyngoesophageal [PE] segment), into the food tube (esophagus), and down into the stomach. I explain that these structures comprise one set of plumbing that is designed, primarily, for food intake. Also, I mention that the important biologic function of the larynx and vocal folds is to

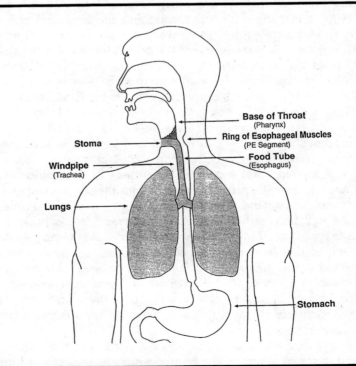

Figure 13–1. Anatomy and physiology associated with total laryngectomy.

prevent food and water from entering the lungs. When the larynx is no longer available to serve as a trap door, the windpipe (trachea) must be diverted and an opening into the trachea (stoma) must be created. The trachea and lungs function as a second set of plumbing designed for breathing in and out to stay alive. Finally, I show him that when the windpipe is connected to the larynx, air from the lungs can pass through the vocal cords and cause them to vibrate for the production of vocal sound. Without the larynx, a substitute sound source is necessary in order to produce voice. The sound source may be a speech aid (an artificial larynx) or the ring of muscles (PE segment) at the top of the esophagus. At this point, I am ready to discuss the three methods of alaryngeal speech.

Using mechanical, lay terminology is very important here!

Artificial Larynx Speech

I explain that most speech aids are battery-operated devices, which, when activated, produce a sound. If an intraoral device is used, the sound is transmitted through a mouth-tube into the oral cavity. If a neck-type device is used, the sound is transmitted through the neck tissue into the pharynx and oral cavity (see Figure 13–2). In either case, the artificial larynx sound is modified by the resonators and is shaped into artificial larynx speech by the articulators.

These instruments are not as easy to learn to use as some people might think. However, unless demented or retarded, most patients can acquire intelligible artificial larynx speech if they receive appropriate speech therapy. You should assure the patient that you will help him select a device from the variety that is available and begin teaching him how to use it as soon as his feeding tube is removed. The goal is for him to be able to express intelligibly a few short, functional phrases by the time he leaves the hospital.

Esophageal Speech

Next, I explain how standard esophageal speech is attained. On the line drawing, I point out the area of the PE segment and talk about the importance of it for the production of esophageal voice. By opening and closing my fist, I illustrate how the PE segment instantaneously opens to allow air from above it to enter the esophagus for insufflation. Then, with a rapid opening and closing of my fist, I illustrate how this ring of muscles can be activated to vibrate and produce sound when air is expelled from the esophagus and passed upward through the segment (see Figure 13–3). The esophageal sound (voice) is transmitted into the pharynx where it is altered by the resonating cavities and formed into esophageal speech by the articulators.

Esophageal speech cannot be attained by everyone. In fact, it is estimated that about 60% of all laryngectomees do not or cannot use esophageal speech as their sole means of oral communication. Some people are highly motivated to learn it because they want to speak without having to depend on any type of prosthetic device.

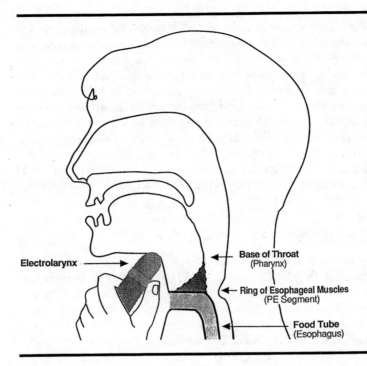

Electrolarynx

Base of Throat
(Pharynx)

Ring of Esophageal Muscles
(PE Segment)

Food Tube
(Esophagus)

Figure 13–2. Artificial larynx speech.

Tracheoesophageal Fistula Speech

Finally, I explain how esophageal voice is attained when a tracheo-esophageal fistula (TEF) procedure has been performed. The TEF can be done either at the time of laryngectomy, as a primary procedure, or at a later date as a secondary procedure. I indicate that after the larynx is removed and a tracheostoma has been created, the surgeon will make a small tunnel (fistula) through the tracheal wall into the esophagus. After several days for healing, the surgeon or speech pathologist will insert a small voice prosthesis into this opening (Figure 13–4). When the patient uses his thumb or a finger to occlude his tracheostoma, air from the lungs will be shunted through the voice prosthesis and into his esophagus. This air will cause vibration of the PE segment that results in sound. The esophageal sound that travels into his oral and nasal cavities can be used to articulate speech.

While I am explaining these steps, I try to underscore the patient's eventual responsibilities for removing, cleaning, and reinserting the prosthesis. Then, I present a list of the criteria for TEF candidacy and,

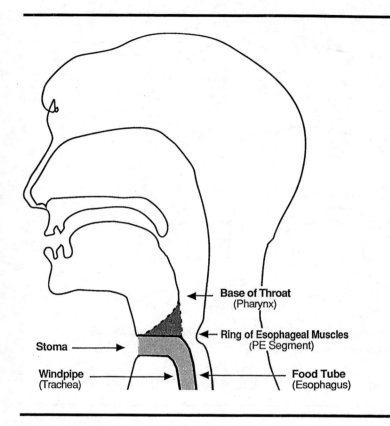

Base of Throat
(Pharynx)

Ring of Esophageal Muscles
(PE Segment)

Stoma

Windpipe
(Trachea)

Food Tube
(Esophagus)

Figure 13–3. Esophageal speech.

together, we appraise his abilities to meet them. The criteria may differ slightly from those originally established by Singer and Blom (1980). Requirements may include (a) patient motivation with the ability to comprehend the method of voice production and a willingness to accept responsibility for care of the voice prosthesis; (b) sufficient manual dexterity and visual acuity to insert the prosthesis and occlude the stoma; (c) ability to generate adequate pulmonary pressure to activate the voice prosthesis; (d) sufficient hearing acuity to detect and monitor phonations; and (e) no evidence of alcohol abuse. Patients who elect TEF as a secondary procedure, after they have been laryngectomized, must meet four additional requirements. They are (a) adequate size and shape of the stoma so it can accommodate the puncture and be totally occluded by the patient's thumb or finger, (b) stoma occlusion does not elicit sustained coughing, (c) patient is

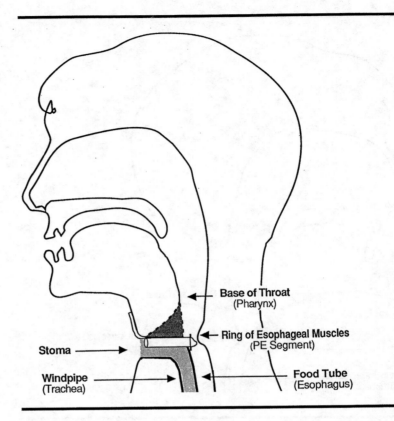

Figure 13–4. Tracheoesophageal fistula speech.

3–6 months postirradiation, and (d) patient performs satisfactorily on an esophageal air insufflation test described by Blom, Singer, and Hamaker (1985).

Before terminating the preoperative session for those who will undergo total laryngectomy, I make an effort to relieve some immediate concerns that are discussed at length in the literature (Salmon, 1986, 1999). I tell the patient and spouse that it is not at all likely that he will die on the operating table and that he will be well cared for by a competent nursing staff. Pain medication will be available; however, most patients report that the pain is no worse than a sort throat and a stiff neck—when radical neck dissection is required. I mention that trained, well-rehabilitated laryngectomized individuals and their spouses from the New Voice Club are available to make pre- and postoperative visits. Because there is controversy about whether such a visit should be scheduled before or after surgery, I let the patient and spouse decide.

I advise all patients that staples or insoluble stitches will be used to close the incisions. Because the sutures need time to heal, the patient will not be allowed to swallow food or liquids. Instead, a feeding tube will be in place for 7–10 days. Dressings and other tubes may also be present, but their use is routine and should not be considered extraordinary.

If the spouse expects to visit the patient in his room immediately prior to surgery, I suggest she be there at least an hour before his operation is scheduled. Otherwise, he may already have been sedated and/or taken to the operative area before she arrives. Also, I indicate how long the surgery might take. I suggest she may want someone to wait with her during a relatively long day. I note the day of surgery and plan a short visit with her in the surgical waiting room.

Last, you will want to determine which means of communication might be most appropriate immediately following surgery. When he wakes up in the recovery room, he will not be able to make sound for talking. Is the patient literate? If not, after surgery, he may have to mouth words, use a picture communication board, or be taught to use an artificial larynx. If he is literate, obtain a sample of his writing to determine legibility. He will require a pad and pencil or magic slate on which to write. Unless the patient or spouse requests additional information, I usually terminate the session at this point. I do so by saying I will be at the patient's bedside 3–4 days postoperatively.

Postoperative Counseling

Postoperative contacts with laryngectomized patients and significant others usually begin in the hospital within 3 to 4 days following surgery. The nature of these contacts will depend on the extent of surgery, the type of communication and swallowing problems exhibited, and whether the patient received preoperative counseling. If the patient was seen preoperatively, I review the material previously discussed and move on from there. If he was not seen preoperatively, I present the initial material in more detail except for that concerning the surgery and the immediate impact it has on breathing, coughing, and voicing. According to Casper and Colton (1998), "It is not necessary to cover all the material that might have been included in a presurgical contact, because the patient has already gone through the surgery and is now ready to go beyond it" (p. 43). I try to see patients at least twice per day and include the family members whenever possible; there is a lot for them to learn in the short time between surgery and hospital discharge.

In general, the initial sessions are purely educational. I provide patients with written descriptions about their type of surgery so they can read about it at their leisure and share the information with family and friends. Many descriptions are published by the American

The address: American Cancer Society, 1599 Clifton Rd. NE, Atlanta, GA 30329.

Cancer Society (ACS), the International Association of Laryngectomees (IAL), and others referenced under *Recommended Readings* at the end of this chapter. Also, when appropriate, I explain resuscitation procedures for neck-breathers. I show videotapes or play audiotapes that demonstrate the method(s) of speech that might be used. If the patient has undergone total laryngectomy, I arrange, with his permission, an appointment with trained visitors from the New Voice Club. These people can serve as an inspiration and present a walking, talking example of how a near-normal life can be resumed following laryngectomy.

Partial Laryngectomy Appraisal

Patients who have undergone a partial laryngectomy typically have a tracheostomy so they are breathing through the hole (stoma) in their neck. Generally, they are aphonic and are communicating by whispering and writing. Some still have a nasogastric feeding tube in place. If not, they may complain of frequent choking when swallowing food or liquids. Sometimes the swallowing problems are transitory. When they persist, there is a risk of aspiration and pneumonia. Decisions must be made about continuing dysphagia therapy, subjecting the patient to long-term feedings through a stomach tube, or performing a total laryngectomy. A tracheostomy also may be permanent or transitory, so you may need to teach the patient to occlude his stoma to produce voice. Initially, with or without a tracheostomy, the patient may be voiceless or exhibit a breathy voice quality. Determine if the patient achieves improved voice quality when you instruct him to vary pitch and loudness. You should encourage the positive changes in follow-up voice therapy. If only a short time has elapsed between surgery and your first postoperative contact, velopharyngeal closure and some tongue movements may be affected by a nasogastric feeding tube. If so, one does not usually need to delay formal assessment, but the effects of the feeding tube should be taken into account when the patient's articulation and speech rate are assessed. Usually, a reduced rate of speaking tends to provide more pulmonary support for increased volume, and more deliberate articulation will improve intelligibility. During the assessment, determine whether changes in these parameters have a positive influence on the patient's voice and speech. If so, they should receive more attention in your follow-up therapy.

Total Laryngectomy Appraisal

There are several reasons why a speech pathologist might not interact with a laryngectomee and family member for either pre- or postoperative counseling within a hospital setting. According to Graham (1997), the time between the diagnosis and surgery may be limited, a referral may not be made, the patient may choose not to follow through with the surgeon's referral, or the patient may have been counseled by a speech pathologist in a major cancer center and, then, referred for ongoing therapy to a clinician located closer to his home community. Therefore, the first meeting with a laryngectomee could well be after hospital discharge and take place in a hearing and speech clinic, a convalescent home, or the office of a speech pathologist who is in private practice.

The laryngectomized individual may know little or nothing about alaryngeal speech, in which case he might be mouthing words, using gestures, writing, or exhibiting any combination thereof. He may know about all three of the methods, but use only one type. If so, he might be genuinely interested in additional therapy to improve his communicative skills using the one method more effectively. Another individual might be interested in learning how to use a different type of alaryngeal speech as a secondary or backup method. Well rehabilitated laryngectomees who speak effectively and are trained to make hospital visits to newly laryngectomized patients frequently want to demonstrate more than one type of speech and, so, they seek additional training. Another individual may have lived with a laryngectomy for several years, adjusted to it, and be interested in sharing his experiences with schoolchildren, nursing students, emergency personnel, and others in the community as an educational service. This type of person would want to refine his communicative skills and, perhaps, seek your endorsement. As a final example, consider a laryngectomee who might be encountering several problems when trying to acquire a new method of speaking or to use a particular type of alaryngeal speech more effectively. Such problems usually occur with those trying to learn esophageal speech or with those trying to achieve or maintain successful voicing with tracheoesophageal speech. So, it is possible to see people for evaluation who exhibit varying conditions and are in different stages of rehabilitation. Their presenting symptoms will vary based on time since surgery, past experiences, communication goals, and expectations for total rehabilitation, both now and in the future.

As a speech pathologist, my primary goal is to help the laryngectomee develop a functional communication system that he can accept and, hopefully, feel downright proud about having acquired. If this goal is met, I believe that person will have a good chance of being accepted in his social circles and of resuming a lifestyle that he considers worthwhile.

My first responsibility is to explain the three types of alaryngeal speech and consult with the patient as he considers these alternatives. When he has determined a method of choice, we will together establish a therapy program designed to help him achieve functional communication. Later, we may broaden the therapy program if the patient wishes to fine tune his skills or learn another method.

Artificial Larynx Speech

I encourage all laryngectomized patients to learn to use an artificial larynx. My immediate goals are to talk with the patient and family about the advantages and disadvantages of artificial larynx devices, to acquaint them with the various types and assortment of devices available, and to guide them in their selection as well as their learning to use such an instrument. I display as many devices as are available by placing them on a table and discussing the distinctive features of each (see Figure 13–5). I assist patients in holding and operating them. I give each patient a list of supply sources and current prices for later reference. There is no set formula for helping a person select a device; suitability must be determined on an individual basis. The following are some factors to consider when helping patients select an instrument.

An intraoral device may be used if the patient undergoes postoperative radiotherapy and his neck becomes too sore to tolerate the pressure of a neck-type device. Also, if radical neck surgery has been performed that substantially changes the neck structure, a neck-type device may not work well. In both instances, an oral adaptor for a neck-type instrument, an interdental speech aid, or an intraoral artificial larynx that requires use of a mouth tube would be appropriate. Figure 13–5 illustrates the variety of speech aids currently available.

Various types of the neck-type electrolarynx differ in terms of weight, shape, size, and diameter of the vibrating head. Obviously, there are differences among patients with respect to neck size and density. A thick, fleshy, or swollen neck will absorb rather than transmit sound delivered by the device, so an instrument that produces a more powerful sound should be selected. A person with a small, thin neck may be able to use a less powerful device. Soft, supple tissue is required to embed the vibrating head; when none can be located around the neck or chin area, cheek placement may be necessary.

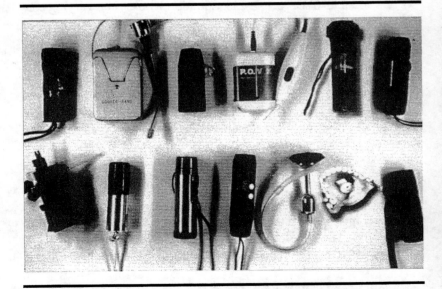

Figure 13–5. An assortment of artificial larynx devices representing different types available (intraoral, interdental, and neck-type).

In addition to these considerations, one should take into account differences in cost, ease of manipulation, cradling comfort, and subjective preferences of patient and spouse. In many clinics, when the final selection is made, a loaner device of that type is made available. Then, therapy should be initiated prior to hospital discharge.

Use of artificial larynx devices has steadily increased over the last 15–20 years (Morris, Van Demark, Smith, & Mayes, 1992; Salmon, 1999). Approximately 40% of laryngectomees use speech aids either as a primary means of communication or as a backup (Gelman, 1995). Unless a person is demented or severely retarded, he should be able to learn to use such an instrument quite satisfactorily provided the therapy is appropriate.

Tracheoesophageal Fistula (TEF) Speech

Criteria to be met by those interested in TEF have been discussed previously. Recovery time differs for these patients, depending on whether the TEF was performed as a primary or secondary procedure and whether other related surgery was performed also. While patients are recovering, they can meet individuals who use TEF speech or view them on videotape (Figure 13–6). Even if the patient viewed it preoperatively, I like to show him a videotape of a patient demonstrating the removal, cleaning, inserting, and taping of his voice prosthesis. At that time, we use a mirror to examine the shape of the patient's stoma and estimate whether he will use finger or thumb occlusion. Also, we look

> Successful use of the TEF procedure requires considerable cooperation by the patient and the family.

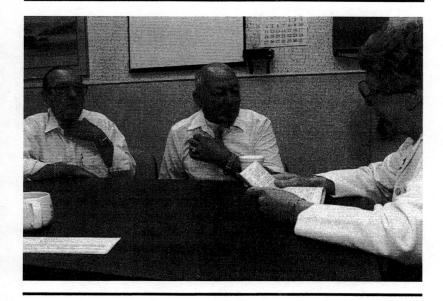

Figure 13–6. Therapy with two laryngectomized individuals using TEF speech.

at the surface surrounding his stoma and discuss the likelihood of his being able to wear a tracheostoma valve (which eliminates the need for finger or thumb occlusion). I want to appraise these factors and to stimulate the patient's thinking about his responsibility in the speech rehabilitation process. When he is scheduled for voice prosthesis placement, his feeding tube is removed from the puncture site, the functioning of the pharyngoesophageal (PE) segment is tested, and an appropriately sized voice prosthesis is inserted. At this point, treatment begins during which the patient must be taught how to maintain and use his prosthesis.

The percentage of laryngectomees who have a TEF procedure is increasing yearly. Extrapolating from the available data (Gelman, 1995; Morris et al., 1992), a good estimate is that in the U.S.A. approximately 40% of those having undergone laryngectomy within the last 15 years use tracheoesophageal speech. However, some patients are not able or willing to maintain and use a voice prosthesis satisfactorily. Sometimes, the reasons can be easily determined and remedied in therapy. For example, the fistula may need to be remeasured and the prosthesis resized. Other times, the problems are more complex, such as a migrating fistula or leakage of swallowed material into the trachea causing aspiration. Proper diagnostic procedures and proposed solutions for these more complex problems must be carried out by speech pathologists or surgeons who have received special training associated with TEF speech. One should consult these specialists, usually at major medical centers, whenever the problems become worse or persist after reasonable efforts have been made to correct them during diagnostic therapy.

Esophageal Speech

The surgeon determines when patients can begin esophageal speech therapy. Some prefer the instruction be delayed for 30 days postoperatively; others believe it can begin after the patient is able to swallow solid foods. While still recovering in the hospital, the patient should be taught the basic skills of using an artificial larynx and be encouraged to use one during his initial esophageal speech training. He can meet esophageal speakers or view them on videotape.

I explain that whether he has adequate "plumbing" to produce esophageal voice will need to be determined later, in trial therapy, or with an esophageal air insufflation test. When he is able to swallow, I assess tongue, lip, and jaw movements since they are used, typically, to insufflate the esophagus. I also talk with the patient to assess his willingness to persist and his understanding that acquisition of proficient esophageal speech generally takes at least 6 months. Within the last 20 years, there has been a marked decrease in the number of laryngectomees using esophageal speech for their primary means of communication (Gelman, 1995). The average length of time taken to acquire it, the associated costs, and the option since 1981 of tracheoesophageal speech are no doubt reasons for its decline. Still, there are those interested in learning to use it as a primary or secondary method of alaryngeal speech. When patients fail to progress, there are a number of physiological reasons that should be investigated, such as hypertonicity or hypotonicity of the P-E segment. Specialists at the major medical centers are familiar with the assessment procedures appropriate for such cases and should be consulted whenever patients' failure to show progress in therapy cannot be explained and persists beyond a reasonable time frame of 4–6 sessions.

Not all laryngectomees are candidates for esophageal speech training. Motivation is an important factor in the ability to acquire esophageal speech (Shanks, 1986). Other psychological or physiological characteristics that have a positive effect are extroversion, independence, age, adequate hearing, and sufficient tongue mobility. All of these factors must be considered in your appraisal. However, you must consider also the plea by Shanks (1986, p. 346) who wrote, "it has not been said that if someone fails to meet the different criteria, that person should be denied the chance to try to speak [with esophageal speech] after laryngectomy. It is a person's right to talk."

Section Summary

In this section, I have discussed surgical procedures and ramifications associated with laryngeal cancer. I have suggested ways to counsel patients and their significant others so their acquired knowledge might lessen the emotional impact of their losses. Speech pathologists must not ignore the physiological, psychological, economic, and social factors associated with the surgery. Fears or problems related to these factors can interfere with a patient's ability to benefit from any rehabilitation efforts. According to Casper and Colton (1998), "It is the responsibility of the speech-language pathologist to be aware of these problems; to provide a supportive, open, nonjudgmental atmosphere in which they can be discussed; and to offer referral to appropriate personnel or agencies" (p. 47). Finally, I have offered suggestions you may incorporate when observing and assessing behaviors to enhance your appraisal process. The evaluation process is ongoing because patient behaviors and needs are ever-changing. When patients fail to improve in therapy or exhibit new and unexplainable problems, they should be referred to appropriate specialists.

SUMMARY

The speech-language pathologist is an important member of the team providing services to the patient with head and neck surgery and to the patient's family. Our major goals with these patients are to assess the impact of the disease and its treatment on the communication skills of the patient and to provide means for rehabilitation of those skills.

There is considerable diversity among these patients in range of disease, residual capabilities, and personal characteristics. As a consequence, frequently, diagnostic and treatment methods must be planned on an individual basis.

REFERENCES

American Cancer Society. (1992). *Cancer Facts & Figures—1992.* Atlanta, GA: Author.

Blom, E. D., Singer, M. I., & Hamaker, R. C. (1985). An improved esophageal insufflation test. *Archives of Otolaryngology, 111,* 211–212.

Casper, J. K., & Colton, R. H. (1998). *Clinical manual for laryngectomy and head/neck cancer rehabilitation* (2nd ed.). San Diego, CA: Singular Publishing Group.

Fairbanks, G. (1960). *Voice and articulation drillbook* (2nd ed.). New York: Harper & Row.

Fisher, H., & Logemann, J. (1971). *Fisher-Logemann Test of Articulation Competence.* Boston, MA: Houghton Mifflin.

Gelman, J. (1995). Trends in alaryngeal speech. *Advance for Speech-Language Pathologists and Audiologists, 5,* 15.

Graham, M. S. (1997). *The clinician's guide to alaryngeal speech therapy.* Newton, MA: Butterworth-Heineman.

Imai, S., & Michi, K. (1992). Articulatory function after resection of the tongue and floor of the mouth: Palatometric and perceptual evaluation. *Journal of Speech and Hearing Research, 35,* 68–78.

Landis, S. H., Murray, T., Bolden, S., & Wingo, P. A. (1998). Cancer statistics, 1998. *CA A Cancer Journal for Clinicians, 48*(1), 6–30.

Leonard, R., Goodrich, S., McMenamin, P., & Donald, P. (1992). Differentiation of speakers with glossectomies by acoustic and perceptual measures. *American Journal of Speech-Language Pathology, 1,* 55–63.

Logemann, J. A. (1989). Speech and swallowing rehabilitation for head and neck tumor patients. In E. N. Myers & J. Y. Suen (Eds.), *Cancer of the head and neck* (2nd ed., pp. 1021–1043). New York: Churchill Livingstone.

Morris, H. L., Van Demark, D. R., Smith, A. E., & Mayes, M. D. (1992). Communication status following laryngectomy: The Iowa experience 1984–1987. *Annals of Otology, Rhinology, and Laryngology, 101,* 503–510.

Salmon, S. J. (1986). Adjusting to laryngectomy. In W. H. Perkins & J. L. Northern (Eds.), *Seminars in speech and language: Current strategies of rehabilitation of the laryngectomized patient, 7,* 67–94. New York: Thieme.

Salmon, S. J. (Ed.). (1999). *Alaryngeal speech rehabilitation: For clinicians by clinicians.* Austin, TX: Pro-Ed.

Shanks, J. C. (1986). Essentials for laryngeal speech: Psychology and physiology. In R. L. Keith & F. L. Darley (Eds.), *Laryngectomee Rehabilitation* (2nd ed., pp. 337–349). Austin, TX: Pro-Ed.

Singer, M. I., & Blom, E. D. (1980). An endoscopic technique for restoration of voice after laryngectomy. *Annals of Otology, Rhinology, and Laryngology, 89*, 529–533.

Skelly, M., Donaldson, R. C., Fust, R., & Townsend, D. (1972). Changes in phonatory aspects of glossectomy intelligibility through vocal parameter manipulation. *Journal of Speech and Hearing Disorders, 37*, 379–389.

Weber, R. S., Ohlms, L., Bowman, J., Jacob, R., & Goepfert, H. (1991). Functional results after total or near total glossectomy with laryngeal preservation. *Archives of Otolaryngology—Head and Neck Surgery, 117*, 512–515.

RECOMMENDED READINGS

American Cancer Society. (1994). *Primeros pasos: Palabras de ayuda para laringectomizados* [Brochure]. Atlanta, GA: Author.

American Cancer Society. (1995). *First steps: Helping words for the laryngectomee* [Brochure]. Atlanta, GA: Author.

Gargan, W. (1969). *Why Me? An Autobiography.* New York: Doubleday & Company.

International Association of Laryngectomees. (1998). *Rehabilitating laryngectomees* [Brochure]. 7440 N. Shadeland Ave., Suite 100, Indianapolis, IN: Author.

Lanpher, A. (1965). "Hello, Tallulah." In W. Ross (Ed.), *The climate is hope* (pp. 35–50). Englewood Cliffs, NJ: Prentice-Hall.

Lauder, J. (Ed.). (1998). *Self-help for the laryngectomee* (1998–1999 ed.). 11115 Whisper Hollow, San Antonio, TX: Lauder Enterprises.

Moss, D. G. (1988). *Why didn't they tell me?* Seattle, WA: Laryngectomee Supply Company.

Nicholson, E. (1975). Personal notes of a laryngectomy. *American Journal of Nursing, 75*, 2157–2158.

CHAPTER

14

Cleft Palate

Sally J. Peterson-Falzone, Ph.D.

This chapter deals with the diagnostic questions, methodology, and decisions relative to patients with clefts at all developmental and treatment stages. The special diagnostic procedures that are generally available only in medical settings are discussed briefly. The majority of the information is about the assessment tasks faced by the speech-language pathologist who functions in nonmedical settings such as public schools and private practice. The discussion is based on a wide variety of research studies, some of which are listed in the References and Resources Bibliography, and on the *Parameters for the Evaluation and Treatment of Patients with Cleft Lip/Palate or Other Craniofacial Anomalies* as published by the American Cleft Palate-Craniofacial Association in 1993 (this document is currently being revised).

AN OVERVIEW

It's highly possible that you know someone with cleft lip and palate but may not know much about the disorder. Briefly, it is a birth defect that occurs once in about 650 live births. It is a highly variable defect, expressed as cleft lip, cleft palate, or both, and in a complete form (extending through all of the affected structures) or incomplete form (only a partial extension). In any case, the cleft is the result of incomplete development of the structures early in fetal life. We do not yet have a full understanding of all the many genetic and environmental factors that can cause clefts, but new information on causation is being gathered virtually on a daily basis.

If there is a cleft lip, there will be some facial disfigurement, although often mild in degree. If the cleft extends through the gum ridge (the alveolus), there will be dental problems ranging from missing teeth to a marked misfit (malocclusion) between the upper jaw (the maxilla) and the lower jaw (the mandible). If the cleft extends through the palate (the roof of the mouth), the baby will initially have problems sucking and, later, will not be able to direct the air stream through the mouth during the first speech attempts. The resulting "nasal leak" will take the form of nasal emission during the production of consonants requiring the buildup of intraoral air pressure, and hypernasal voice quality on vowels and vocalic segments. (This is an oversimplified description of speech in individuals with clefts, but one that will be helpful for our purposes here.)

With this brief background, we now proceed to discuss the matter of diagnosis of communication problems in children and adults with clefts.

THE FIRST FEW MONTHS OF LIFE

The speech-pathologist on a cleft palate/craniofacial team typically meets the child and family during the first critical weeks of life. At this stage, our diagnostic concerns include (1) the effects of the cleft on prelinguistic vocal output, (2) how the presence of the cleft may

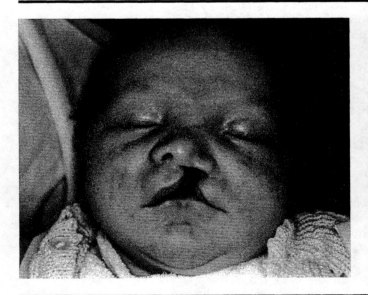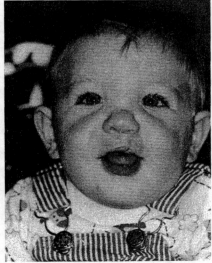

Figure 14–1. Infant with unilateral cleft lip and palate before and after lip repair. (Center for Craniofacial Anomalies, University of California-San Francisco, William Y. Hoffman, surgeon)

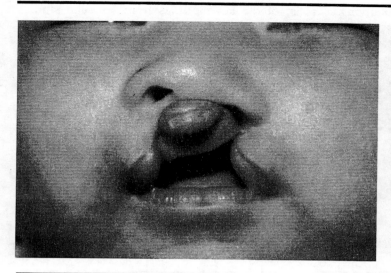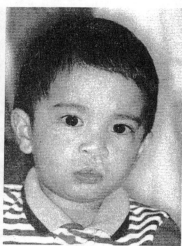

Figure 14–2. Child with incomplete bilateral cleft (complete on left side, incomplete on right) before and after lip repair. (Center for Craniofacial Anomalies, University of California-San Francisco, William Y. Hoffman, surgeon)

affect the family emotionally and thus influence their stimulation of the child, (3) the high probability of middle ear fluid and hearing loss, and (4) the possibility of associated malformations and/or syndromes (over 50% of children with clefts have at least one associated minor or major malformation).

When you see the child and family at this early stage, you have an excellent opportunity to prevent or minimize later problems in communication development. This text contains chapters on assessment of various aspects of communication behavior in infants and young children. Depending on both the time available and the particular setting in which you meet with the child and family, you may use a variety of tools to assess early development. As an example, the *MacArthur Communicative Development Inventory* (Fenson et al., 1993) consists of two parent-inventory scales, one for infants up to the age of 15 months and one for toddlers aged 16 to 30 months. Scales are also available for families whose dominant language is not English. The information derived with this tool can predict later problems in language development, and investigators have found it to be useful in identifying deficits in children with cleft palate.

In the last decade or so, there has been a welcome burst of studies of prelinguistic vocalizations and of early phonetic and phonologic development in children with clefts. Investigators have studied the differences between the early vocalizations of babies with clefts and those of babies without clefts and offered theories about how these differences influence later speech development.

Most infants in the United States and Europe do not undergo surgical closure of the palatal cleft during the first 6 months of life. So most of these studies are of children with open cleft palates.

Following is a list of the key findings from six such studies (Chapman, 1991; Chapman & Hardin, 1992; Grunwell & Russell, 1987; O'Gara & Logemann, 1988, 1990; O'Gara et al., 1994; Philips & Kent, 1984):

■ In their reduplicated babbling (e.g., "bababa"), babies with clefts show a relative lack of the normal acoustic cues for the differences between consonants and vowels. Parents of babies with clefts often report that their babies were late in babbling, perhaps because the parents simply cannot recognize the babbling behavior due to the lack of normal acoustic cues.

■ Babies with clefts produce many more sounds made at the boundaries of the vocal tract, that is, the lips and the vocal

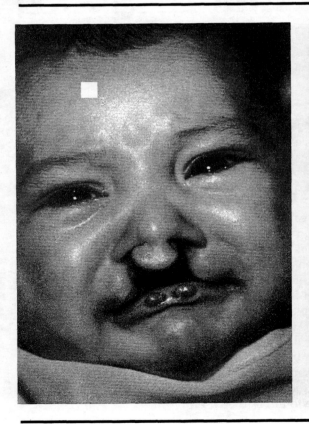 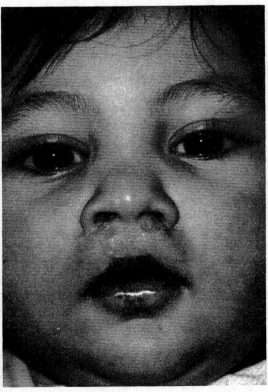

Figure 14–3. Pre- and postoperative pictures of an infant with an incomplete bilateral cleft (complete on the left side, incomplete on the right) and lower lip mounds. The mounds signal the presence of Van der Woude syndrome, a condition combining lower lip pits or mounds with various forms of clefting. This syndrome is autosomal dominant, meaning the risk for recurrence in the family, or in this child's own children, is 50%. (Center for Craniofacial Anomalies, University of California-San Francisco, William Y. Hoffman, surgeon)

cords, as opposed to sounds made within the mouth, and, at 6 months of age, they do not show the "takeover" of alveolar consonants heard in noncleft babies by this age.

- Babies with clefts use more nasals, glides, and the glottal fricative /h/ than the stop-plosives that are preferred by noncleft babies.
- Babies with clefts also use fewer syllables in their early vocalizations than do noncleft babies.

Clinically, these findings tell us that there will be some early, unavoidable differences in speech sound development in infants with clefts. Our first diagnostic task is to assess the infant's general communicative development, to be certain that it is in line with his or her overall development. Second, we want to study early vocalizations carefully so that we can explain to parents (1) what they are hearing from their child, (2) how this may be different from early speech sound development in normal infants, and (3) ways in which they may help to promote normal speech and language development in their child.

Some infants have been fitted with palatal plates prior to surgical closure of the palate to try to promote more normal articulation development. This is technically difficult to do, especially if the child advances to the toddler stage and removes the plate at will, usually feeding it to the dog!

AFTER PALATE CLOSURE

Surgeons, speech pathologists, orthodontists, and other members of cleft palate/craniofacial teams are still trying to determine an optimum age range for surgical closure of the palatal cleft. Currently, the most common ages of palatal surgery in the United States fall in the range of 9 to 18 months. Within the team context, postoperative evaluations typically begin 2 to 3 months after surgery and are carried out periodically as the child grows. Specifically, we want to determine whether palatal surgery has been successful in providing the child with velopharyngeal closure. We also want to determine whether language and speech development are within normal limits and, if not, in what way. One obvious possibility is that the child may have learned some abnormal speech production patterns in her attempt to compensate for the open cleft palate.

We are still trying to determine the best time for palatal surgery to promote normal speech development without causing problems in later growth of the midface. A lot of data have been put forth, but the argument is far from over.

Children with repaired clefts who show significant delays in speech development before the age of 2 years often show "catch-up" in the sounds they produce (Chapman & Hardin, 1992). O'Gara Logemann, and Rademaker (1994) strongly emphasized the factor of time, stating "time is an even stronger variable than age of palatoplasty for development of palatal, alveolar and velar place features, oral stops, and oral fricatives." Although these authors used the word "time," they were not implying that the passage of time alone, without intervention, should produce the changes that they had documented. All of the children in their study (1994) had been consistently monitored and treated by an interdisciplinary craniofacial team, and the treatment included active intervention in the form of parent counseling to increase stimulation in the home.

Determining Adequacy of Velopharyngeal Function in Toddlers

If you have the equipment, *videotape* your evaluations of infants and toddlers. The information you get will be even more valuable than from audiotaped samples.

In the very young child, we are usually entirely dependent on perceptual evaluation of speech in determining whether the palatal surgery has "worked." Most instrumental assessments of the function of the velopharyngeal mechanism *for speech* are not applicable since the patient's cooperation is required and small children typically do not! Because standardized articulation tests (do not confuse these with tests of language development) are unlikely to elicit sufficient output in children under the age of 3 years, clinicians have generally resorted to toys or other objects selected to elicit the particular speech sounds of concern (e.g., the stops, fricatives, and affricates, which require high intraoral pressure) and to observations of the child's verbal interactions with a parent.

As you carry out these examinations, you must be familiar first of all with the normal sequence of development of speech sounds in order to compare the output of the individual child with other children of his age. For example, it is important to remember that voiced consonants precede voiceless consonants in normal acquisition. Speakers with inadequate velopharyngeal function may have difficulty making the normal contrasts between voiced and voiceless consonants, but if more voiced than voiceless consonants are heard in a toddler with a repaired cleft, this may simply reflect his developmental stage, not residual velopharyngeal inadequacy. Of equal importance when you are assessing a child with a repaired cleft is your experience in distinguishing consonants produced with correct placement but nasal emission from those produced with inappropriate articulatory placement. It is a troublesome but relatively common finding that young children may persist in nasal emission of the airstream on pressure consonants even if the surgery has provided them with a functional or potentially functional velopharyngeal system, particularly if the surgery was performed well after the child started producing meaningful speech. In these cases, it is helpful to explore the child's ability to direct the airstream orally in play activities and "nonsense" speech play.

You need to be particularly concerned about the presumably compensatory articulations that appear in some children with clefts in the early stages of speech sound development and frequently persist after a functional velopharyngeal system has been provided through surgery or prosthetic care. These errors may be the most frequent examples of the effects of early articulatory/phonetic constraints on phonologic development, discussed in the following section. Textbooks on cleft palate have described glottal stops and pharyngeal fricatives for decades. Pharyngeal stops, pharyngeal affricates, velar fricatives, middorsum palatal stops, and the "posterior nasal fricative" have been described as additional types of errors that seem to be heard more often in speakers with cleft palates than in noncleft individuals. Trost-Cardamone (1994) also added pharyngeal affricates (pharyngeal fricative + glottal or pharyngeal stop) to the list. Other clinicians have verified the occurrence of these misarticulations in children with either current velopharyngeal inadequacy or a history of such inadequacy. Glottal or pharyngeal articulations may occur either as substitutions or as coarticulations, that is, as simultaneous articulatory maneuvers with other places of production. Fortunately, Trost-Cardamone's 1994 instructional videotape provides practical experience in listening for and transcribing these errors.

Performance on stimulability tasks is revealing when you are trying to decide on the adequacy of velopharyngeal closure. A young child's response to direct imitation of nonsense syllable repetition or other tasks that do not use real words already incorporated into his vocabulary (and therefore vulnerable to habituated sound production patterns) may provide you with a different insight into the potential for velopharyngeal closure in speech. That is, in imitating nonsense syllables after you, the child is less likely to be restricted by previously learned patterns, in contrast to what he may do in words already in his glossary. Also, his first response to a picture stimulus may be characterized by nasalization (nasal air emission) on a plosive or fricative, but on imitation of the examiner that nasal emission may disappear. If so, he may well have the physiologic capability for velopharyngeal closure, but simply has not learned that he can, in fact, make the sound without nasal emission.

A Word About Examination of Oropharyngeal Structures

Optimally, any child with a cleft is already being followed by a cleft palate or craniofacial team and thus receives periodic assessments of the integrity of oropharyngeal structures. But, even in these cases, you will have to make your own evaluation of the child's current status. Assessment of the oral structures has been discussed in Chapter 5. With respect to children with repaired clefts, the following points should help you:

1. The repaired lip is rarely of consequence in the speech problems in individuals with clefts. However, if the lip is abnormally short, bilabial consonants may be produced as labiodentals. A more frequent problem is a discrepancy in position of the upper and lower lips due to retrusion of the maxilla. If the upper lip is significantly behind the lower lip, labiodental targets may be produced with the lower incisors against the upper lip, or may be produced as bilabials. Tip-dental consonants may become "tip-labials," for example, contact between the tongue-tip and the upper lip for /t/, /d/, and /n/.

2. In any child, forceful pressure on the dorsum of the tongue with a tongue depressor can elicit a gag and/or a cessation of cooperation for the rest of the exam. In the child with a repaired cleft,

the muscular link between the tongue and the velum—the palato-glossus muscle—may be tighter than normal, and pushing down on the tongue dorsum may interfere with upward movement of the velum, thus giving false information about velar movement and, inferentially, movement patterns of the velopharyngeal structures.

3. In virtually any speaker, "velopharyngeal closure" is not visible on the intraoral view because the site of closure is hidden behind the velum itself. In the young child, with or without a cleft, velopharyngeal closure is actually velum-adenoid closure, that is, the velum is closing against the adenoid pad and not directly against the posterior pharyngeal wall. The adenoid pad is not normally visible on the direct intraoral examination.

4. Precisely because the direct intraoral view limits what the examiner can see and understand about velopharyngeal closure, it is important to remember the "nonvisible" factors that can influence velopharyngeal closure, that is, factors that cannot be adequately assessed on this view. These include mechanical interference with velar movement (such as by enlarged tonsils or pharyngeal webbing), a deficiency of muscle mass on the nasal surface of the velum, abnormal direction of pull of the velar musculature, and inadequate movement of pharyngeal musculature towards closure.

Effects of Early Phonetic Constraints on Postclosure Phonetic, Phonologic, and Language Development

Most of the studies described above regarding early vocalizations and phonetic development in children with clefts were longitudinal studies, providing information on development in these children following palatal closure. These studies, together with those of other studies limited to postsurgery communication development, provide us with critical information about what to expect in children with clefts during their toddler and preschool years. Following are some of the important findings:

- A higher percentage of glottal placements (glottal stops and the glottal fricative /h/) than heard in noncleft children.
- A delay in the appearance of "oral stop predominance" and also in the use of oral fricatives.
- A preference for midvowels over high or low vowels.
- A sort of chain reaction from early phonetic constraints to phonologic problems to influences in early language development. For example, toddlers targeted and produced more words beginning with nasals, vowels, and approximants, and infrequently targeted words beginning with stops, fricatives,

or affricates (Estrem & Broen, 1989). In essence, they selected words that contained the sounds they were capable of producing.

- Limited phonetic inventories and differences in phonologic process usage that may become more apparent with increasing age, or more likely, with the increasing language output of the child.
- An apparent decrease or disappearance in the above differences as children mature.

The results of the studies that provided us with these generalizations serve as a warning to us regarding assessment of phonologic development and expressive language development in children with clefts. These children are subject to structural influences that do not affect other children and that may exert an effect long after the structural problem has been eradicated. Be careful to examine phonetic and phonologic aspects of speech sound development separately and also to place your observations of early language development within the context of these influences. There are, of course, other factors that can affect language development in children with clefts: adverse reactions of adults and peers to facial appearance, increased vulnerability to ear disease and hearing loss, interruptions in social and educational development due to hospitalizations, and so on.

FOLLOW-UP EVALUATIONS IN THE TODDLER AND PRESCHOOL YEARS

Within the team context, regular follow-up evaluations of children in this age range are typically scheduled every 6 to 12 months since this is a period of rapid development. Now the child can cooperate more fully for instrumental evaluation of velopharyngeal function. Nasopharyngoscopy is feasible in many children as young as 4 years, and multiview videofluoroscopy may be used with even younger children so long as they are able to cooperate sufficiently and perform the tasks appropriately so that clear views may be obtained with a minimum of radiation exposure. Aerodynamic studies and acoustic studies using instrumentation such as the Nasometer are also feasible with fairly young children. An important warning here is that no instrumental technique can prove that a velopharyngeal system is capable of adequate closure if the child is "bypassing" the system, that is, if he is relying exclusively on glottal placements or other speech sounds that do not require velopharyngeal closure. The validity of the information is dependent not just on the phonemes modeled by the examiner, but on the child's own phonologic "matches" to those targets.

When you are examining a child with a cleft in the toddler and preschool years, the accuracy of your assessment will depend in

Be wary of deciding on the size of a fistula based only on your visual inspection of the palate. Fistulas are often irregular in shape not just in the horizontal plane (i.e., on the surface of the palate), but in the vertical plane (going from the oral surface of the palate upward towards the nasal cavity). A fistula may be either larger or smaller than what you see on the palatal surface, and probing it is not recommended unless you are in a medical setting.

large part on a knowledge of the particular problems to which these children may be vulnerable: hypernasal resonance on vowels and vocalic segments, nasal air loss on pressure consonants, use of compensatory articulations and other atypical backed articulations, phonetic errors that may be related to structural problems in the developing dental and jaw relationships, and errors in placement that may be related to a palatal fistula. A palatal fistula is an opening between the oral and nasal cavities, which may be either the result of a surgical breakdown or an intentionally unrepaired area if the surgeon decided there would be too little tissue or too much tension across the line of repair to allow for good healing and sustained closure of that particular part of the cleft. Depending on size and location, a fistula results in nasalization of speech in somewhat the same way, though usually to a lesser extent, as dysfunction of the velopharyngeal mechanism.

With specific regard to nasal air loss on pressure consonants, a key diagnostic question is related to consistency: if the air loss is present on all pressure consonants, there is most likely a physical inadequacy in the function of the velopharyngeal mechanism. If the air loss is heard on pressure consonants produced at all oral placements but is not consistently audible on each token, the velopharyngeal system may be closing inconsistently, subject to such factors as phonetic context. If the air loss is limited to anterior pressure consonants, a palatal fistula may be present, or, conversely, the lack of air loss on velar stops may simply reflect a lingual assist to the velum in closure. If the air loss is limited to a specific consonant or class of consonants, the speaker may be exhibiting phoneme-specific nasal air loss. This loss, like the compensatory articulations that may persist after physical management of velopharyngeal inadequacy, reflects an error in learning and should not be taken as indicative of a velopharyngeal mechanism that is truly incapable of closure.

Since assessment will vary with the child's age, and with linguistic and cognitive functioning, your testing may include a sample of connected speech (preferably spontaneous), a speech sound inventory such as that typically elicited through picture articulation tests, and stimulability testing. It is a good idea to audiotape the entire speech sample so that you can replay it as often as necessary to facilitate your accurate, reliable transcription and also to provide you with a baseline for later comparisons. Your analysis of the speech sample should include an estimate of overall intelligibility, comparison of productions to developmental norms, a phonetic inventory, and a phonological pattern analysis. According to Trost-Cardamone and Bernthal (1993), "The main goal in all evaluations is to distinguish speech errors that may be due to faulty velopharyngeal or other structural deviations from speech errors that are compensatory or developmental in nature" (p. 317). These authors provide a chart of guidelines for deciding on appropriate management, depending on the results of the assessment of the child's sound system.

Some clinicians have reported that problems in velopharyngeal function can lead to secondary problems in laryngeal function, specifically overdrive or "hyperfunction" of the laryngeal system presumably due to partial loss of the vocal airstream through an inadequate velopharyngeal port. Speech evaluations of children with clefts should include perceptual evaluation of laryngeal function, and referral for medical assessment of the laryngeal system when indicated (Maternal and Child Health Consensus Statement, 1993).

EVALUATION OF VELOPHARYNGEAL FUNCTION

By the time the child has reached the preschool years, and often earlier, parents, surgeons, and speech-language pathologists are concerned about "objective" evaluation of the status of velopharyngeal closure. How can we be certain that the palatal surgery worked, or that further physical management (surgical or prosthetic) of the velopharyngeal mechanism will be needed? Even within the context of the cleft palate/craniofacial team functioning in a medical setting, where elaborate instrumentation is available, evaluation of velopharyngeal function follows a hierarchical approach that begins with a perceptual evaluation.

In nonmedical settings, we can use some simple and safe techniques to obtain a gross index of the presence or absence of air leakage through the nose. A mirror held beneath the nose during production of speech samples containing pressure consonants or a sustained fricative will fog if there is nasal air loss; in the case of a child with a cleft, it is wise to test both sides of the nose because various degrees of nasal obstruction are common in these children. The same is true for the commercially available See-Scape, which consists of a nasal olive connected through a section of flexible plastic tubing to an upright section of rigid, clear tubing containing a small piece of styrofoam. When the nasal olive is held in the naris as the subject produces the desired speech sample, airflow through the tube causes the styrofoam to rise in the rigid tubing. With either this device or the mirror test, the examiner must be cautious to hold the olive or the mirror in place only during the production of oral pressure consonants, not during production of nasal consonants or during normal nasal respiration. An additional problem with the See-Scape is that small children are often delighted to see the styrofoam rise in the tube, and may begin to direct the airstream nasally even though their velopharyngeal mechanisms are functioning adequately. In the "modified tongue-anchor technique," you can use a small piece of sterile gauze to gently hold the tip of the child's tongue outside the mouth, and direct the child to close his lips around the rest of the tongue and inflate his cheeks. The theory behind this approach is that (a) inflation of the cheeks is impossible in the presence of inadequate velopharyngeal function and that (b) anchoring the tongue forward keeps the dorsum of the tongue out of the area of the velopharyngeal port, preventing a lingual assist to the velum for closure. It is critical to bear in mind that each of these techniques is crude and subject to influences that may not be immediately apparent to you; *none are capable of actual measurement of the function of the velopharyngeal system.*

Imaging of the Velopharyngeal System

With rare exceptions, visualization of the velopharyngeal system cannot be accomplished outside a medical setting. However, this brief synopsis of imaging techniques is included to give you a feel for the more sophisticated ones that are available. For a detailed discussion, please see Moon (1993).

Still Cephalometric X Rays

Orthodontists use lateral, frontal, and oblique films to assess craniofacial structure and growth in their patients. These films are taken with the head in a fixed position and a standardized X–ray tube-to-focal-plane distance. A lateral film focused at the midsagittal plane may be used for assessing the size and relationship of velopharyngeal structures at rest and perhaps during sustained production of a pressure consonant. The advantages of this approach are the relatively low dose of radiation, about .01 rads for a single film (Moon, 1993); the common availability of the instrumentation; and the standardization. The disadvantages are that the velopharyngeal system cannot be studied during actual speech production, and that the image is a two-dimensional representation of a multidimensional system.

Multiview Videofluorography

Fluorography is essentially "motion-picture X ray." With the advent of videorecorders, it became possible to videotape these examinations, thus using far less radiation than was necessary for the exposure of movie film. Most cleft palate/craniofacial centers now use multiview videofluorography as one means of visualizing the velopharyngeal mechanism. The typical views are lateral, frontal, and a base which gives a cross-sectional or horizontal view of the velopharyngeal port. In the lateral view, the examiner can see the movement of the velum and any forward excursion of the posterior pharyngeal wall. The amount and level of medial movement of the lateral pharyngeal musculature can be studied in the frontal view. The base view shows the contribution of all of these structures—the velum, lateral walls, and posterior wall—towards closure, but the vertical level of movement of each structure is obscured. Oblique views are useful if asymmetric movement is suspected. (Please see Witzel and Stringer, 1990, for a description of additional useful views.) The major disadvantages of multiview videofluorography are the lack of a standardized head position (although some facilities have added head-holders to their units) and the radiation exposure. The amount of exposure varies, of course, with the specific equipment and the length of the study, but dosage estimates offered by Skolnick and Cohn (1989) indicated that a multiview workup could reach as much as 2.5 rads. This is not inconsequential in a small child.

Computerized Tomography

To date, there has been relatively little application of CT scans or cine-CT scans to the study of the velopharyngeal mechanism, quite likely because of the expense involved and also the limitations of the procedure. We may see more research using this instrumentation, but routine clinical use for study of the velopharyngeal mechanism even in large craniofacial centers does not seem imminent. The same is true for magnetic resonance imaging, which does not involve radiation; future advances in MRI technology could lead to wider application in the imaging of the velopharyngeal mechanism.

Ultrasonography

In the 1970s there were a few investigations on the use of ultrasonography to study the movement of the lateral pharyngeal walls in speech. The interest in this technique was sparked by problems in imaging the lateral walls with other techniques, and also by the fact that ultrasound does not involve radiation. Moon (1993) discussed the limitations of this instrumentation in the study of the speech mechanism and pointed out that there are no published reports of its use with patients exhibiting problems in the function of the velopharyngeal mechanism.

Oral Endoscopy

A rigid endoscope, inserted orally, was used in the 1960s for evaluating velopharyngeal function but has such severe limitations that the technique is now rarely used. One limitation is that when the velum elevates and closes against the posterior pharyngeal wall, the oral view can provide little information. Another is that, even in the rare instance in which the mechanism for closure is visible on this view, the presence of the rigid scope in the mouth obviously limits the speech sample.

Nasopharyngoscopy

Nasal endoscopy for study of the velopharyngeal mechanism was first reported by Pigott (1969), who used a rigid, side-viewing endoscope of small diameter. Nasal endoscopy allows study of the velopharyngeal system from above, without interfering with speech production. Flexible fiberoptic nasopharyngoscopy (Karnell, 1994) is more widely used than oral endoscopy and, together with multiview videofluorography, has become a fairly common technique of assessment in cleft palate/craniofacial centers. Technical advances have led to endoscopes of decreasing diameter, allowing for greater patient comfort and compliance. The quality of the information derived is at least as dependent on the expertise of the examiner as it is on the characteristics of the individual scope. The use of nasopharyngoscopy is not recommended in a nonmedical setting because of the invasive nature of the technique and because a topical anesthetic is usually needed for comfortable insertion of the scope.

Measuring the Function of the Velopharyngeal System

The major approaches to measuring the consequences of velopharyngeal closure or lack of closure during speech can generally be classified into acoustic and aerodynamic studies. The instrumentation is noninvasive but can be very expensive.

Spectrography

Researchers first began to understand the effects of inadequate velopharyngeal function on the acoustic energy distribution of speech through the use of spectrographic analysis. These studies began to appear in the mid-1950s, and spectrography remained a popular research tool into the mid-1980s. However, spectrography is not a practical or commonly used clinical tool in the evaluation of velopharyngeal function.

Accelerometry

Accelerometers are small, vibration-sensitive transducers. In the study of nasality in speech, one accelerometer is placed on the side of the nose and another on the thyroid lamina. The accelerometric "index" of oral-nasal coupling is the ratio of output of the two transducers. Nasal accelerometry has been advocated as a useful tool in the assessment of speakers with suspected problems in velopharyngeal closure, and the relatively small amount of published data seem to indicate a significant relationship between accelerometer ratios and the amount of nasality heard by listeners. The instrumentation can be used outside a medical setting, but the technical requirements (transducers, amplifiers, rectifiers, computer or oscilloscope screens, etc.) have limited its use.

Measurement of Sound Pressure Level

For several decades, researchers have tried to compare the pressure level of the sound signal emitted from the nose to that emitted from the oral cavity and to use this comparison as an index of velopharyngeal function. Currently, the most popular instrument for making these measurements is the Nasometer™, a commercially available, computer-based device, which is the outgrowth of the earlier TONAR I and TONAR II devices developed by Fletcher (1970, 1972). There has been a recent flourish of studies correlating Nasometer™

measurements to listener judgments of nasality as well as to other indices of velopharyngeal adequacy. Many clinicians are currently using this instrument to corroborate their perceptual judgments of hypernasality. However, the cost of the instrumentation may be prohibitive for many potential users.

Aerodynamic Studies

Historically, clinicians and researchers used various approaches to detecting nasal airflow (the mirror test and See-Scape, described previously), measuring nasal or oral airflow (pneumotachographs), and measuring oral air pressure (e.g., the oral manometer). Warren and Dubois (1964) developed a quantitative technique of using measurements of nasal air flow, nasal air pressure, and oral air pressure to calculate the cross-sectional area of the velopharyngeal orifice area during speech. This approach has been used to categorize patients into adequate closure, adequate/borderline closure, borderline/inadequate closure, and inadequate closure groups based on pressure-flow estimates of VP orifice size. Investigators have not been in complete agreement about the correlation of listener judgments to pressure-flow estimates of orifice size, but active research continues. There is a commercially available hardware and software package for pressure-flow studies, the PERCI-PC (Microtronics Corporation, Carrboro, NC). As stated by Warren (1989, p. 234), "This system is used to collect pressure-flow data and the software provides analysis modes for measuring the pressure, air flow, volume, sphincter area, resistance, conductance, and timing variables associated with palatal closure and breathing." Either the full laboratory instrumentation array or the PERCI-PC is in use in several cleft palate/craniofacial centers around the world. Both are noninvasive. The instrumentation and hardware for the PERCI-PC are less formidable than the laboratory array, but nevertheless require considerable financial investment and training for the examiner.

A Further Note on Instrumental Assessment

Other types of instrumentation have been used in investigations of velopharyngeal activity, but generally only in laboratory settings as opposed to clinical assessments. Please see Moon (1993) for a discussion of electromyography, phototransduction, and mechanical-electrical "movement transduction." Of the three, there does seem to be a potential for clinical applicability for the photodetector.

THE SCHOOL–AGED CHILD

Due to improvements in surgical care and also to earlier diagnosis and intervention for communication problems in young children with clefts, it is now far more common for these children to reach school age exhibiting good velopharyngeal closure for speech and age-appropriate articulation skills. For example, 2 decades ago,

Morris (1973) surveyed the published data and estimated that approximately 25% of the children who had repaired cleft palates had inadequate velopharyngeal closure for speech requiring further surgical or prosthetic treatment. In a retrospective analysis modeled after Morris's study but limited to personal experience with 240 children treated in three major cleft palate/craniofacial treatment centers, I found this percentage to have dropped to 16% (Peterson-Falzone, 1990). Chapman (1993) reported "catch-up" in phonologic development in children by the age of 5 years that would not have been expected based on results of earlier studies of articulation competency in school-aged children with clefts, and attributed the discrepancy to changes in management. Nevertheless, in dealing with children in this age group, you will be faced with at least four diagnostic questions: (1) What are the possible effects of adenoid involution and of natural craniofacial growth on velopharyngeal closure? (2) What are the effects of changing dental and occlusal factors on articulation, and to what extent should these alter decisions about therapy? (3) What surgical procedures may be taking place in a child of this age, and what may be the impact on plans for therapy? (4) What goals are appropriate in therapy?

Adenoid Growth and Involution

The adenoid pad is visible on radiographic views of the nasopharynx by 6 weeks of age and increases in size thereafter until it reaches a peak size and begins to involute (atrophy). Investigators disagree regarding the age at which the maximum size is reached, indicating two possible peak ages: around 5 years (Linder-Aronson & Leighton, 1983), and 9 to 10 or 11 years (Subtelny & Koepp-Baker, 1956). In any child under the age of 5 years, the adenoid pad is probably increasing in size. At any age over 5 years, the pad may be either still growing or undergoing natural resorption. While there have been very few reported cases of the onset of velopharyngeal inadequacy secondary to natural involution of the adenoids in children without clefts (Peterson-Falzone, 1985), the gradual disappearance of the adenoids in children with clefts, combined with the natural downward-and-forward growth of the face, can lead to late onset of velopharyngeal inadequacy in a child whose original palatoplasty had provided him with good velopharyngeal closure. The number of such reported cases is small, but certainly enough to alert us to the possibility of changing velopharyngeal status in the school-aged child.

Dental and Occlusal Factors

As in every other child in the early school-age years, the sequenced loss of deciduous dentition and eruption of the permanent dentition may temporarily interfere with articulatory accuracy in children with clefts. However, children with clefts may also have (1) absence of the lateral incisor and/or canine on the side of the cleft, (2) malalignment of the dentition in the area of the cleft, (3) lateral crossbite on the side of the cleft, and (4) anterior crossbite due to maxillary retrusion. In addition to the natural changes in dental status, there may be changes secondary to dental, orthodontic, or prosthetic intervention. It is impossible to predict how an individual child will respond to these fluctuating states. Some children adapt well to even multiple missing teeth and an accompanying malocclusion; others seem unable to improve articulatory placement in the presence of a relatively minor dental anomaly. Such problems are more likely to cause problems in speech if they are present in combination (e.g., missing teeth plus a crossbite) rather than as isolated entities, and if they occur during the child's speech-learning years as opposed to adult years. You have to decide if the articulation problems you are trying to eradicate are due to a dental/occlusal anomaly for which the child cannot realistically compensate, at least for the present. Stimulation testing provides part of this answer; response to therapy over a specified time period should provide the rest. Depending on the child's maturational status and motivation and also on the schedule of therapy (individual versus group, intensity, length of sessions), if production does not improve over a predetermined time frame, you should reconsider whether therapy is a good idea. In any case, consultation with the craniofacial team and specifically with the child's dentist and/or orthodontist is critical before therapy is initiated. It is possible that time spent in therapy may be time lost, either because progress is temporarily impossible or because the "misarticulation" will spontaneously improve once the dental/occlusal situation improves.

A related problem may be the presence of a residual defect through the alveolus (gum ridge) on the cleft side. In most cleft palate treatment centers in the United States, bone grafting of this defect is not done until the ages of 9 to 12 years, depending on the dental development of the child. If the defect is large enough, there may be a patent opening from the oral cavity into the buccal sulcus or even up into the nasal cavity. In the former case, the child may exhibit a slight puffing out of the lip on production of /p/ and /b/. If the opening extends into the nose, there may be nasal air loss on all anterior pressure consonants. If this constitutes a significant speech problem for the child, you can consult with the cleft palate/craniofacial team or the child's dentist regarding the possibility of the use of a dental plate constructed to close the space. The same is true, of course, for fistulae through the palate into the nasal cavity.

Surgical Procedures

Surgical repair of a residual alveolar defect (discussed above) or a palatal fistula may take place during the child's school-age years. The effect of these defects on speech varies with size and location, and is not predictable from child to child. Successful repair of even a small palatal fistula can be much more difficult than one would expect.

If secondary management of the velopharyngeal system is needed, the options are (1) a prosthetic speech bulb, (2) a variety of surgical techniques for lengthening the soft palate, and (3) a variety of surgical procedures, generically termed pharyngoplasties, for altering the configuration of the velopharynx. The decision that such management is needed should be the result of collaboration between the cleft palate/craniofacial team and the treating speech-language pathologist, particularly because the child's history of progress in therapy will play a key role in that decision.

Selecting Appropriate Goals for Therapy

For the child with a repaired cleft palate, the critical questions regarding appropriateness of therapy center on the compensatory articulations and other atypical "backed" placements. Certainly therapy to teach correct oral placements is indicated if the repaired velopharyngeal mechanism is intact. However, therapy to teach correct placements may also be appropriate even in the presence of an inadequately functioning velopharyngeal mechanism. The modification of placements from glottal and pharyngeal to oral may actually result in a change in the behavior of the velopharyngeal mechanism in speech, in the optimum case completely eliminating the need for further surgical or prosthetic management. In any event, if a child is producing nothing but glottal and pharyngeal placements, secondary surgery on the mechanism should not be performed until an attempt has been made to modify these placements through therapy.

Elimination of compensatory articulations can be quite difficult. Again, a key question is the amount of time over which these efforts should be made. If production does not improve over a predetermined time frame, the efficacy of therapy should be reconsidered. That time frame should be specified in weeks or months, not years. Burnout on the part of the child is always a possibility, and becomes inevitable once he knows that therapy is not making it easier for him to make himself understood.

With regard to therapy to eliminate nasal emission, the decision for or against therapy is simplest when the problem is one of phoneme-specific nasal emission. This is a problem that will not be eradicated by anything other than speech therapy. If nasal emission and hypernasality are consistent but mild in degree, clinicians in medical settings may use nasopharyngoscopy to provide biofeedback to the speaker in the effort to modify velopharyngeal closure. However, this is not applicable in other professional settings. Finally, if nasal emission and hypernasality are consistent and severe in degree, consideration must be given to further physical management of the velopharyngeal mechanism.

Other Related Concerns
in the School-Aged Child

Research into the psychological status, emotional adjustment, and educational achievement of children with clefts has been ongoing for over 5 decades. It is has long been known that these children showed a higher prevalence of reading problems than their noncleft peers. However, we have only recently become aware of the high frequency of educational problems in this population. In a recent study on nonsyndromic children from two large cleft palate treatment centers, nearly half had deficient educational progress as evidenced by learning disabilities or low school achievement, and over one quarter had repeated at least one grade (Broder, Richman, & Matheson, 1998). These findings are both disturbing and motivating for professionals who care for these patients and their families.

THE TEENAGER AND YOUNG ADULT

Although most of the habilitative procedures that a youngster with a cleft palate will need are accomplished prior to her teenage years, there are some "end-stage" phases of management that can still affect her communication skills. Completion of orthodontic therapy usually takes place during this time. If congenitally missing teeth have not been replaced by implants prior to this age, replacement either by implants or a fixed bridge will probably be accomplished in the teenage years. If a surgical advancement of the midface is needed to bring the upper and lower jaws into good alignment, that surgery will most likely take place after completion of facial growth (age 15 to 16 in girls, a year or so later in boys). This surgery can have a beneficial effect on speech if there were preoperative misarticulations related to malalignment of the jaws. However, in some cases, the forward movement of the midface may result in inadequate velopharyngeal closure. If this postadvancement inadequacy does not disappear spontaneously over time, further physical management of the velopharyngeal system will be necessary.

Throughout this chapter, I have assumed that the child with a cleft palate is under appropriate multidisciplinary care from the early days of life. This assumption leads, in turn, to the assumption that the habilitative process is essentially complete by the late teenage or early adult years. In reality, there are still significant numbers of teenagers and young adults who come to cleft palate/craniofacial centers for the first time in their lives with incomplete, inadequate care. In the worst cases, the cleft has not been successfully repaired, and speech is characterized by severe hypernasality, pervasive nasal air loss, and often a heavy reliance on compensatory articulations. These individuals become "salvage" cases for the team and for the treating speech-language pathologist alike. Although the team surgeons may be able to repair the velopharyngeal mechanism suc-

Some important aspects of treatment will not be completed by this time, such as follow-up genetic counseling as the teenager prepares for his own family life.

cessfully, it is more than likely that extensive and intensive therapy will be required to improve speech. Although successful habilitation is not impossible, the multiple difficulties in communication and social acceptance experienced by these late-presenting patients constitute the ultimate justification for early referral of infants with clefts to multidisciplinary teams for timely intervention and rigorous longitudinal monitoring.

SUMMARY

We have reviewed the principle points of diagnosing speech problems in children with clefts from the early months of life through the early adult years. The information presented here should serve as an introduction that leads the clinician to sources of more detailed, advanced material on diagnosis and treatment such as that found in professional journals and graduate-level texts. Information prepared specifically for patients, families, and the general public may be obtained through the American Cleft Palate–Craniofacial Association, 1829 East Franklin, Suite 1022, Chapel Hill, NC, 27514; telephone 800-24-CLEFT.

REFERENCES

*Parameters for the Evaluation and Treatment of Patients with Cleft Lip/Palate or Other Craniofacial Anomalies. Maternal and Child Health Consensus Statement. *Cleft Palate-Craniofacial Journal, 30,* (Suppl. 1), 1993.

The First Few Months of Life

Chapman, K. L. (1991). Vocalizations of toddlers with cleft lip and palate. *Cleft Palate-Craniofacial Journal, 28,* 172–178.

Chapman, K. L., & Hardin, M. A. (1992). Phonetic and phonologic skills of two-year olds with cleft palate. *Cleft Palate-Craniofacial Journal, 29,* 433–441.

Fenson, L., Dale, P. S., Reznick, J. S., Thal, D., Bates, E., Hartung, J. P., Pethick, S., & Reilly, J. S. (1993) *MacArthur communicative development inventories.* San Diego, CA: Singular Publishing Group.

Grunwell, P., & Russell, J. (1987). Vocalizations before and after cleft palate surgery: A pilot study. *British Journal of Disorders of Communication, 22,* 1–17.

O'Gara, M. M., & Logemann, J. A. (1988). Phonetic analyses of the speech development of babies with cleft palate. *Cleft Palate Journal, 25,* 122–134.

O'Gara, M. M., & Logemann, J. A. (1990). Early speech development in cleft palate babies. In J. Bardach & H. L. Morris (Eds.), *Multidisciplinary management of cleft lip and palate* (pp. 717–721). Philadelphia, PA: W. B. Saunders.

O'Gara, M. M., Logemann, J. A., & Rademaker, A. W. (1994). Phonetic features by babies with unilateral cleft lip and palate. *Cleft Palate-Craniofacial Journal, 31,* 446–451.

Philips, B. J., & Kent, R. D. (1984). Acoustic-phonetic descriptions of speech production in speakers with cleft palate and other velopharyngeal disorders. In N. J. Lass (Ed.), *Speech and language: Advances in basic research and practice* (Vol. II, pp. 113–168). New York: Academic Press.

After Palate Closure

*Chapman, K. L., & Hardin, M. A. (1992). Phonetic and phonologic skills of two-year olds with cleft palate. *Cleft Palate-Craniofacial Journal, 29,* 433–441.

Estrem, T., & Broen, P. A. (1989). Early speech productions of children with cleft palate. *Journal of Speech and Hearing Research, 32,* 12–23.

*O'Gara, M. M., Logemann, J. A., & Rademaker, A. W. (1994). Phonetic features by babies with unilateral cleft lip and palate. *Cleft Palate-Craniofacial Journal, 31,* 446–451.

Trost-Cardamone, J. E. (1994). *Cleft palate misarticulations: A teaching tape* [Videotape]. Northridge, CA: Instructional Media Center, California State University, Northridge.

Follow-up Evaluations in the Toddler and Preschool Years

*Parameters for the Evaluation and Treatment of Patients with Cleft Lip/Palate or Other Craniofacial Anomalies. Maternal and Child Health Consensus Statement. *Cleft Palate-Craniofacial Journal, 30,* (Suppl. 1), 1993.

Trost-Cardamone, J. E., & Bernthal, J. E. (1993). Articulation assessment procedures and treatment decisions. In K. T. Moller & D. C. Starr (Eds.), *Cleft palate: Interdisciplinary issues and treatments* (pp. 307–336). Austin, TX: Pro-Ed.

Evaluation of Velopharyngeal Function

Fletcher, S. G. (1970). Theory and instrumentation for quantitative measurement of nasality. *Cleft Palate Journal, 7,* 601–609.

Fletcher, S. G. (1972). Contingencies for bioelectronic modification of nasality. *Journal of Speech and Hearing Disorders, 37,* 329–346.

Karnell, M. P. (1994). *Videoendoscopy: From velopharynx to larynx.* San Diego, CA: Singular Publishing Group.

Moon, J. B. (1993). Evaluation of velopharyngeal function. In K. T. Moller & C. D. Starr (Eds.), *Cleft palate: Interdisciplinary issues and treatments* (pp. 251–306). Austin, TX: Pro-Ed.

Pigott, R. W. (1969). The nasoendoscopic appearance of the normal palato-pharyngeal valve. *Plastic and Reconstructive Surgery, 43,* 19–24.

Skolnick, M. L., & Cohn, E. R. (1989). *Videofluoroscopic studies of speech in patients with cleft palate.* New York: Springer-Verlag.

Warren, D. W. (1989). Aerodynamic assessment of velopharyngeal performance. In K. Bzoch (Ed.), *Communicative disorders related to cleft lip and palate* (3rd ed., pp. 230–245). Boston, MA: College-Hill Press.

Warren, D. W., & Dubois, A. (1964). A pressure-flow technique for measuring velopharyngeal orifice area during continuous speech. *Cleft Palate Journal, 1,* 52–71.

Witzel, M. A., & Stringer, D. A. (1990). Methods of assessing velopharyngeal function. In J. Bardach & H. L. Morris (Eds.), *Management of cleft lip and palate* (pp. 763–776). Philadelphia, PA: W. B. Saunders.

The School-Aged Child

Broder, H. L., Richman, L. C., & Matheson, P. B. (1998). Learning disability, school achievement, and grade retention among children with cleft: A two-center study. *Cleft Palate-Craniofacial Journal, 35,* 127–131.

Chapman, K. L. (1993). Phonologic processes in children with cleft palate. *Cleft Palate-Craniofacial Journal, 30,* 64–72.

Linder-Aronson, S., & Leighton, B. C. (1983). A longitudinal study of the development of the posterior pharyngeal wall between 3 and 16 years of age. *European Journal of Orthodontics, 5,* 47–58.

Morris, H. L. (1973). Velopharyngeal competence and primary cleft palate surgery, 1960–1971: A critical review. *Cleft Palate Journal, 10,* 62–71.

Peterson-Falzone, S. J. (1985). Velopharyngeal inadequacy in the absence of overt cleft palate. *Journal of Craniofacial Genetics and Developmental Biology, 1*(Suppl.), 97–124.

Peterson-Falzone, S. J. (1990). A cross-sectional analysis of speech results following palatal closure. In J. Bardach & H. L. Morris (Eds.), *Management of cleft lip and palate* (pp. 750–757). Philadelphia, PA: W. B. Saunders.

Subtelny, J. D., & Koepp-Baker, H. (1956). The significance of adenoid tissue in velopharyngeal function. *Plastic and Reconstructive Surgery, 17,* 235–250.

RECOMMENDED READINGS

The First Few Months of Life

Brookshire, B. L., Lynch, J. L., & Fox, D. R. (1980). *A parent-child cleft plate curriculum: Developing speech and language.* Tigaard, OR: C. C. Publications.

Dorf, D. S., Reisberg, D. J., & Gold, H. O. (1985). Early prosthetic management of cleft palate. Articulation development prosthesis: A preliminary report. *Journal of Prosthetic Dentistry, 53,* 222–226.

After Palate Closure

Chapman, K. L. (1993). Phonologic processes in children with cleft palate. *Cleft Palate-Craniofacial Journal, 30,* 64–72.

Estrem, T., & Broen, P. A. (1989). Early speech productions of children with cleft palate. *Journal of Speech and Hearing Research, 32,* 12–23.

Lynch, J. L., Fox, D. R., & Brookshire, B. L. (1983). Phonological proficiency of two cleft palate toddlers with school age follow-up. *Journal of Speech and Hearing Disorders, 48,* 274–285.

O'Gara, M. M., & Logemann, J. A. (1988). Phonetic analyses of the speech development of babies with cleft palate. *Cleft Palate Journal, 25,* 122–134.

O'Gara, M. M., & Logemann, J. A. (1990). Early speech development in cleft palate babies. In J. Bardach & H. L. Morris (Eds.), *Multidisciplinary management of cleft lip and palate* (pp. 717–721). Philadelphia, PA: W. B. Saunders.

O'Gara, M. M., Logemann, J. A., & Rademaker, A. W. (1994). Phonetic features by babies with unilateral cleft lip and palate. *Cleft Palate-Craniofacial Journal, 31,* 446–451.

Powers, G. R., Dunn, C., & Erickson, C. B. (1990). Speech analyses of four children with repaired cleft palates. *Journal of Speech and Hearing Disorders, 55,* 542–549.

Trost, J. E. (1981). Articulatory additions to the classical description of the speech of persons with cleft palate. *Cleft Palate Journal, 18,* 193–203.

Follow-up Evaluations in the Toddler and Preschool Years

McWilliams, B. J., Morris, H. L., & Shelton, R. L. (1990). *Cleft palate speech* (2nd ed.). Toronto: B. C. Decker.

Morris, H. L. (1990). Clinical assessment by the speech pathologist. In J. Bardach & H. L. Morris (Eds.), *Management of cleft lip and palate* (pp. 757– 762). Philadelphia, PA: W. B. Saunders.

Trost, J. E. (1981). Articulatory additions to the classical description of the speech of persons with cleft palate. *Cleft Palate Journal, 18,* 193–203.

Trost-Cardamone, J. E. (1994). *Cleft palate misarticulations: A teaching tape* [Videotape]. Northridge, CA: Instructional Media Center, California State University, Northridge.

Evaluation of Velopharyngeal Function

Dalston, R. M. (1982). Photodetector assessment of velopharyngeal activity. *Cleft Palate Journal, 19,* 1–8.

Dalston, R. M., Warren, D. W., & Dalston, E. T. (1991). Use of nasometry as a diagnostic tool for identifying patients with velopharyngeal impairment. *Cleft Palate-Craniofacial Journal, 28,* 184–189.

Fox, D. R., & Johns, D. (1970). Predicting velopharyngeal closure with a modified tongue-anchor technique. *Journal of Speech and Hearing Disorders, 35,* 248–251.

Horii, Y. (1983). An accelerometric measure as a physical correlate of perceived hypernasality in speech. *Journal of Speech and Hearing Research, 26,* 476–480.

Karnell, M. P., & Morris, H. L. (1985). Multiview endoscopic evaluations of velopharyngeal physiology in 15 normal speakers. *Annals of Otology, Rhinology, and Laryngology, 94,* 361–365.

Karnell, M. P., Seaver, E. J., & Dalston, R. (1988). A comparison of photodetector and endoscopic evaluations of velopharyngeal function. *Journal of Speech and Hearing Research, 31,* 503–509.

Redenbaugh, M., & Reich, A., (1985). Correspondence between an accelerometric nasal/voice amplitude ratio and listeners' direct magnitude estimations of hypernasality. *Journal of Speech and Hearing Research, 18,* 273–281.

Shprintzen, R. J. (1989). Nasopharyngoscopy. In K. Bzoch (Ed.), *Communicative disorders related to cleft lip and palate* (3rd ed., pp. 211–229). Austin, TX: Pro-Ed.

The School-Aged Child

Hoch, L., Golding-Kushner, K. J., Siegel-Sadewitz, V. L., & Shprintzen, R. J. (1986). Speech therapy. In B. J. McWilliams (Ed.), Current methods of assessing and treating children with cleft palates. *Seminars in Speech and Language, 7,* 313–325.

Morris, H. L., Wroblewski, S. K. M., Brown, C. K., & Van Demark, D. R. (1990). Velar-pharyngeal status in cleft palate patients with expected adenoidal involution. *Annals of Otology, Rhinology, and Laryngology, 99,* 432–437.

Peterson-Falzone, S. J., & Graham, M. S. (1990). Phoneme-specific nasal emission in children with and without physical anomalies of the velopharyngeal mechanism. *Journal of Speech and Hearing Disorders, 55,* 132–139.

The Teenager and Young Adult

Kummer, A. W., Strife, J. L., Grau, W. H., Creaghead, N. A., & Lee, L. (1989). The effects of Le Fort I osteotomy with maxillary movement on articulation, resonance, and velopharyngeal function. *Cleft Palate-Craniofacial Journal, 26,* 193–199.

Vallino, L. D. (1990). Speech, velopharyngeal function, and hearing before and after orthognathic surgery. *Journal of Oral and Maxillofacial Surgery, 48,* 1274–1281.

MRI

McGowan, J. C., Hatabu, H., Yousem, D. M., Randall, P., & Kressel, H. Y. (1992). Evaluation of soft palate function with MRI: Application to the cleft palate patient. *Journal of Computer Assisted Tomography, 16,* 877–882.

Wein, B. B., Drobnitzky, M., Klajman, S., & Angerstein, W. (1991). Evaluation of functional positions of tongue and soft palate with MR imaging: Initial clinical results. *Journal of Magnetic Resonance Imaging, 1,* 381–383.

Yamawaki, Y., Nishimura, Y., Suzuki, Y., Sawada, M., & Yamawaki, S. (1997). Rapid magnetic resonance imaging for assessment of velopharyngeal muscle movement on phonation. *American Journal of Otolaryngology, 18,* 210–213.

* These references are repeated because they contain material pertaining to more than one developmental or treatment stage.

CHAPTER

15

Disordered Swallowing

Adrienne L. Perlman, Ph.D.

Many speech-language pathologists (SLPs) work with patients who have problems chewing or swallowing. This problem is called "dysphagia," which comes from the Greek word *phagein*, meaning "to eat." Although dysphagia can occur anywhere along the path from the lips to the stomach, speech-language pathologists are primarily concerned about problems in the oral cavity, pharynx, or larynx. And so, to be precise, SLPs treat oropharyngeal dysphagia. Similarly, gastroenterologists (physicians who diagnose and treat disorders of the esophagus, stomach, and intestinal tract) also use the term dysphagia when referring to esophageal dysphagia.

Because patients with dysphagia are frequently identified in association with other medical problems, the majority of speech-language pathologists who diagnose and treat dysphagia work in the hospital setting. Although physicians are the most likely to identify a patient with dysphagia, it is not uncommon for a parent, teacher, nurse, occupational therapist, or speech-language pathologist to observe or suspect problems with swallowing.

Once dysphagia is suspected, the adult or child should be referred to a physician. The physician can then refer the patient for special examinations. Because schools and nursing homes do not have the equipment necessary for a complete dysphagia diagnosis, patients usually go to hospitals for their diagnostic workups. After the hospital evaluation, school clinicians and clinicians who work in nursing

/dɪsfeɪʒə/ is the commonly accepted pronunciation; although some people insist upon saying /dɪsfɑʒə/.

homes can then become responsible for the therapy that is recommended for their patients.

Because initial identification of the problem can occur in any of the environments in which one finds an SLP, a background in dysphagia is important for all clinicians. Much of the basic information you need to begin understanding normal and disordered swallowing is presented in your courses on anatomy, speech science, neuropathologies, and voice disorders. However, to be qualified to work with this population, you will need advanced courses specific to the physiology and pathophysiology of swallowing, as well as on diagnosis, treatment, and team management.

This chapter is intended to provide you with introductory information about the normal swallow, identifying a swallowing problem, techniques currently used by SLPs for diagnosis of swallowing problems, and some of the other professions that are involved in management of dysphagic patients.

> This chapter is intended to provide beginning students with no more information than they can safely "swallow!"

NORMAL SWALLOWING

In your anatomy course you were introduced to the sensorimotor function of the cranial nerves and the role of those nerves in innervating the muscles of speech and voice production. The cranial nerves that innervate the muscles of speech and voice production (V, VII, IX, X, and XII) also contribute to the sensory and motor function of the face, mouth, larynx, and pharynx during chewing and swallowing. A thorough discussion of the cranial nerves and the mucosa and muscles they innervate is presented elsewhere (Perlman, 1991; Perlman & Christensen, 1997). If you choose to read those papers, I suggest that you have a textbook by your side that shows the origins and insertions of the muscles of the face, mouth, pharynx, and larynx as well as the paths of the cranial nerves.

> It is important for you to learn this information. It will relate directly to your work, particularly with adults and children who have experienced acquired or congenital neuromuscular diseases or disorders, stroke, certain systemic diseases, or head and neck cancer.

Certain structures play a particularly significant role in the assessment of swallowing disorders. These structures are identified in Figure 15–1. The following sections will try to describe the function of the mouth, pharynx, and larynx during the oral and pharyngeal stages of swallowing.

The Oral Stage of Swallowing

The oral stage of swallowing can be divided into the oral preparatory and the oral transport phases (Figure 15–2). During the preparatory phase, the lips, jaw, tongue, soft palate, muscles of mastication, and buccal muscles all work to move the bolus (food or liquid) around in the mouth. This phase can last for extended periods if the taste is particularly good, but be very short if the flavor of the bolus is unpleasant. Along with taste, other factors that may influence the duration of this phase among individuals with normal oral function are

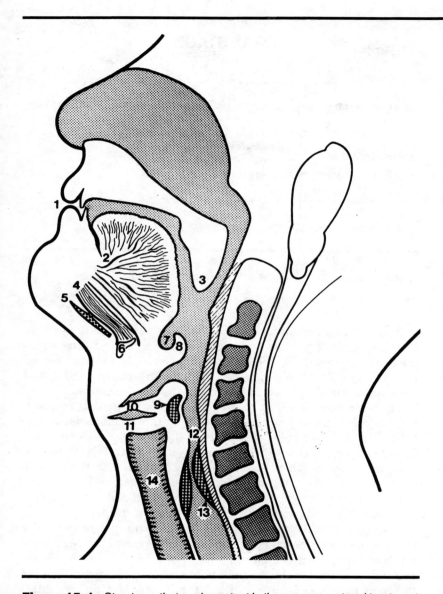

Figure 15–1. Structures that are important in the assessment and treatment of disordered swallowing:

1. lips
2. tongue
3. soft palate
4. geniohyoid m.
5. mylohyoid m.
6. hyoid bone
7. vallecula
8. epiglottis
9. arytenoid cartilage
10. false vocal fold
11. true vocal fold
12. pyriform sinus
13. cricopharyngeus m.
14. trachea

the temperature, viscosity, and size of the bolus. Factors such as degree of oral sensitivity, rate of secretion of saliva, the viscosity of saliva, and whether the patient is edentulous (toothless), can also affect this phase of swallowing.

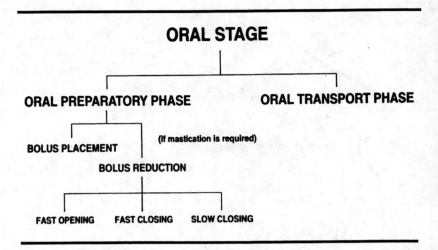

Figure 15–2. Phases of the oral stage of the swallow.

If the food bolus requires mastication, the oral preparatory phase includes a reduction phase, which is simply the phase during which the food is chewed. The bolus is placed between the molars, chewed until it is broken into small pieces, mixed with sufficient saliva, and then appropriately placed on the tongue for oral transport.

The reduction phase can be divided into a fast opening, fast closing, and slow closing phase, all a reflection of mandibular movement. The fast opening stage occurs as the mandible descends, the fast closing stage occurs as the mandible ascends, and the slow closing phase begins when the teeth make contact with the food in preparation for the grinding process. And so, the muscles of mastication must be strong and very well coordinated and the jaws must be reasonably well aligned for chewing to occur properly.

During the oral preparatory phase, the soft palate generally touches the posterior tongue. As the oral transport phase begins, the lips and buccal muscles contract, the posterior tongue depresses, and the remainder of the tongue performs a stripping action against the hard palate as it propels the bolus (mass of food or liquid) toward the oropharynx. The muscles of the floor of the mouth contract and the soft palate elevates.

The Pharyngeal Stage of Swallowing

After the bolus enters the oropharynx, the pharyngeal stage of the swallow begins. This stage consists of a series of rapid, coordinated motions that work to propel the bolus into the esophagus. The pharyngeal stage is very complex and it may be difficult for you to follow these actions with just one reading of the following paragraphs. I suggest that you suck on a piece of hard candy or sip a favorite beverage while reading (and rereading) the following two paragraphs. The purpose is not to keep you awake, but to make it easier for you to do repeated swallows. Keep swallowing and try to visualize the actions that are described. Refer to Figure 15–1 or a favorite anatomy book if you need to.

During the oral transport phase, the muscles of the floor of the mouth begin to contract. As these muscles contract, the hyoid bone is pulled into a more anterior-superior position and the larynx also elevates and moves somewhat forward. The movement of these two structures helps to open the entrance to the esophagus at the level of the cricopharyngeus muscle. This is the muscle that must also relax when patients use esophageal or tracheoesophageal puncture speech.

Once the bolus enters the oropharynx, the false vocal folds and true vocal folds contract and the other adductory muscles of the larynx help to close the laryngeal aditus (entrance). That closure protects the airway from penetration of the food or liquid. Additionally, the epiglottis covers the entrance to the larynx, providing further protection for the airway, reshaping the anterior portion of the pharynx, so that the pharynx becomes more cylindrical, and diverting the bolus toward the pyriform sinuses which are just above the entrance to the esophagus. As the larynx closes, there is a period of apnea (absence of respiration) which is usually followed by an expiration.

It takes less than 1 second (about 800 milliseconds) from the time the bolus enters into the oropharynx until it passes into the esophagus. Considering the precise coordination needed during swallowing, it is easy to understand why so many individuals develop swallowing problems. On the other hand, given this complex organization, it is impressive that so many of us do so well.

CAUSES AND EFFECTS OF OROPHARYNGEAL DYSPHAGIA

Oropharyngeal dysphagia generally results from neuromuscular or structural changes in the oral cavity, pharynx, or larynx. Among infants and children, the more frequent causes of dysphagia include developmental or traumatic neuromotor disorders and congenital anatomical defects. Problems in feeding and swallowing in the pediatric population can be different than those of adult populations (Arvedson & Brodsky, 1993).

Among the adult population, dysphagia is most commonly associated with stroke, neurologic disease, systemic disease, head and neck cancer surgery, radiation therapy for head and neck cancer, traumatic brain injury, and cervical spine disease. Changes in the efficiency of the swallow have been found to occur as a result of certain medications. Also healthy individuals of advanced age can demonstrate swallowing problems that are reflective of the general changes that occur in the sensorimotor system with aging. And, just like a speech or language disorder, dysphagia may be a symptom of a yet undiagnosed disease.

The astute student will recognize from the previous list that many of the causes of dysphagia in both children and adults are also causes of communication disorders. And so, some of the patients who are treated by speech-language pathologists for disordered swallowing may also be treated for communication problems. Two examples are patients with Parkinson's disease who may have dysarthria as well as dysphagia and patients who have had all or a portion of their tongue removed (total or partial glossectomy) for oral cancer.

Respiratory complications, malnutrition, and dehydration are critical health problems that can result from dysphagia. Along with these potential physical health problems, the inability to eat normally often limits the social interactions that so frequently center around food in our society. Not being to able to share a meal with family and friends can have serious emotional effects on swallowing-impaired individuals.

> Imagine having to take all nourishment through a tube in your stomach and never again eating a pizza or Grandma's cookies, or even drinking a glass of water.

THE SWALLOWING EVALUATION

As indicated earlier, the complexity of dysphagia and associated disorders and diseases requires study and treatment by a number of specialists. Consequently, a thorough examination and accurate diagnosis often requires the participation of several different healthcare professionals. Here, we are most interested in the role of the SLP, but we will consider also the role of other specialists.

Case History

The evaluation begins by reading the patient's hospital chart or whatever other records are available. The intent is to learn about the individual's past medical history as well as the current medical diagnosis; coexisting problems; medications taken by the patient; respiratory status; nutritional, dietary; and hydration status; and the general physical condition of the patient. We are looking for indicators that suggest that the patient may be at risk for malnutrition, dehydration, or aspiration (the penetration of food or liquid into the trachea) as well as for clues as to the cause of the dysphagia.

Information about the respiratory status is important because we will want to know if the patient has a history of aspiration pneumonia or other respiratory complications. A patient with a history of such problems is generally treated more conservatively that one who has a healthy, robust set of lungs.

Of special interest is whether the patient has a tracheotomy and, if so, what type of tracheostomy tube has been placed. If a patient requires an inflatable tracheostomy tube to protect his lungs from the aspiration of oral secretions, then it is highly unlikely that he can safely swallow food or liquid. These patients are usually examined clinically and are carefully followed but not tested with radiologic imaging techniques until the tracheostomy cuff can be deflated. Patients who are on ventilators for assistance with breathing are usually in special ventilator units and their special needs are beyond the scope of this chapter.

We will likely learn from the clinical records whether the patient has been losing weight, how the patient receives his nutrition (by mouth or by an alternative feeding method such as a nasogastric tube or gastrostomy tube), and laboratory values related to the patient's nutritional status. These laboratory values are usually interpreted by a physician or a dietitian. Three values most commonly used to ascertain nutritional status are serum albumin, total lymphocyte count, and prealbumin. An albumin of 3.5 or greater, a total lymphocyte count of 1500 or greater, and a prealbumin ranging from 16–36 are generally considered normal. It is always wise to talk with the local dietitians and learn what laboratory tests and ranges they use to indicate the various levels of severity of malnourishment. If the patient is taking his meals by mouth, the clinical records should state if he is on a regular or a special diet.

Patient/Family Interview

After the history has been obtained from the available documentation, we are now ready to interview the patient and family. In our context, the term "family" is used loosely; a family member may actually be a nonrelated caregiver or significant other. The questions asked of the patient and family are intended to help decide how to proceed with the proper method of evaluation and/or referral. Also, much of the information will be important when treatment options are considered.

As with any other history taking, it is important to record who is providing the information. If the patient is unable to answer for himself, then it is important to know how close the informant is to the patient and the probable accuracy of the information that is provided.

Throughout this interview we observe the patient's speech and language status and look for any indications of impaired judgment or memory or signs of attention deficit. Obviously, any such problems will influence decisions about testing procedures and therapy techniques associated with the possible dysphagia. Also, we need to be alert to the need to follow-up at another time with formal testing of speech, language, cognition, or hearing.

History taking begins with open-ended questions such as asking the patient or informant to describe the swallowing problem and describe what makes swallowing better or worse. We want to know when the problem began and of any incidents that occurred at that time that could account for the onset. We also ask whether the onset was sudden or if the dysphagia developed gradually. Additionally, we need to know whether the problem has become progressively worse or has remained at the same level of severity for an extended

Some patients live in a nursing home or other care facility. Many of these institutions are short of staff, and that will have an influence on what your final recommendations can be for the patient.

Talk, listen, and observe your patient. Pay attention to speech, voice, language, and behavior.

period and if the problem is always present or if it is intermittent and comes and goes with no particular pattern. Prognosis for the patient who has experienced a recent surgery or neurological insult resulting in dysphagia may be very different than for a patient whose dysphagia is of gradual onset and may be an early sign of degenerative neurological disease.

Once the preliminary questions have been asked, it is time to begin with more specific questions about whether there are any of the following symptoms during or after eating:

1. food/liquid from the nose (nasal reflux)

2. drooling

3. food residue found in the mouth after eating

4. dry mouth (xerostomia)

5. coughing/choking during or after eating or drinking

6. the sensation of a lump in the throat

7. a sticking sensation in the throat

8. pain or discomfort on swallowing (odynophagia)

9. voice changes

10. heartburn

11. frequent regurgitation or vomiting

12. frequent burping

13. taste problems

14. appetite changes

The most obvious cause of nasal reflux is failure to close the velopharyngeal port during swallowing. If the velopharyngeal disorder is so severe as to result in nasal reflux, it is likely that the patient's speech will be nasalized. Because that patient may be a candidate for management by dental prosthesis or possibly surgery, a referral to a special management team is needed. If the cause of the velopharyngeal disorder is not already known, a neurologic referral is certainly indicated to determine whether the velopharyngeal disorder is symptomatic of a neurologic disease. Ideally, cancer patients who are to undergo a partial or total palotectomy (surgical removal of part or all of the hard and/or soft palates) should be seen by a prosthodontist preceding the surgery.

Drooling or residue in the mouth after eating are often symptomatic of neurological impairment. These findings are common with patients who have strokes and in children with certain neuromuscular disorders. Drooling does not necessarily mean that the individual cannot eat safely, but it is a "flag" that suggests that the patient may be at risk for poor oral control of a liquid or food bolus. The "squirreling" of food in the cheeks due to decreased sensation or buccal muscle weakness can result in spillover into the unprotected airway causing that person to choke on the residue some time after eating.

A dry mouth (xerostomia) can affect the oral stage of the swallow and decrease taste sensation. Xerostomia can occur from certain systemic diseases, radiation treatment to the mouth or neck, or any other cause that decreases salivary gland production such as various medications. Also, with advanced age, the amount of saliva that is produced is decreased. If there is decreased secretion of mucus in the pharynx, it can be difficult for a food bolus to travel smoothly into the esophagus and portions of the bolus may stick in the pharynx. There are "artificial saliva" products on the market that may be helpful. Depending on the patient's history, it may be appropriate to refer the patient to a dentist who is accustomed to treating xerostomia or it may be necessary to refer the patient to a physician for a medical examination.

Individuals who cough or choke during or after meals may describe the problem as a tickling in the throat or the sensation of something going down the wrong pipe or falling into the windpipe. Such a description cues the clinician that, when proceeding to a visual imaging examination (usually radiologic), which we will be discussing later in this chapter, the clinician should be on the lookout for penetration of food or liquid into the larynx. Just because a person coughs does not mean there is aspiration; rather, the cough may be a successful defense that prevents penetration into the trachea. Likewise, just because someone does not choke or cough does not mean that they do not aspirate; that person may have decreased sensation and be a "silent aspirator." Silent aspiration is a commonly occurring event, and the conscientious clinician knows that the absence of a cough provides no information regarding the safety of a swallow.

This is important because many dysphagic patients are silent aspirators.

The underlying cause for the complaint of a sensation of a lump in the throat or of something sticking in the throat after swallowing can be difficult to diagnose. One cause for this complaint is the reflux of contents in the stomach or esophagus; that is, the contents "come up again." Of course, the complaint can be because food is indeed sticking in the patient's throat. Visual imaging techniques that are used for evaluation and which will be discussed later help to identify the cause for this sensation. If, on visual imaging, there is no food sticking in the throat, a consult with a gastroenterologist is generally warranted.

The report of voice changes needs to be followed up with additional questions. If the voice change occurs just after eating or drinking, it may be the result of food or liquid entering the laryngeal vestibule and either settling on or penetrating the vocal folds. The additional material on the vocal folds will change their vibratory pattern. On the other hand, a history of voice change may be indicative of a laryngological problem such as weakness or paralysis of a vocal fold or laryngeal cancer. Differential diagnosis is then performed with laryngoscopy by an otolaryngologist.

When patients report that they have experienced taste changes, appetite changes, odynophagia (pain on swallowing), heartburn, vomiting, or excessive stomach gas, it is important that a physician be consulted. These are not symptoms associated with oropharyngeal dysphagia, rather they are symptoms of a variety of possible medical problems that require a physician's attention. Some of the medical problems can be life threatening and so a referral should not be delayed.

Examination of the Patient

Discussion with the patient, family, or significant others provides the basis for an informal assessment of speech, language, and cognition. Although specific problems will not be discussed in this chapter, it is sufficient to suggest that, if the patient has significant cognitive or linguistic deficits, those problems can influence the decisions that will be made regarding task instructions, the type of diagnostic tests to perform, and recommendations for treatment.

The sensorimotor examination is performed to determine if there is any impairment of the face, mouth, pharynx, or larynx that can affect chewing or swallowing. The impairment can be sensory, motor, or structural. When a portion of the mouth, larynx, or pharynx has been altered (such as partial pharyngectomy or laryngectomy) or is malformed (such as Pierre Robin syndrome), the condition is considered structural. If the impairment is sensorimotor, the examiner then determines if the breakdown in function is in the peripheral or central nervous system. When assessing swallowing it is very important to assess sensory as well as motor function.

The oromotor examination and a complete discussion of the evaluation of swallowing is described elsewhere (Perlman et al., 1991). Nevertheless, it seems useful at this point to discuss certain observations that should be made during the examination.

Face

Sensory. For a qualitative estimate of facial sensation, ask the patient to close his eyes and to touch the locations where you have applied very light touch and then deep pressure, perhaps with a manicure stick or a feather. Test the upper and lower lips and the perioral region.

Motor. Note the symmetry, strength, and tone of the muscles of the face. Assess the lower face at rest, during conversation, on lip rounding, and when smiling. Most patients can swallow adequately even if the lips are weak; however, the complexity or severity of a patient's disease or disorder is more fully understood if the facial muscles are assessed. Although the upper face does not contribute to speech or swallowing, a complete cranial nerve examination would include observation of the muscles of the eyes and forehead.

Mouth

Look at the oral mucosa for the presence or absence of oral secretions. Generally, the oral mucosa will glisten; but if a patient has xerostomia, the mucosa will appear dry. Excessive secretions suggests that the patient is unable to manage his saliva satisfactorily. Too much saliva, particularly if it can be seen pooling in the oropharynx, is generally indicative of a serious swallowing problem.

Note the condition of the teeth and whether any are absent. If the molars are missing or if they are exceptionally worn down, the patient may not be able to chew solid foods satisfactorily.

Sensory. As with the lips and perioral region, touch the tongue and the hard and soft palates lightly and ask the patient to indicate when he senses the touch. You can use a sketch of the lips, tongue, and palate and instruct the patient to point to the location you touched. A diagram adapted from that used by Silverman and Elfant (1979) may be a useful way for obtaining and recording this information.

Because the sensory innervation of the tongue comes from cranial nerves V, VII, and IX, taste and sensation may be affected along with the motor function to the face and muscles of mastication. If taste or sensation is found to be selectively impaired, you can use this information to the patient's advantage when performing radiologic examination and when making decisions regarding treatment. For example, if sensation is present only on the left side, be sure to place the food bolus on the left side of the tongue.

Also, look for the squirreling of food in the lateral sulci. This is suggestive of decreased sensation and can also indicate weakness of the cheek or tongue muscles.

Motor. Observe the soft palate at rest, during vowel prolongation, and during a gag. It is my policy to let the patient know that I am going to try to make him gag because it generally builds trust and allows me to do other things in the patient's mouth without causing adverse reactions. On some occasions this can work against me, in that the patient pulls away or overreacts. Although the absence of a gag can mean that the cranial nerve IX–X reflex is impaired, there are many people who just do not have a gag reflex but who have good palatal movement that can be seen when they produced the prolonged /a/. Also, do not forget that the presence of a gag tells you *nothing* about the safety of the swallow. It only tells you that the reflex is intact.

> The absence of a gag *may* be indicative of a swallowing problem. The presence of a gag does not tell you anything about the safety of the swallow.

Look at the tongue at rest and on protrusion. Note if the tongue is symmetrical and if the size is within normal limits. Note also if there is a reasonable range of tongue motion adequate for touching the hard palate, retruding the tongue as is necessary for swallowing, and moving it to manipulate a food bolus as described earlier in this chapter. Look for fasciculations or tongue atrophy, particularly in dysarthric patients. Be attentive if there has been partial or total glossectomy since these patients are at high risk for dysphagia.

Respiration, Speech, and Voice

We need to determine whether the respiratory, phonatory, articulatory, or resonatory systems are impaired. Patients with respiratory problems may not be able to clear their lungs of foreign material as well as patients with normal lung function. Also, they may not be able to safely coordinate respiration and swallowing. Consequently, they need to be treated with caution when nutritional options are considered.

Problems with the articulatory system may be indicative of weakness or incoordination of the muscles that are used for chewing and swallowing as well as for speech. Resonance problems may be suggestive of velopharyngeal incompetency or incoordination which can also have an impact on the efficiency of the swallow.

If the patient exhibits a wet hoarse voice quality or if the voice is perceived as breathy or of weak intensity, it is important that a laryngoscopy be performed. Some individuals with paralysis or paresis of the vocal folds aspirate because an important valve protecting the airway has been compromised. When a laryngoscopy reveals excessive secretions in the hypopharynx or if a patient's voice is wet sounding, it is likely that the patient is an aspirator. However, it is important to remember that a clear voice does not mean that the patient swallowed without aspiration.

Once the clinical examination is completed, the clinician decides how to proceed. It is possible that the SLP will decide that the problem is not within his or her domain and that the patient should be referred to another specialist such as an otolaryngologist, gastroenterologist, or neurologist. For example, a referral to a gastroenterologist would be appropriate, if, after a careful interview, it becomes evident that the clinical signs suggest that the patient may be experiencing gastroesophageal reflux. Another example for the need to refer a patient would be if the patient's complaints of dysphagia are part of a cluster of symptoms such as hoarseness and/or odynophagia; in that case, the patient should be referred to an otolaryngologist. At times the patient needs to be seen by both the SLP and another specialist.

> Reports indicate that only about 42% of the patients who aspirate are identified by clinical examination. This strongly reinforces the need for dynamic imaging of the swallow.

If the problem is in the domain of the SLP, then it is necessary to decide which instrumental procedures should be used for further diagnosis. Because the clinical examination neither reliably identifies patients who aspirate (Splaingard, Hutchins, & Chaudhuri, 1988) nor provides adequate information for treatment planning, it is advisable to proceed with additional diagnostic procedures.

DIAGNOSTIC PROCEDURES

Several objective diagnostic procedures are available to the SLP. Because the type of information obtained is not necessarily the same for each, you need to be able to decide which procedure will provide you with the most appropriate information while causing your patient the least risk or discomfort.

In many institutions, videofluoroscopy is the only diagnostic procedure for the assessment of swallowing, and, in the majority of instances, it may be the only objective procedure that needs to be performed. More information is available on the application and interpretation of videofluoroscopy than any of the other procedures. Nevertheless, it is important for you to know about the other techniques.

Videofluoroscopy

This procedure is also commonly referred to as the modified barium swallow (MBS), the cookie swallow test, test of oropharyngeal function (OPSF), or a dysphagia swallow study (DSS). Other terms that have been used include deglutition study and oropharyngeal motility study (OPMS). No matter which term is used, the examination is essentially the same. My personal preferences are DSS or OPSF because they provide some explanation as to what the examination is about.

I choose to avoid use of the term modified barium swallow because the first word can easily get "lost in the shuffle," resulting in a patient inadvertently receiving a traditional barium swallow which is a totally inappropriate test for evaluating oropharyngeal swallowing and, at times, can be dangerous for a dysphagic patient.

The problem with the term "cookie swallow" is that it does not provide any information as to the purpose of the examination; also the majority of patients at acute care hospitals never get far enough along in the examination to take a bite of cookie or other solid food, so the term seems inappropriate in most instances. Also, I am aware of too many episodes where medical staff have referred to female clinicians as the "cookie lady," not a particularly professional title.

OPSF is a moving picture X-ray examination of swallowing *function*. Although there are times when a portable fluoroscopy unit may be taken to a patient's bedside, generally patients are seen in radiology departments.

The patient is examined in the lateral (Figure 15–3a) and anterior-posterior (AP) (Figure 15–3b) planes. Most of the information is obtained in the lateral plane, but the AP view provides information relating to the symmetry of the swallow, the presence of a pocket that is called a diverticulum, and often permits gross observation of the movement of the vocal folds. Although some clinicians prefer to shorten the examination to a lateral view only, I strongly believe that this is a big mistake. Even one swallow in the AP plane can provide very important diagnostic information; and so, the AP plane should always be examined.

The patient is given radiopaque material (barium) and as the fluoroscopy camera images the patient during the oral and pharyngeal

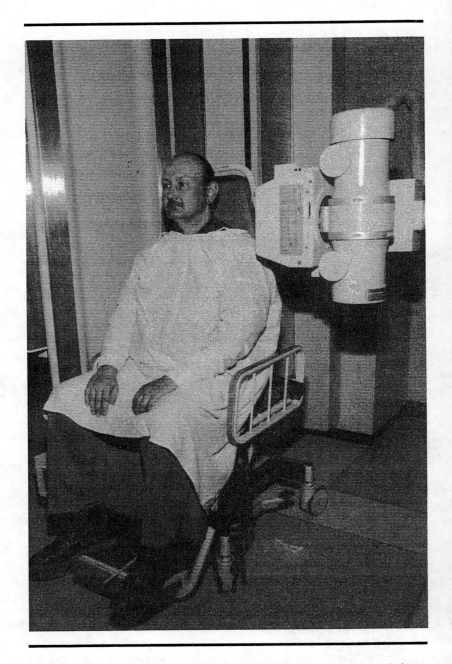

Figure 15–3A. Position of patient for video examination in the lateral plane.

stages of swallowing, that image is recorded on videotape. This examination is not intended to identify lesions or structural abnormalities. The identification of a lesion or a structural abnormality falls within the responsibility of the radiologist.

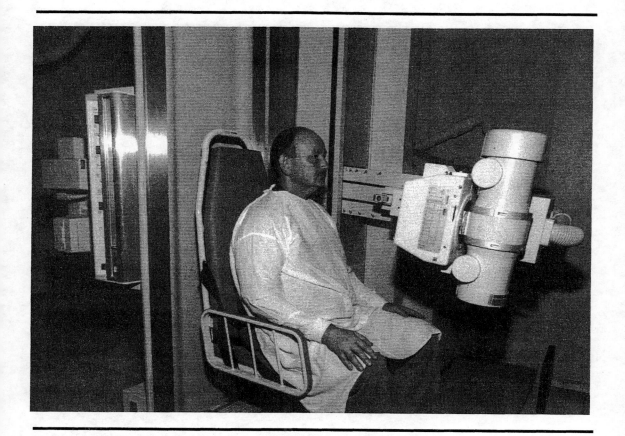

Figure 15–3B. Position for examination in the anterior-posterior plane.

Figure 15–4 shows the lateral and AP views of an individual with a normal swallow. As you can tell, there is very little barium remaining in the mouth or pharynx. Figure 15–5 shows the residuals from the swallow of a dysphagic patient. On the lateral view there is significant barium residue in the pyriform sinuses and aspiration; note the barium on the vocal folds as well as in the trachea. The AP view of another swallow from the same patient shows bilateral vallecular and pyriform sinus stasis; barium can be seen in the trachea.

Following the examination, the clinician can look at the videotape of the swallow in slow motion or even frame by frame. The purpose of this careful examination is to identify oral, pharyngeal, or laryngeal events that may be contributing to the patient's dysphagia. The technique can assist in determining not only if the patient is aspirating, but why he is aspirating. Information on performing the videofluoroscopic examination is available in many sources, but I particularly recommend the descriptions provided by Logemann (1993, 1998).

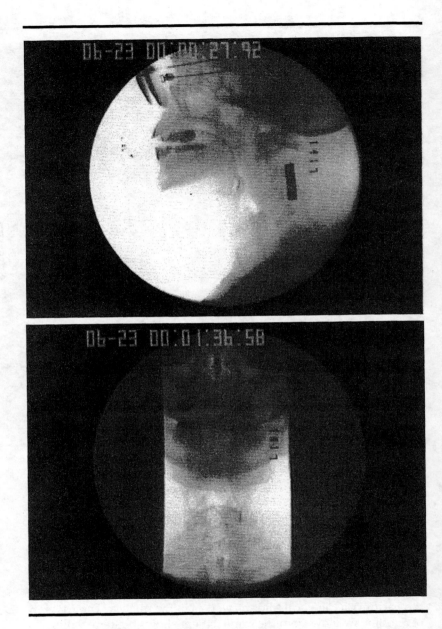

Figure 15–4. A fluoroscopic image in the lateral (top) and A–P (bottom) planes, showing no oropharyngeal dysphagia.

The videofluoroscopic procedure is an extremely informative examination technique, but the examiner needs to remember that this is an X–ray procedure and therefore the patient is exposed to all the hazards of radiation. For that reason, the procedure should not be used indiscriminately. The procedure is generally contraindicated when no new or useful information will be obtained, if the patient

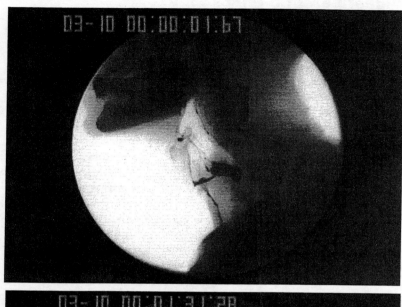

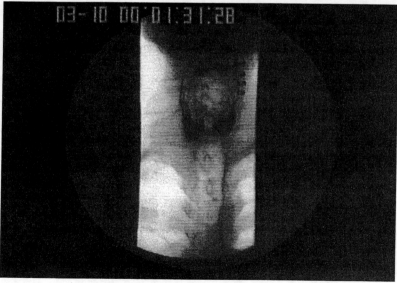

Figure 15–5. A fluoroscopic image in the lateral (top) and A–P (bottom) planes, showing significant barium residue.

has no swallow, or if a patient's level of alertness is such that the individual cannot be safely nourished by mouth. If a patient is extremely ill, the decision to proceed with an examination needs to be considered very carefully; if the physician feels the evaluation is necessary, then either a nurse or physician, and possibly a respiratory therapist, should be in attendance during the examination.

Videofiberoptic Endoscopy

Traditionally, fiberoptic endoscopy has been used by laryngologists and speech pathologists to assess laryngeal and velopharyngeal function during phonation. With the addition of a small camera onto the endoscope, these images can be videorecorded. The procedure can also be used to observe the swallowing process, although the information obtained from endoscopy is more restricted than that obtained from a videofluoroscopic examination.

During the examination, the endoscope is passed transnasally until the valleculae, epiglottis, hypopharynx, pyriform sinuses, and larynx can be viewed. The patient is given something to swallow such as milk, water, or applesauce with a few drops of food coloring added, and the examiner records the swallowing events onto videotape. By coloring the food or liquid, it is easy to identify the test material and to determine if there is residue after the swallow. Clinicians generally avoid the use of yellow or red coloring; green is most frequently used.

The larynx, pyriform sinuses, epiglottis, and base of tongue are shown in Figure 15–6. This is the standard "starting point" when doing an endoscopic evaluation of swallowing.

This procedure permits visualization of the pharynx and larynx (from above) before and after the swallow; during the swallow the video image is obliterated. It is the best procedure for examining the larynx. By pulling the endoscope back until it is above the soft palate, the action of the velum can be observed throughout the swallow. Obviously, information is obtained on the oral stage of the swallow with this procedure. The methodology for fiberoptic endoscopic examination of swallowing has been described by Langmore, Shatz, and Olson (1988).

Ultrasound

This imaging technique is used to track the movement of the tongue and the hyoid bone during swallowing and is therefore limited to assessing oral function. The ultrasound transducer is held under the patient's chin; high frequency waves are transmitted and the reflected waves are received and transformed into a video image and then recorded on tape. Whereas the soft tissues of the tongue allow for passage of most of the ultrasound wave, the hyoid bone is so dense that it resists the passage of the waves and the reflected waves from the hyoid produce a shadow. Thus, the examiner can observe the movement of the tongue during the oral phases and can observe the movement of the shadow representing the motion of the hyoid bone during the pharyngeal stage of the swallow. Some investigators have used ultrasound to look at other aspects of the swallow, but that requires not only very special expertise but also highly sophisticated ultrasound equipment. Additional information about ultra-

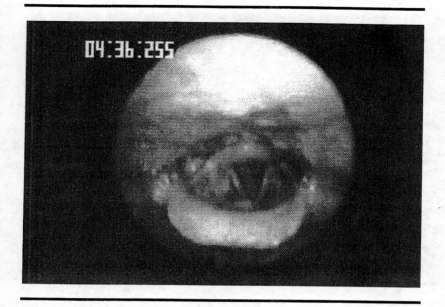

Figure 15–6. A fiberoptic endoscopic view showing the larynx, pyriform sinuses, base of tongue, and epiglottis.

sound can be obtained from Sonies (1991), Perlman (1997), and by Watkin and Miller (1987). Figure 15–7 shows the ultrasound machine and the transducer placed submentally.

Electromyography (EMG)

When a muscle fiber or group of fibers contract, the fibers generate a very small electrical signal and, like a signal generated by a radio transmitter, that signal can be picked up with the right type of antenna. In the case of EMG, the antenna is called an electrode. When fine wire electrodes are placed in a laryngeal, pharyngeal, or oral muscle and the individual performs a motor act that causes the muscle to contract, the small electrical signal emitted from the muscle is picked up by the electrodes, passed through an amplifier, and can be recorded. If the muscle is paralyzed, then no signal or an aberrant signal will be transmitted. An example of a rectified EMG signal from the superior pharyngeal constrictor muscle of a normal subject and from a patient with pharyngeal constrictor paralysis is shown in Figure 15–8.

Electromyography is not only used to determine if a muscle is paralyzed; neurologists also use EMG in the differential diagnosis of various neuromuscular diseases. For a heavy dose of reading about the use of EMG in the assessment of certain aspects related to swallowing, refer to the latter portion of the chapter by Cooper and

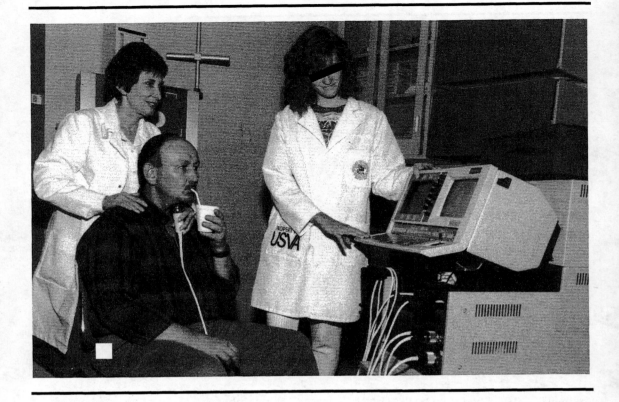

Figure 15–7. The ultrasound machine as it is used for obtaining information on the tongue and hyoid bone during swallow.

Perlman (1997). Probably of greater interest to you, the student, is the information relative to the use of surface EMG as a form of biofeedback in the treatment of certain aspects of dysphagia. For information on that technique see the work of Crary (1995).

Respiration

The common pattern of healthy, young adult respiration during deglutition consists of expiration, deglutition apnea, and expiration. Work is presently underway to ascertain if such a pattern is also noted in persons of various ages as well as in persons with neuromuscular or respiratory disorders. Also of interest is the issue as to whether or not a patient who is likely to aspirate during eating is more likely to exhibit a respiratory-swallowing pattern different from an individual who is not likely to aspirate. The assessment of respiration can be easily performed with a Respirodeglutometer (Klahn & Perlman, in press); however, other instrumental tech-

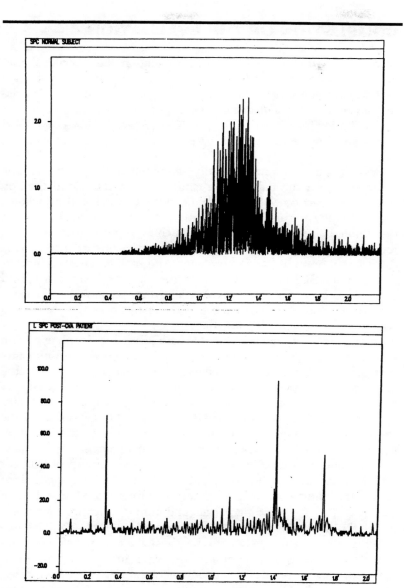

Figure 15–8. An example of a rectified EMG signal from the superior pharyngeal constrictor muscle, during swallow by a healthy individual and an individual with paralysis of the pharyngeal constrictor muscle.

niques have been used for this purpose. Depending on the findings of research in progress, the use of respirodeglutometry may become commonplace as one of the tools used for the assessment of patients with dysphagia.

This technique is new and so there is little quantitative information available at this time. Selley has published some interesting descriptive studies which you may find interesting (Selley et al., 1990, 1994).

COMPLETION OF THE EVALUATION

At the completion of the swallowing evaluation, the clinician should be in a position to describe the severity of the patient's dysphagia and the symptoms that result in dysfunction. One method of describing severity is the *Functional Assessment Scale* developed by the Rehabilitation Institute of Chicago (RIC–FAS, 1992). This scale is used to rate swallowing function on a 7-point scale from normal to severe impairment.

When the clinician has carefully evaluated all findings, it is time to determine if the patient is a candidate for behavioral therapy under the direction of the SLP or a candidate for dental prosthetic, medical, and/or surgical intervention. The final decision may be determined after consensus has been achieved with input from various specialists who are part of a structured or unstructured, interdisciplinary or multidisciplinary team. And so, it is extremely important that the SLP be well versed in the anatomy, physiology, and pathophysiology of oropharyngeal swallowing. Additionally, of course, the clinician must be able to interpret the results from the procedures used to assess swallowing function.

In most institutions, it is the SLP who heads the dysphagia team or who serves as the key component in the diagnosis and management of patients when no formal team is in operation. Although the scope of this chapter does not include discussion of team management, there are certain responsibilities that a dysphagia clinical management team can assume that are worth mentioning. Some of the responsibilities include: (1) establishing protocols for identification of patients with dysphagia and for routing patients through the necessary clinics involved in assessment; (2) developing protocols for patient management and nourishment; (3) developing a method for chart entry and record keeping that is meaningful to all members of the team; and (4) providing patient and family education and ongoing staff training. Consequently, it is important that the SLP be able to communicate effectively with the physician and other health care professionals, as well as with families, when interpreting examination results and recommending treatment options that have been determined as a result of the complete dysphagia evaluation. The importance of this cross-discipline communication cannot be overemphasized.

SUMMARY

The diagnosis and treatment of patients with oropharyngeal dysphagia has become a major portion of the caseload of many speech-language pathologists. Although the greater number of clinicians who work with this population are in hospitals, nursing homes, or rehabilitation centers, SLPs are frequently responsible for management of dysphagic children and adults in other environments as well.

Thorough examination begins with a review of the patient's history, an interview with the patient and/or significant others, clinical examination, and generally at least one objective technique. The clinical examination should consist of an informal assessment of speech, language and cognition, and an in-depth sensorimotor examination of those structures important to deglutition.

The most frequently used objective method for assessing swallowing is the videofluoroscopic examination of swallowing function. There are other techniques that are appropriate depending on the question that is being asked about the patient. At the completion of the swallowing evaluation, the clinician should be in a position to describe the severity of the patient's dysphagia and the causes of dysfunction, and to make recommendations for treatment or for further evaluation. Diagnosis and management of dysphagia are generally most efficient and effective when there is team management. The configuration of the team is dependent on the type of institution and the patient population. It is often the SLP who heads the dysphagia clinical management team; so it is important for the SLP to be able to communicate effectively with physicians, other health care professionals, and families when interpreting examination results and recommending treatment options that have been determined as a result of the complete dysphagia evaluation.

REFERENCES

Arvedson, J. C., & Brodsky, L. (Eds.). (1993). *Pediatric swallowing and feeding.* San Diego, CA: Singular Publishing Group.

Cooper, D. S., & Perlman, A. L. (1997). Electromyography in the functional and diagnostic testing of deglutition. In A. L. Perlman & K. Schulze-Delrieu (Eds.), *Deglutition and its disorders,* San Diego, CA: Singular Publishing Group.

Crary, M. A. (1995). A direct intervention program for chronic neurogenic dysphagia secondary to brainstem stroke. *Dysphagia, 10,* 6–18.

Klahn, M., & Perlman, A. (in press). Temporal and durational patterns associating respiration and swallowing. *Dysphagia.*

Langmore, S. E., Shatz, M. A., & Olson, N. (1988). Fiberoptic endoscopic examination of swallowing safety: A new procedure. *Dysphagia, 2,* 216–219.

Logemann, J. A. (1993). *Manual for the videofluorographic evaluation of swallowing* (2nd ed.). Austin, TX: Pro-Ed.

Logemann, J. A. (1998). *Evaluation and treatment of swallowing Disorders* (2nd ed.). Austin, TX: Pro–Ed.

Perlman, A. L. (1991). The neurology of swallowing. *Seminars in Speech and Language, 12,* 171–183.

Perlman, A. L. (1997). Application of instrumental procedures to the evaluation and treatment of dysphagia. In B. C. Sonies (Ed.), *Dysphagia: A Continuum of Care.* Gaithersburg, MD: Aspen Publishing.

Perlman, A. L., & Christensen, J. (1997). Topography and functional anatomy of the swallowing structures. In A. L. Perlman & K. Schulze-Delrieu (Eds.), *Deglutition and its disorders*. San Diego, CA: Singular Publishing Group.

Perlman, A. L., Langmore, S., Milianti, F., Miller, R., Mills, R. H., & Zenner, P. (1991). Comprehensive clinical examination of oropharyngeal swallowing function: Veterans Administration procedure. *Seminars in Speech and Language, 12,* 246–253.

RIC–FAS, Version 3. (1992). Rehabilitation Institute of Chicago (p. 71).

Selley, W. G., Ellis, R. E., Flack, F. C., Bayliss, C. R., & Pearce, V. R. (1994). The synchronization of respiration and swallow sounds with videofluoroscopy during swallowing. *Dysphagia, 9,* 162–167.

Selley, W. G., Flack, F. C., Ellis, R. E., Ellis, R. E., & Brooks, W. A. (1990). The Exeter dysphagia assessment technique. *Dysphagia, 4,* 227–235.

Silverman, E. H., & Elfant, I. L. (1979). Dysphagia: An evaluation and treatment program for the adult. *American Journal of Occupational Therapy, 33,* 382–392.

Sonies, B. C. (1991). Ultrasound imaging and swallowing. In M. Donner & B. Jones (Eds.), *Normal and abnormal swallowing: Imaging in diagnosis and therapy* (pp. 109–119). New York: Springer-Verlag.

Splaingard, M. L., Hutchins, B., Sulton, L. D., & Chaudhuri, G. (1988). Aspiration in rehabilitation patients: Videofluoroscopy vs. bedside clinical assessment. *Archives of Physical Medicine and Rehabilitation, 69,* 637–640.

Watkin, K. L., & Miller, J. L. (1997). Instrumental imaging technologies and procedures. In B. C. Sonies (Ed.), *Dysphagia: A continuum of care*. Gaithersburg, MD: Aspen Publishing.

RECOMMENDED READINGS

Any of the textbooks listed in the references above.

Beck, T. J., & Gaylor, B. W. (1990). Image quality and radiation levels in videofluoroscopy for swallowing studies: A review. *Dysphagia, 5,* 118–128.

Dysphagia Journal.

Gritzmann, N., & Fruhwald, F. (1988). Sonographic anatomy of the tongue and floor of the mouth. *Dysphagia, 2,* 196–202.

Langmore, S. E. (1991). Managing the complications of aspiration in dysphagic adults. *Seminars in Speech, Language, and Hearing, 12.*

CHAPTER

16

Adults With Mental Retardation

Louise Kent, Ph.D.
Betty J. Price, M.S.

PURPOSE

The purpose of this chapter is to acquaint you with current trends in the assessment of communication for adults with mental retardation (MR). Specifically, our job is to present the attitudes, skills, and information that we want you to own before finishing a clinical practicum with adults with MR. We hope you will take these perspectives to heart when you serve individuals with MR and their families.

BACKGROUND

Unless you have a family member or a close friend or neighbor who has MR, you probably do not know much about it. All of my knowledge about the subject has been acquired since receiving my M.A., and none has been acquired in formal courses. I first learned about MR as a child from neighbors, and I learned more about it from children and their parents in a small, university-based speech clinic. After earning my doctorate, I continued to learn as I worked in two large Michigan residential facilities for people with MR.

The challenge to find and to integrate the best practices for people with MR has led me through a fascinating and fulfilling career in speech-language pathology and behavior analysis. The point of this is to impress on you my belief that the field of mental retardation has a great deal to offer you as a specialty area. But, because this area lacks strong representation in academic and clinical programs in speech-language pathology, you may need to gain your expertise primarily through direct experiences with people with MR, their families, and the clinicians who work with them.

Before we move on, you and I need to agree on what we mean by *adult*, and I need to make you aware of the current definition of mental retardation. For purposes of our discussion here, adults with MR are 22 years of age or older who are no longer receiving services from public school special education programs. The current definition of mental retardation, approved by the American Association of Mental Retardation in 1992, is as follows: "Mental retardation refers to substantial limitations in present functioning. It is characterized by significantly subaverage intellectual functioning, existing concurrently with related limitations in two or more of the following applicable adaptive skill areas: communication, self-care, home living, social skills, community use, self-direction, health and safety, functional academics, leisure, and work. Mental retardation manifests before age 18." This definition is intended to influence how we serve people with mental retardation and the services we offer them.

Further information about definitions of MR can be obtained from the AAMR, 17199 Kalorama Road NW, Washington, DC 20009.

Perspectives on Mental Retardation

I want to share with you some perspectives that professionals in the field of MR embrace as standards for services, and I hope that you will embrace them, too. The overarching perspective is one of dignity in intervention. The goals for intervention are independence and inclusion. We want people with MR to have chances to become as independent as possible in every way. When there are barriers, we want to remove them through instruction and through the use of *adaptations*. We want individuals with MR to have chances to be included in normal living environments; to be included in typical employment settings, as shown in Figure 16–1; to have access to all services and entertainment in our communities, as shown in Figure 16–2; and to have friends in the same way that you and I have friends.

Adaptations are changes we make that allow people to do things that would otherwise be more difficult or impossible.

To help achieve these goals, we apply certain standards. These standards can be applied to recommendations that we make regarding communication intervention, to specific activities, or to just about anything that pertains to adults with MR, including, for example, the kind of telephone we think is appropriate for a particular MR consumer. I'm going to list and describe some of these standards here,

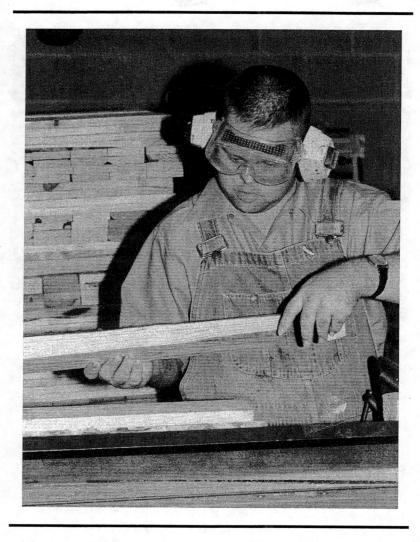

Figure 16–1. Robert Hirsch at work. People with MR deserve the opportunity to learn useful job skills for gainful employment. (Courtesy of Bill Walker, Executive Director of the Center for the Retarded, Houston, TX, where Mr. Hirsch is a client.)

but it will be up to you to apply them in each context in which you work with people with MR.

Social Significance

Typically, people value some things more than others. We tend to prefer the things we perceive as valued in our society. For example, we value the opportunity to work for pay and to spend our money as we choose.

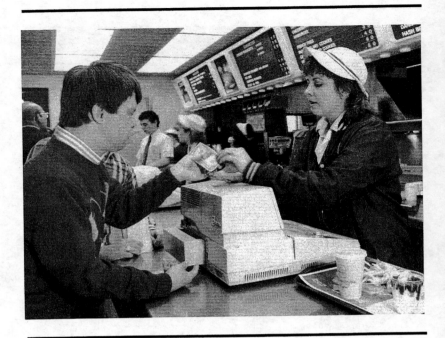

Figure 16–2. Wayne Crouse places his order: "Two all-beef patties, special sauce, lettuce, cheese, pickles, onions on a sesame seed bun." People with MR deserve the opportunity to learn useful interactive skills for everyday life, including visits to a fast food restaurant! (Courtesy of TARGET, Inc., Westminster, MD, From the brochure *Everyone Has to Live Somewhere*.)

Functional

This is a term we use to describe activities that we consider essential in our society. In other words, if we think an activity *must* be performed, it is deemed functional. Doing the laundry is an activity that most of us view as essential, hence, *functional*.

Social Interaction and Communication with Nondisabled People

Treat adults with MR-like adults.

For individuals with mental retardation, social interaction and communication with nondisabled people are viewed as essential for inclusion in the mainstream of society. Activities that encourage such interaction and communication are valued over those that do not.

Age-Appropriate

This term describes what is appropriate for typical adults. For example, adults wear adult-styled clothing even though they may be small in stature.

Durability

Durability refers to skills that have use and value over a long period of time. For example, telephone skills are useful indefinitely, provided there are phones to use. Furthermore, using the phone is functional, age-appropriate for adults, and of high social value.

Practical

This term refers to just how many opportunities there will be to do, or to use, something. If there are opportunities everyday to engage in an activity, we say that learning to perform that activity is practical. For example, most of us eat at least three meals each day; so, good table manners are practical and they have high social value as well. Laundry may not need to be done daily, but doing the laundry is also viewed as practical since there are frequent opportunities for practice. Notice that it's a durable skill also.

Preference

All of us want to express our preferences in the things we do and have. We attach a high value to the opportunity to make our own choices. People with MR have preferences, too.

Everyone appreciates opportunities to make choices.

Culturally Correct

We are most comfortable in our own culture. Those traditions and practices that are valued and accepted in a person's culture are considered culturally correct for that person. We live and work in a multicultural society today; and we should be sensitive to the cultural traditions and practices of those we serve.

What Is an Ecological Assessment?

Best practice says that the most effective way to teach adults with MR is to provide instruction in the environments in which the individuals are expected to function. Best practice also says that the most effective way to teach communication skills to adults with MR is to teach them in the context of activities in which they are embedded. The same is true for assessment.

Best practice favors ecological assessments.

Best practice says that assessments of communication skills should be conducted "in the field," in the environments in which individuals live, work, play, and transact the business of daily life. This means that assessments should be done in the home, on the job, on the bus, in the supermarket, at the pharmacy, at McDonald's, at the snack bar, at the post office, at K-Mart, at the bank, etc. And we should be assessing the communication skills that are embedded in activities that typically occur in these environments, for example, buying bus tokens, buying donuts, ordering a pizza, cashing paychecks, renting a video, getting a haircut, or attending worship.

You can see that ecological assessments of communication represent a departure from assessments conducted in clinic environments. Ecological assessments are time intensive but productive in that they identify goals that meet the standards just presented. For now, though, we need to concentrate on performing a *primary* assessment of communication, and this is done appropriately in a clinic environment. The ecological assessment is an important form of *secondary* assessment that may be recommended after the primary assessment has been completed.

What Is an Augmentative/Alternative Communication (AAC) Assessment?

An AAC assessment is another kind of secondary assessment you may want to recommend or to learn to perform yourself. When a consumer is unintelligible or does not speak, it is becoming more and more common practice to assess that person's potential to communicate effectively by using augmentative/alternative communication systems. AAC systems sometimes provide individuals with greater independence and participation in functional activities of daily living. For this reason, it is sometimes important to include an AAC assessment as part of a consumer's communication assessment.

What Is an AAC System?

As defined by the American Speech-Language-Hearing Association, an AAC system is "an integrated group of components, including the symbols, aids, strategies, and techniques used by individuals to enhance communication" (ASHA, 1991). As used in this definition, and to further quote directly from the definition, the term *symbol* refers to the methods used for "visual, auditory, and/or tactile representation of conventional concepts (e.g., gestures, photographs, manual sign sets/systems, picto-ideographs, printed words, objects, spoken words, Braille)" (ASHA, 1991). It is important to note that, according to this definition, the use of gestural communication (including, for example, facial expressions, eye gaze, and body postures, in addition to hand gestures) is within the overall definition of AAC. This means that interventions designed to increase the ability of persons with the most severe intellectual disabilities (e.g., profound mental retardation) to communicate through gestures and other natural modes fall within the scope of the AAC specialist's domain. The term *aid* is used to refer to "a physical object or device used to transmit or receive messages (e.g. communication book, board, chart, mechanical or electronic device, or computer.)" (ASHA, 1991.). In this context, the terms *aid* and *device* are used interchangeably. A *strategy*, in the ASHA definition, is a "specific way of using aids, symbols, and/or techniques more effectively for enhanced communication" (ASHA, 1991). Finally, the term *technique* refers to "a method of transmitting messages (e.g., linear scanning, row-column scanning, encoding, signing, and natural gesturing)" (ASHA, 1991). These four components—symbol, aid, strategy, and technique—are the critical elements that comprise all AAC interventions (Beukelman & Mirenda, 1993, p. 3). A thorough understanding of this definition and familiarity with its components is essential to conducting an adequate AAC assessment and for devising a successful plan of intervention.

THE ASSESSMENT PROCESS

The Speech-Language Pathologist (SLP) as a Member of an Assessment Team

Because an individual with MR presents a variety of needs, interdisciplinary teams are needed to provide comprehensive assessments. More often than not, the SLP is a member of such a team. Minimally, the team includes a psychologist, social worker, and a physician, who may be represented by a nurse. Other service providers, such as SLPs, may also serve on such teams. My bias, of course, is that every team should include an SLP since communication skills contribute heavily to a person's success in any environment.

How to Begin the Assessment Process?

A review of whatever background information is available introduces you to the consumer as a person. (I often use the term *consumer*, rather than patient or client, because it is preferred by the Texas Department of Mental Health and Mental Retardation. In Tennessee, the consumer is referred to as *the citizen*.)

To make efficient use of your preparation time, record your notes and questions in the appropriate sections of an outline of your written report. One important question is whether or not a reliable informant will be with the consumer at the time of the assessment. Other questions will arise. Acronyms such as TRC (Texas Rehabilitation Commission) will appear in the text of reports without clarification. Diagnostic codes may be used that are foreign to you. You may have questions about the purposes of medications that the consumer is receiving. And you may find discrepancies between reports with respect to anything from date of birth to case number. In every instance, you will want to know what opportunities the individual has to interact with nondisabled people outside the family. You will want to know what they do during a typical day and how they spend their weekends.

Critical information may be missing from the file! You may need to gather information about the consumer. You will need school records, a reliable developmental story, a medical history, a current

> You need a reliable informant in order to obtain the needed information.

physical, and a social history including a description of the present living arrangement and programming during the day. You may be able to get some of this information from informants. To obtain copies of documents, however, you will need to request and obtain permissions for their release.

When you finish your review of the background information, organize what you have learned into the relevant sections of your report. Be sure to highlight any specific questions to be asked of the informant(s) during the assessment in the sections where the information will be reported.

Plan Your Interaction With Informants

The outline for your written report can serve as a guide for how you will spend your assessment time with the consumer. Right away, however, you will encounter a challenging problem: How are you, a stranger, going to engage an adult with MR in a conversation that will allow you to gather the kind of information you need? And, what if the person does not talk at all? You will need one or more informants who know the consumer well. Identify your informants and make arrangements to talk with them on the same day and at the same place where you will assess the consumer. Plan to interview the informant(s) *before* you interview the consumer. Parents and family members or direct care staff who have known the consumer for at least 6 months can provide you with reliable information about how the consumer communicates.

When you talk with informants, ask them to tell you about the consumer as a person: What makes her laugh? How does she show anger? How does she communicate what she wants? How does she handle frustration? Does she have a job? What does she like about it? How does she get to work? Does she have a best friend? Is she interested in the opposite sex? Does she eat out? What does she do on Saturdays? Does she do her own hair? Does she do her own laundry? Can she cook? Does she like games? Does she like sports? Does she belong to the "Y" or to a health club? How does she exercise? How much time does she spend with people without disabilities? What do they do together? Does she have adult brothers and sisters? How are they involved in her life? Who is she really close to? Does she get many phone calls?

You do not need to address all of these questions, and you do not just ask questions. Listen. If the informants are talkative, let them talk as long as they stay on a topic. Informants can help prepare you for your consumers. Plan to spend 30–45 minutes with informants before you interview consumers.

Listen to informants. Practice your interviewing skills!

Plan a Functional Communication Interview

Based on what you learn from reviewing the available information, plan how you will interview the consumer. You probably will have a fairly accurate picture of how the person communicates. If the person talks at all, you will be able to informally assess articulation, voice, rate, fluency, pitch, loudness, pragmatics, expressive vocabulary, and suprasegmental aspects of speech such as melody, stress, and inflectional patterns.

You will need to include an oral examination in the assessment (see Chapter 5). This is an important part of the assessment and is always expected. The consumer will be more likely to cooperate if you perform the examination midway through the interview, rather than at the beginning or at the end. Treat the person with the same respect you would accord any other adult person and expect the same in return. Demonstrate what you want the consumer to do. Let them look in your mouth. And let them examine any instruments or props you use. Be aware that as you conduct the oral examination it is possible to assess language at the same time: "Let me see your teeth." "Show me how you chew." You are performing an oral examination, but you are also communicating with the consumer.

> The oral exam is a must. Don't forget it.

In some instances, consumers may have difficulties swallowing or chewing. When this is the case, teams often depend on the SLP for assessments, referrals, and recommendations regarding adaptive equipment and management techniques. Additional material about these aspects is presented in Chapter 15. When you need this kind of expertise on the job, you can turn to more experienced SLPs and other professionals for advice. It is your professional responsibility, however, to seek continuing education in this area if you find that you continue to need expert help.

Regardless of whether or not the consumer talks, you need to record the interview. Even though you are doing all the talking, the recording will help you remember what you do and how the consumer responds.

If the person does not talk, you will still be able to assess social routines, the communication of personal ID information, receptive language, language-related concepts such as time, and language-related cognitive skills such as visual memory and sequencing. There may be an art to talking with people who do not talk. If it is an art, I'm confident that it is one you can master. I'll give you some tips to get you started later on. For now, let's focus on how to set an adult tone for the interview and how to make it informative for you and fun for both you and your consumer.

> Communication doesn't require speech.

The substance of communication assessments for adults with MR is quite different from speech and language examinations for children or for adults with other types of histories and diagnoses. As you begin the interview, you will need to introduce yourself and make some small talk to help the consumer feel relaxed and at ease with you. Plan this. Rehearse it. It is part of the assessment. You are interested in how the consumer responds to these social approaches.

Next, move into a more formal attitude toward the consumer. Tell him that you are now going to be asking some questions that will help you assess how he communicates. Under the pretext of completing a form, inquire about basic ID information such as full name, address, telephone number, birthdate, age, marital status, employment, etc. Ask the consumer to print his name on the form. Show the consumer a calendar for the year and ask him to find his birthday. Ask him to guess how old you are. Locate today on the calendar and ask him how long it will be until Christmas or his birthday.

After gathering the ID data, compliment the consumer on something: shoes, purse, eyes, hair, anything that catches your eye as especially nice. Observe closely how the consumer responds to this sort of social gesture. Just as you might ask any new acquaintance, ask about what the consumer does during his day. Be sure to assess denial, an important form of negation. For example, even though you may know that the consumer has never been married, ask. Why? Many times professionals working with adults with MR are asked whether an individual is capable of giving informed consent or, less often, whether or not an individual is competent to stand trial. People dealing with such issues may look to you for help. Documentation showing that a person can reliably deny the truth value of statements, ranging from concrete to abstract, can be helpful in this regard. Do not confuse denial with forms of negation such as rejection or nonexistence. Denial requires the person to indicate that a statement about an object, person, place, time, event, plan, and so on is false.

> How would you assess a person's ability to give informed consent for surgery?

Give the consumer generous amounts of time to respond. Rephrase your comments or questions to give the consumer the benefit of every doubt. Supply prompts and encouragers including starters such as "Your first name is Charlie and your last name is . . . ." Pause. Be prepared to keep the interview going on your own. Even though consumers may never say a word, they usually will participate. Typically, adults with MR appreciate the respect and attention you give them; and when family members are present, *they* appreciate it, too.

> People who don't speak can still communicate.

Most adults with MR work at jobs in the community or in workshops run by agencies. Ask questions you can confirm or that require explanations and demonstrations. For example, "How do you get to work in the morning?" "Do you drive?" "What day of the week do you get paid?" Ask questions that reveal the consumer's memory, his language, and his language-related concepts such as money, measurement, time, health, and safety. "What do you do when you get tired?" "What do you do when you run out of work?" "What time do you get to work in the morning?" "What do you do on your break?" "Show me here on the map where you live." "What do you do when you get home?"

Point to the emergency numbers in the front of the phone book and ask what they are for. Before you put the telephone book aside, wonder out loud how much it weighs. Ask how we could weigh it. Ask the consumer to guess how much *you* weigh. You are interested in how the consumer responds and in whether she seems to understand you and the situation.

Switch the conversation to leisure activities. Show a TV guide and ask the consumer to tell you about a favorite show. Ask about shopping. "Where did you buy those shoes?" "What size are they?" Compare your shoe size with hers. Wonder which is larger. Wonder about the price of shoes generally. "I have some money here." Put 75 cents in change on the table. "Do you think this is enough money for a pair of shoes?" "How about a Coke? Could we buy a Coke with it?" "Show me how you could use this money to get a Coke out of a machine." Ask which coin is largest, which one is worth most. Ask which is the larger of two identical coins. Ask whether the consumer can count and then ask him to count the coins. Find out whether he knows the names of the coins. "This is a quarter and this one is. . . ." Or, "Give me the nickel. You may keep the quarter."

Most adults with MR can tolerate at least 45 minutes of this kind of interview. When the consumer begins to show signs of tiring, tell him that you are almost finished. Ask him to estimate how long you have been talking. Give him a pad of paper and a pencil and say something like, "Up 'til now I've been asking all the questions. Now, it's your turn. Ask me something." Give several prompts as needed. Whisper, "Ask me what my favorite color is." "Ask me my middle name." "Ask me where I'm going when we finish here." Thank the consumer for her participation. Compliment her again. Observe what she does when you tell her that the interview is finished.

Tips on Talking With a Person Who Does Not Speak

Just because someone does not talk, we may not safely assume that she or he does not hear or is not listening or does not comprehend what is being said. Communication does not require speech. When a person does not talk back to you, continue to try to establish eye contact with her as you try to engage her in some sort of give and take of communication. Pause frequently, sometimes with a questioning intonation and sometimes not. Do things as you talk. For example, take out your billfold and open it. Look at some of your own family snapshots or photos of pets or friends. Then start to talk about the photos. "This is my dog. His name is Manfred. He was stolen out of my car one time when we went hunting. He was a good dog." Then look up, "Do you have a dog?" Pause. "Maybe you have some pictures."

Move on to something else. Take out your driver's license and show it to the person. "This is my driver's license." Pause. "That's me. Look at that. What a face." Pause. "Do you have any ID?" When you pause, you are giving the person an opportunity to "jump in" and you are observing how she is reacting. Does she look up, look away, smile, show interest in any perceptible way? Does she seem to understand how she is supposed to behave during a conversation? Pursue other directions. Take out some folding money or change. Talk about what you can do with it, count it, name it, make it work for you!

> People who don't speak aren't necessarily without language.

Think receptive. Do not ask the person to talk. Ask him to show you objects that you name. Ask him to show you what you do with things and how they work. Ask him to do things that will reflect his language skills. For example, "Would you hand me the phone book, please?" No response. Pause. Pick it up yourself. Pause. Drop it on the floor. "Wow! It's heavy!" "How much do you think it weighs?"

Use things you wear and carry on your person as props: your car keys, a ballpoint pen, billfold, change, family pictures, handkerchief, rings, watch, glasses, earring, shoes, socks. If you carry a briefcase, stock it with pens, pencils, highlighters, paper, small spiral notebooks, a small magnifying glass, napkins, city map, TV guide, and other things that might serve as interesting conversational referents.

Think memory. "Where did I put my keys?" "Could you show me where the water fountain is?" Think visual. "Let's see, here. I'm all turned around. Can you show me how to put a stamp on this letter?"

INTERVIEW PROTOCOLS

I got the idea for interviewing adults with MR from Audrey Holland's *Communicative Abilities for Daily Living* (CADL; 1980), a test that she authored for adults with aphasia. She included a small group of adults with hearing impairments and adults with MR in the norming sample. Interestingly, the performance of the adults with MR was similar to that of her group with anomic aphasia. Although the CADL is suitable, as is, for some people with MR, my experience has been that it is very difficult for the majority of the group. It's impossible for some. I want you to take a look at it, however, because it captures the essence of what we want to do in an interview with adults with MR. It is functional, it covers a range of communicative functions, it's fun, it is socially interactive, it has engaging props, and it poses common everyday situations.

Based on my awareness of the CADL and with the help of another SLP, I included an interview protocol for people with MR in *Shop Talk* (Kent-Udolf & Sherman, 1983). It will not rescue a hopeless situation, but, if you have access to it, you may find it useful. You have the publisher's permission to copy it, and you do not need anyone's permission to adapt it for use with your consumers. The truth is that we are not going to find or create an interview protocol that will suit all adults with MR. The abilities, modes of communication, interests, cultures, and life histories of these individuals vary drastically. It is more reasonable for us to individualize the interview protocol than to expect the consumer to accommodate us!

The AAC Assessment

When an augmentative/alternative communication assessment is appropriate, the assessment should minimally include an assessment of the individual's strengths and weaknesses related to motor/postural, cognitive, speech-language/communication, and sensory skills; the individual's daily routine and environmental settings; and barriers that may interfere with the successful use of an augmentative communication system.

Assessment of the Person

Motor/Postural Skills. This assessment includes an assessment of mobility (whether the person walks independently, with assistance, or is nonambulatory and uses a manual or powered wheelchair); fine motor skills (whether the person can use fingers to point to pictures or to press keys); seating/positioning (whether the person can sit upright in a regular chair or wheelchair and whether sitting supports [pelvic, shoulder, etc.], or other adaptive positioning equipment is currently used or needed); head control; muscle tone and reflex patterns that may interfere with voluntary control; limitations in range of motion; the individual's tolerance for a motor task; and how easily he or she becomes frustrated.

The motor assessment will provide valuable information regarding the person's motoric ability to effectively use a communication system, electronic or otherwise. From this assessment, you should learn which body part(s) the person can use most effectively to activate a communication system, the most optimum position for control of hands, head, or other body parts for system access, and whether a mount or other adaptive equipment will be needed to support use of the communication system.

Cognitive Status. If you are a team member, you will probably have access to the psychological report, which will give you information regarding the consumer's cognitive abilities. In reviewing the report, be sure to focus on the individual's skills/abilities rather than his or her IQ score, for as Beukelman and Mirenda (1992, p. 130) point out, there are currently no formal tests that can predict an individual's ability to meet the cognitive requirements of various AAC techniques. Knowing this, it becomes your responsibility to understand the cognitive requirements of the various AAC techniques/systems and to assess the individual's ability to meet those requirements.

Through informal observation, you assess the individual's attention, ability to understand and follow directions, memory/ability to recall symbols and commands, and problem-solving abilities. Also, assess understanding of causality (cause and effect)—the individual's understanding of a tool, such as a communication board/device or switch to obtain the response of others; and assess understanding of symbolic representation (object/symbol association)—understanding that an object or picture can represent an object or concept that one can communicate and receive. A widely used procedure to assess object/symbol association was cited by Baumgart,

Johnson, and Helmstetter (1990, p. 90). In this procedure, "the person is shown a real object and then asked to choose between two line drawings, one of the object that is present and one of a different object. For example, you might show a real ball and then present two line drawings, one of a ball and one of a wagon. The person is then asked to find the picture of the ball." An excellent description of other techniques that can be used to assess understanding and use of symbols can be found in Beukelman and Mirenda (1992, pp. 131–134).

Information gained from the cognitive assessment will assist you in selecting and/or developing a communication system in keeping with the individual's intellectual capabilities. Be aware that some investigators contend that individuals with mental retardation should not receive augmentative communication systems until sensorimotor stage V (mental age between 12 and 18 months) is reached. However, Calculator and Bedrosian (1988, p. 316) report that there appears to be little if any evidence to support "the practice of withholding augmentative instructions from clients until they demonstrate a specific level of cognitive functioning."

Speech-Language/Communication. Simply put, you want to know *how* the person communicates (facial expressions, eye gaze, pointing/gestures/signs, vocalizations, speech, or written/printed/typed communication); their level of receptive and expressive vocabulary/language (including formal test results, if possible); and their pragmatics or social interaction skills. In regard to social skills, pay particular attention to the consumer's understanding of turn-taking, his ability to establish and maintain eye contact with listeners, and his ability to maintain joint attention with a listener to a common object or event, because these skills have been found to be predictive of success in using AAC systems (Calculator and Bedrosian, 1988, p. 317). Other areas to assess include reading and spelling ability, whether the person makes choices, and whether the person desires to communicate or initiate interaction. Finally, inquire about communication systems that have already been tried, how the consumer accessed the system, how long the consumer used it, and whether it did or did not work.

Perceptual Problems. Note whether the person has any known visual and/or auditory impairments. Questions you might ask yourself to assess visual abilities include: Does the person wear glasses? Can the person fixate on a stationary object? Can the person look right and left without moving his or her head? Does the person recognize people, common objects, photographs, symbols, or pictures? Which symbols or pictures does the individual recognize and what size and what color (color or black and white)? Questions to assess auditory abilities might include whether the person attends to sounds, discriminates among sounds, understands speech, and whether the person passed his or her last audiological screening. Try to obtain reports completed by other professionals (occupational therapist, audiologist, etc.), if any exist, regarding the individual's visual-perceptual and auditory abilities.

Information regarding existing perceptual problems is important in planning the design of your consumer's communication system. For example, if your consumer has a visual impairment, the size and spacing of symbols on the communication board or device may need to be made larger. If the individual is auditorily impaired, yet able to read, a visual display for written feedback may be needed to supplement the picture display and auditory feedback signal on the communication device.

Combine the results of the ecological inventory already described with what you have learned about the person during your AAC assessment. This will help you design an AAC system that is based on real-life situations and thus make the communication system as functional as possible for the consumer.

Barriers to Success

As you conduct your AAC assessment, identify factors (related to the individual or environment) that may "prevent, restrict, or limit" (Levin & Scherfenberg, 1990, p. 15) successful use of an AAC system. Barriers related to the individual might include chronic behavior problems, aggression, self-stimulation, lack of interest in communicating with others, resistance to learning new tasks, low frustration level, and problems related to mobility, cognition, and sensory abilities. Barriers related to the environment might include limited opportunities for system use in social situations, lack of family support, and lack of support in the day program environment. Prior to recommending a communication system, you should consider all existing barriers and plan strategies to minimize or eliminate their interference with AAC intervention.

What Communication System Should You Recommend?

AAC systems are either low tech (nonelectronic) or high tech (electronic). Low-tech systems range from simple picture boards, to picture wallets/books, to letter/word boards. The symbols used on such boards and books for individuals with MR are usually, but not limited to, photographs or pictographic symbols (line drawings, either in black and white or in color). "The user simply indicates (by pointing, or by some kind of signal when someone else does the pointing) a choice of one or more picture symbols in order to communicate a message" (Woltosz, 1994, p. 2). "If a person can turn pages, then a communication book is often used to allow access to more than one page of symbols. If not, a single communication board is used with a reduced symbol set" (Woltosz, 1994, p. 1). Low-tech communication systems are relatively inexpensive and easy to construct, and they have been found to be effective with MR adults who need a simple communication system. *Easy to construct*, however, does not mean that you can expect to put together a quality system quickly. Even the simplest system requires thoughtful planning; and you may find yourself returning to the drawing board, literally, several times before you are pleased with the result.

High-tech systems include electronic communication devices, computers, simple technology (i.e., switches, environmental control units), and other technological aids. There are a wide variety of high-tech systems; for additional information, you can contact equipment distributors or technology consultants in private practice. Also, AbleNet publishes a list of commercial sources of assistive technology for people with disabilities (AbleNet, Inc., 1994). You can call or write to any vendor to obtain catalogues. You can also obtain information through workshops and conferences on AAC systems.

To give a general overview, electronic communication devices range from large devices with large display screens to lightweight devices with small display screens. They vary in terms of the number of locations available for symbols/messages and the type of speech output (synthesized vs. digitized speech). Synthesized speech allows a user to create and choose what they want to say and digitized speech is a recording of human voice which is saved on a communication device and played back when needed. Some electronic communication devices have dynamic displays, "a computer screen with electronically produced visual symbols representing messages" (Beukelman & Mirenda, 1992, p. 56). These devices allow access to thousands of symbols by simply touching the display which activates various screens linked together. They are most often used by individuals with mild mental retardation. Some devices have fixed or static displays (which do not change when a user operates the device) and allow access to a specific number of symbols. For individuals with severe cognitive difficulties, because of language difficulties, these devices are programmed with one meaning assigned to each symbol on the display. For individuals with higher cognitive abilities, multimeaning icons (pictures assigned more than one meaning) are used in conjunction with levels (the display shows a single set of symbols but there are two or more levels) and sequencing (combining icon with a limited set) to expand the availability of language.

Simple technology (e.g., switches, environmental control units) is often used in conjunction with high-tech systems to provide adults with MR an alternate means to access or operate a communication device. These devices also provide a means by which individuals with varying levels of mental and physical disabilities can participate in functional activities of daily living (domestic, recreation/leisure, vocational). For example, through use of a switch, an individual may be able to complete a domestic task involving a blender or food processor, a recreation/leisure activity such as turning on a radio or playing games, and a vocational task that involves using an electrical device or machinery. Finally, simple technology is an excellent teaching tool and can be used to teach prerequisite skills (e.g., cause and effect) for future use of an AAC device.

In summary, some individual needs may best be met with low-technology systems while others may optimally benefit from high-technology systems, and still others from both "simple and sophisticated forms of technology" (Levin & Scherfenberg, 1990, p. 11). Remember, when you select a communication system, the choice you make may have an enormous impact on the individual's life. Understanding the many issues involved in AAC assessment and remembering the goal of assessment, to determine the most functional communication system to meet the communication and environmental needs of the individual, are extremely important if the decision you make is to be the best one.

THE WRITTEN REPORT

How are you going to organize the information you have collected into a useful report? What you want to achieve is one that clearly describes the consumer's linguistic skills and his prognosis. Part I of the report is an overview that can be presented in tabular or sentence form. Part II presents the results of the interview and any secondary assessments, the ecological assessment, and the AAC assessment, if they are conducted. Part III includes your recommendations and prognosis for improvement in functional communication. Given Part I and Part II, in Part III you make recommendations for skilled intervention and predict the future outcome barring unforeseen events and with the assumption that your recommendations will be followed.

Be prepared for mandated report formats that may require you to write a report that is telegraphic in style and will fit in a space that is about 6 inches wide and 5 inches long. Should this happen, you still have a good outline. Use it. Be neat, write small, and address each point clearly but in as few words as possible. For now, however, we'll assume that this is not going to happen.

Part I

This section should include identifying information about the consumer, a summary of the most relevant aspects of the history, a description of communication modes used and their attributes, and the diagnosis. You should also identify your informants and other sources of information. Summarize the findings of the oral examination and summarize what you think are the consumer's current communicative needs for now and for the immediate future.

Provide a description of communicative modes used by the consumer and characterize their primary attributes. If relevant, this is where you address intelligibility, rate, voice, and so on, as you would for a person without MR. In addition, include information about oth-

Speech is only one mode of communication.

er communicative modes such as body language, gestures, sign, and written language; and describe how they contribute to communication. End with a diagnosis. This is usually, but not always, *developmental language delay secondary to MR*. There may be, of course, more than one diagnosis. For example, there may also be a voice disorder or a hearing deficit. Be aware that you are not being asked to diagnose mental retardation or the consumer's level of cognitive development. Your focus should be on communication: speech, language, hearing, voice, the oral mechanism, or other modes of expression.

Part II

In this part, include the results of the interview and any secondary assessments if any have been completed. I prefer to organize the information obtained from the interview around five categories. Any set of categories is going to be somewhat arbitrary, and there will be overlap among them. Do try to avoid reporting the same information in more than one category.

Social Routines

Describe how the consumer performs in the contexts of social routines. Describe his use of polite forms and his manners in speech and non-speech modes such as gestures, smiling, and eye contact. We are interested in all the ways that the consumer initiates and responds to occasions that for you and me would prompt social routines. For example, how does the consumer acknowledge your introduction? How does he acknowledge your compliments? Is eye contact appropriate and comfortable? Does he return your smile? Does he laugh when you act silly?

Review your notes and the tape. You will be surprised at how much social routine information you have acquired.

Personal ID

Everybody should carry ID.

Describe what the person knows about himself and how he communicates it. Intelligibility is critical here whether the consumer talks, prints, or points. The world has a low tolerance for errors having to do with ID information. If the consumer does not talk, does he produce his ID when asked where he lives? Does he carry ID on his person?

Basic Language Skills

In this category, describe receptive and expressive attributes of vocabulary, basic semantic relations such as possession, attributes, and negation (*especially denial*), morphology, and syntax. If speech is not the primary communicative mode, describe what was communicated and how.

Language-Related Concepts

Describe how the consumer communicates with respect to any *time concepts* (minutes on watches, days on calendars, seasons of the year, and words and phrases such as past, later, after awhile, never, soon, and a long time). It is important to know how and whether people can sequence events in time. For example, to call home using a pay phone, I must pick up the receiver, put the required amount of money in the slot, wait for the tone, and then punch in the correct numbers *in order.*

Number Concepts. Include any meaningful uses of numbers from money to weights and measures. Make note of the use or understanding of words such as first, last, pounds, sizes, inches, in fact, any words that suggest an awareness of *amounts* of things.

Spatial Concepts. Report the consumer's use of concepts ranging from an awareness of her own body in space to the abstract use of space in a game of chess. Report how the consumer reveals her awareness of space through its use. For example, does she remember the way back to the waiting area? Does she ask for directions? If she prints her name on your form, how does she use the space? Can she orient to a map or a globe? Can she draw a clock face and attach the hands in the middle?

Concepts of Safety and Health. These concepts require us to recognize what is dangerous in the here and now and what might be bad for us in the future. Does the consumer express awareness of cause and effect? Is he able to communicate physical complaints? What is the consumer's level of awareness of the relationship between cleanliness and disease? How does he respond when you ask why we should wash our hands after using the bathroom or use a tissue when we sneeze?

Concepts of Change. Include the changes that come about as a function of the seasons, aging, normal growth and development of children, decay, changes in temperature in various contexts, changes due to wear or to exposure to the sun. Does the consumer express or seem to understand references to these sorts of relationships?

Cognitive/Linguistic Concepts

This is a category that includes memory for any and everything from special patterns to tunes and words of songs. Of special importance is the kind of visual memory that allows us to reassemble things. For example, in order to glue the handle back on a cup, we must remember how the cup looked before it was broken. This category also includes the ability to group things by category and to cite examples from categories. Reading and writing are cognitive/linguistic skills as is matching pictures of objects to pictures that suggest their use.

Part III

Part III includes your recommendations and prognosis for improvement in communication. When stating a prognosis, it is critical that you state *prognosis for what*. People expect you to tell them whether you think accuracy and effectiveness of communication will improve. If you only say, "Prognosis is good," your audience will not be certain what you are talking about and they may think you are saying something different from what you intend. *Prognosis for improvement in the accuracy and effectiveness of communication* is quite different from *prognosis for improvement in level of intellectual functioning*.

Prognosis for what?

I base my judgment of prognosis for communication on the existing level of communication, on apparent eagerness to communicate, persistence, variety of modes used, willingness to try novel modes, humor, and opportunity for interaction with nondisabled people in a variety of environments. It is okay to qualify the prognosis with the recommendations. In other words, the prognosis for improved accuracy and effectiveness of communication may be good only if the recommendations are followed.

Sometimes it is important to state a prognosis for intelligibility of speech or for voice or for speech itself. When it is appropriate or requested, I do not let the diagnosis of MR influence my judgment unduly. I know that people with MR can learn and change, and I respect their abilities and the breadth of their accumulated life experiences. I am alert to instances, however, when years of therapy have not produced measurable changes. When intelligibility of speech is an issue, I often qualify the prognosis with a recommendation for instruction in the use of backup systems such as a billfold communication system.

When writing your recommendations, go back to the beginning of your report. State your recommendations in the order in which you have addressed the information on which they are based. For example, if you were unable to obtain reports of prior diagnostics or therapy, recommend that these documents be obtained early in your list of recommendations. If you have questions about hearing, recommend an audiological assessment.

Recommend ecological assessments to refine objectives. Assess performance in the environments where it is expected to occur.

If you have indicated a positive prognosis for communication, conclude with recommendations for intervention that are consistent with your prognosis and refer the consumer to suitable sources for service delivery. To target communication skill deficits that are embedded in high priority activities, I often recommend ecological assessments of communication. Before making specific recommendations for intervention, I hope that you will review the standards for service that were presented earlier in this chapter.

DESCRIPTION OF REFERENCES

I have tried to keep the list of references short in the hope that you will read them. Each one is included for a reason. The Snell (1987) book is, to me, the best text ever published in the field of special education. I particularly recommend that you read the chapters on assessment and on domestic and community skills. The article by Mirenda (1993) describes the best practice in service delivery and reveals some of the passion of those who serve people with severe disabilities. I have included the Wilcox and Bellamy (1987) catalog because it is unique and it explains by example what is meant by "age-appropriate" and "functional." It will give you valuable ideas for assessment and for programming. Holland's CADL (1980) and my own book, *Shop Talk* (1983) are included because they provide examples of functional communication interviews. The references to the AAC literature are included in order to lead you to additional information in this rapidly developing technology and the philosophy of service that provides its foundation.

SUMMARY

In this chapter I have proposed a comprehensive communication assessment procedure for adults with mental retardation. A functional communication interview is suggested as the primary assessment; and two secondary assessments are suggested for use as appropriate: the ecological assessment and the AAC assessment.

Splashed throughout the chapter is a fair amount of preaching about how to treat people with MR. I want to close with just two more thoughts on that subject. When you serve an adult with MR, you are serving more than that individual. You are also serving the consumer's family and everyone else who serves that person. You have the opportunity to make differences that matter to all of these people.

And, finally, as you interact with adults with MR, be aware that you have the power to influence the attitudes and actions of others. Let your performance demonstrate how to show respect for these individuals. One way to show respect is to "give credit for life experiences." What I mean is that age equivalents for test scores do not tell the whole story. Even though a person may be described as having a mental age of 4 years, *that person is not 4 years old* and should not be treated like a 4-year-old child. Make an effort to model the standard of chronological age-appropriateness whenever possible. You might be surprised at the difference this makes.

REFERENCES

AbleNet, Inc. (1994). *Commercial sources of assistive technology for people with disabilities*. Minneapolis, MN.

Baumgart, D., Johnson, J., & Helmstetter, E. (1990). *Augmentative and alternative communication systems for persons with moderate and severe disabilities*. Baltimore, MD: Paul H. Brookes.

Beukelman, D., & Mirenda, P. (1992). *Management of severe communication disorders in children and adults: Augmentative and alternative communication*. Baltimore, MD: Paul H. Brookes.

Calculator, S. N., & Bedrosian, J. L. (1988). *Communication assessment and intervention for adults with mental retardation.* Boston, MA: Little, Brown.

Holland, A. L. (1980). *Communicative abilities in daily living: A test of functional communication for aphasic adults.* Austin, TX: Pro-Ed.

Kent-Udolf, L., & Sherman, E. R. (1983). *Shop talk: A prevocational language program for retarded students.* Champaign, IL: Research Press.

Levin, J., & Scherfenbert, L. (1990). *Selection and use of simple technology in home, school, work, and community settings.* Minneapolis, MN: AbleNet.

Mirenda, P. (1993). AAC: Bonding the uncertain mosaic. *AAC Augmentative and Alternative Communication, 9,* 3–9.

Snell, M. E. (1987). *Systematic instruction of persons with severe handicaps.* Columbus, OH: Charles E. Merrill.

Wilcox, B., & Bellamy, G. T. (1987). *The activities catalog.* Baltimore, MD: Paul H. Brookes.

Woltosz, W. (1994). *Dynamic displays: The changing face of augmentative communication.* Palmdale, CA: Words+, Inc.

CHAPTER

17

Children Who Are Hard of Hearing

Jill L. Elfenbein, Ph.D.

As you begin this chapter, you may ask yourself, "Why is discussion of children with hearing losses included in a book about diagnosis in speech-language pathology?" The answer is simple. Hearing loss affects children's abilities to acquire speech and language skills. The diagnosis and treatment of those problems is well within the scope of practice of speech-language pathologists. Indeed, in many instances speech-language pathologists are the professionals who are best prepared to help children who are hard of hearing develop good communication skills.

In this book, discussion of children who have hearing losses is divided into two categories. The disorders of children who are deaf are described in Chapter 18. In this chapter, we consider the disorders of children who are hard of hearing. These are the children who have hearing losses that fall in the mild-to-severe hearing loss range. You will discover that even a mild hearing loss can have a marked effect on communication skill development.

Figure 17–1 provides an example of how degree of hearing loss is determined. There are some differences of opinion among audiolo-

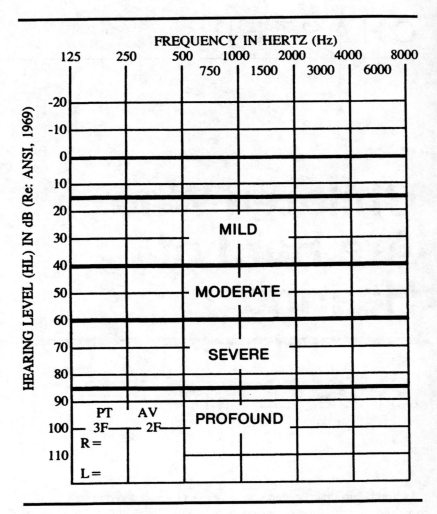

Figure 17–1. Examples of cutoff points used by clinicians to describe degree of hearing loss for children.

gists about the cutoff points between categories. For example, some use 80 dB HL as the cutoff for profound hearing loss/deaf; others use 90 dB HL. The actual cutoff points are of limited importance. The primary basis for the assessment protocol, prognosis, and treatment plan is the child's abilities, not a label of hard of hearing or deaf.

DEFINING THE TERM "HARD OF HEARING"

The capitalized term *Deaf* refers to individuals who belong to a cultural group that shares a signed language (Humphries, 1993).

You will discover that a variety of terms are used to describe the continuum of communication patterns demonstrated by individuals who have hearing losses. These include *hard of hearing, hearing impaired, Deaf, and deaf*. It is important that the terminology we use reflects the personal preferences of our clients and facilitates eligibility for and access to services (e.g., treatment, assistive technology) (Joint Committee of the American Speech-Language-Hearing Association and the Council on Education of the Deaf, 1998).

The term "hard of hearing" covers a large and heterogeneous population. Ross (1990) reports as estimate that 16/1000 school-aged children have average thresholds between 26 and 70 dB HL. He notes that, if we add children with milder but educationally significant hearing losses, the number of children considered to be hard of hearing would be nearer 30/1000.

Figure 17–2 provides a representation of conversational level speech plotted on an audiogram. The most intense speech sounds are the vowels. Consonant sounds are less intense than vowels. Some consonants, such as /s, f, t, tʃ, ʃ/, are characterized by energy focused in the high frequencies.

Individuals who are hard of hearing demonstrate a broad range of speech perception abilities. Figure 17–3 shows audiograms for two 18-month-old children whose hearing losses are newly identified. These children have had vastly different exposure to speech and other sounds in their environments and thus will present different pat-

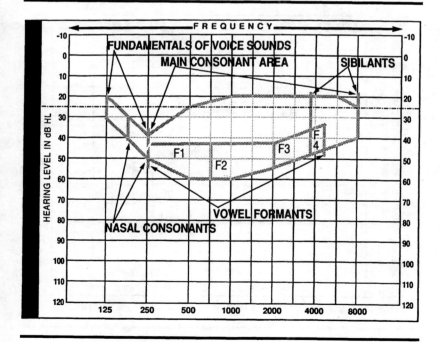

Figure 17–2. Acoustic spectrum of the speech signal plotted on an audiogram. (Reprinted with permission from *Assessment and Management of Nonmainstreamed Hearing-impaired Children*, by M. Ross, D. Brackett, and A. Maxon, 1991, Figure 8–2. Austin, TX: Pro-Ed.)

Child A

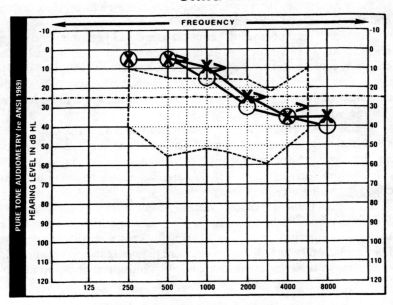

Child B

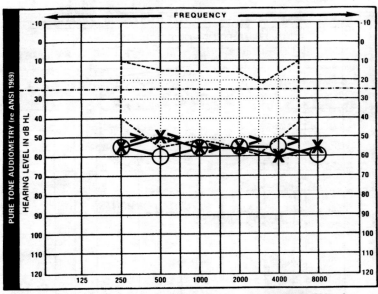

Design © by Bob Essman and the New York League for the Hard of Hearing

Figure 17–3. Pure-tone threshold data for example cases described as Child A and Child B. (Audiogram form used with permission of York Press, Inc., from "Audiological Evaluation of the Mainstreamed Hearing–impaired Child," by J. R. Modell, 1990, p. 41. In *Hearing-impaired children in the mainstream*, edited by Mark Ross, ©1990 by York Press, Inc.

terns of communication skill acquisition. Child A has a mild, high-frequency, sensorineural hearing loss. Her responses to environmental sounds and her level of communication skill acquisition may not differ enough from those of her normally hearing peers to raise the red flags that lead to referral for evaluation. However, she is missing valuable acoustic input, particularly when she is in a poor listening environment such as playing with her brother on the kitchen floor while the dishwasher is running. Child B has a bilateral, flat, moderate, sensorineural hearing loss. He hears only intense environmental sounds and receives little information from conversational speech. It is likely that his communication skills are significantly delayed relative to those of age peers with normal hearing. Both Child A and Child B are hard of hearing.

A different type of graph is used to show how hearing aids help a child to hear speech signals. Figure 17–4 provides an example using data from a third child, Child C. All data are plotted in dB SPL. Normal thresholds are represented by the dashed line at the bottom of the graph. The average speech spectrum is represented by the dotted line. Just above the speech spectrum are the child's unaided thresholds. As you can see, without any amplification, only a portion of the low-frequency range of the speech spectrum is sufficiently intense to

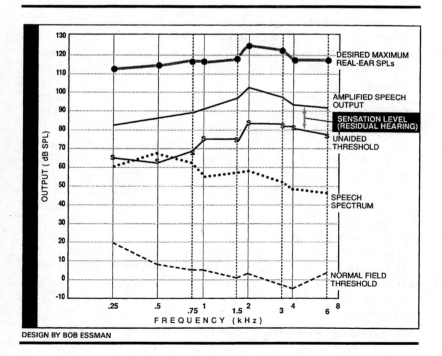

DESIGN BY BOB ESSMAN

Figure 17–4. Example of an SPL gram (SPL-O-GRAM). (Used with permission of Pro-Ed, from *Assessment and management of mainstreamed hearing–impaired children: Principles and practices,* by M. Ross, D. Brackett, and A. B. Maxon, 1991, p. 229. Austin TX: Pro-Ed)

be detected by the child. The solid line shows the average speech spectrum after it has been amplified by the child's hearing aid. With amplification, this child is able to hear sounds across the speech frequency range. Note that the two speech spectrum representations are plots of average data. The energy range extends approximately 12 dB above and 18 dB below these lines. The last bit of information plotted on this graph is the maximum output desired by the audiologist. The goal is to make speech audible without reaching levels that will make the child uncomfortable or put the child at risk for additional hearing loss due to overamplification of the sounds. It is important to remember that amplification of speech signals increases speech audibility, but does not give children normal or even near normal hearing. Data such as those in these figures indicate neither the distortion that may be present nor the difficulty that children will have in coping with background noise.

> Ask your audiology professor about the special techniques used to fit hearing aids on young children.

Distortion or absence of low intensity, high-frequency speech sounds has a marked effect on the information an individual can extract from conversation. The listener may be unable to discriminate among words that have similar phonemic structure, such as *mass*, *match*, and *mash*. It is difficult for young language learners to know whether they are hearing one word with multiple meanings or three separate words.

High-frequency speech sounds also carry significant amounts of information about the morphological markers used in English. Consider the problems that children will have if they don't hear the /t/ that represents "not" in contractions such as "can't," the /s/ that signals that "books" is plural, and the /s/ or /t/ that changes the verb "walk" to the third person singular "walks" or the past tense "walked."

The listening environment is another factor that has a strong impact on the speech perception abilities of individuals who have hearing losses. Background noise and long reverberation times (the time it takes the sound that echoes off of hard surfaces to decay) can cause problems for all listeners. Finitzo-Hieber and Tillman (1978) demonstrated that, as noise and reverberation time increases, the speech recognition abilities of children with hearing losses drop much more sharply than do those of children with normal hearing. When both background noise and reverberation time are high, the ability to recognize speech is severely limited.

> Noise is unwanted sound—it can be anything from a conversation in the hallway outside your door to band practice.

Hawkins (1988) concluded that, in order for a child who is hard of hearing to function adequately, a listening environment should have a reverberation time of 0.5 seconds or less and a signal-to-noise ratio of +15 or greater. That is, the signal level should be at least 15 dB above the noise level and echoes should decay rapidly. Data gathered from typical classroom settings indicate that few classrooms meet either standard.

> Poor signal-to-noise ratio also has a dramatic impact on perception of spoken English by children with normal hearing for whom English is a second language.

The term "hard of hearing" encompasses not only children who have sensorineural hearing losses but also those who have permanent conductive hearing losses, such as hearing loss associated with ossicular chain malformation, and some who have mixed hearing losses. In addition, there is mounting evidence that children who have normal hearing in only one ear (those with unilateral hearing losses) and children who have normal hearing only some of the time (those with fluctuating conductive hearing losses resulting from otitis media) are at a disadvantage in auditory learning situations such as the average classroom. They, too, may be described as hard of hearing.

Hearing loss does not always occur in isolation. Estimates are that as many as 30% of children with hearing losses have at least one other disability (Gallaudet University Center for Assessment and Demographic Studies, 1992). Additional disabilities may be problems such as cerebral palsy, craniofacial anomalies, and mental retardation that affect communication skill development in predictable ways. They may also include problems such as cardiac irregularities that result in prolonged hospitalization and/or may be life threatening. In such instances, we sometimes see an indirect effect on communication skill development. We may also see an effect on parents' perceptions of the importance of communication skill deficits.

ESTABLISHING THE CLINICAL QUESTIONS

In decades past, children who were hard of hearing were often first identified between the ages of 2 and 5 years. As newborn hearing screening gains acceptance, the numbers of children identified and fitted with amplification by the age of 6 months grows. As a result, the youngest of our clients come to us because of risk for, not demonstration of, delays in speech and language skill development.

As is true for the other groups of children that you are studying, it is common for parents to request an evaluation because of concerns that their children's communication skills are different from those of age peers. This is sometimes the reason that a child's hearing loss is first identified.

Other common reasons for assessment include determining the direction of treatment and monitoring progress. For the child who is hard of hearing, treatment may take many forms, including one-on-one sessions focusing on the development of speech articulation or language skills, group discussion of strategies used to cope with communication breakdown, and provision of assistive listening devices for the classroom. In many instances, the breadth of the questions posed will require that a team of teachers and clinicians gather data and consider solutions.

PLANNING THE DIAGNOSTIC PROTOCOL

Children who are hard of hearing often demonstrate communication skills like those of younger children who have normal hearing. Thus, we can use many of the same strategies for both groups. The primary

> Instruments that measure otoacoustic emissions and auditory brainstem responses can be used to screen for hearing loss in newborns.

purpose of this part of the chapter is to identify the ways that protocols must be modified to meet the special needs of children who are hard of hearing.

Team Approach

Although a medical model may be used during the diagnosis of hearing loss, it is more common to see behavioral/educational models and systems models used when clinicians are evaluating speech and language skill deficits that are related to hearing loss. Children who have hearing losses are often followed by a team of professionals with special skills in the areas of hearing loss and/or education. Members typically include speech-language pathologists, audiologists, teachers of the hearing impaired, otologists, psychologists, and classroom teachers. Other support personnel such as reading specialists may also be involved. Whether the team is large or small, it is important to remember that parents are partners in the collaborative effort to identify and meet the child's needs.

As the team begins to outline an assessment plan, you need to consider what types of information each member of the team can add. In some instances, a single evaluation session will be sufficient time for you to gather the data that you will provide. In others, several sessions or a period of diagnostic therapy may be a better alternative. Roush and Matkin (1994) provide an excellent introduction to a wide variety of multidisciplinary team models that are used for evaluating young children with hearing losses.

Environment

When selecting and arranging the room in which you will work, it is important to provide for good transmission of acoustic information. Noise levels must be low. Something as simple as the fan used to cool the room on a hot June day can have a tremendous impact on a child's ability to communicate.

Lighting must be appropriate for transmission of visual cues. The light should be on your face. Avoid sitting in front of a window. If the light source is behind you, your face will be in the shadow making it difficult for the child to speechread. Be sure that the chairs are positioned so that the child does not have to twist or turn to get a good view of your face.

Hearing Aids and Other Assistive Listening Devices

Many children who have hearing losses wear hearing aids. If they do, it is essential to check the hearing aids before beginning the evaluation. Do not assume that, because parents and teachers believe that the evaluation is important, they will ensure that the hearing aids are functioning properly. Equipment does not always cooperate. For example, Elfenbein, Bentler, Davis, and Niebuhr (1988) discovered that 10% of children who were aided monaurally and 52% of children who were aided binaurally each arrived for a daylong psychoeducational and communication skill evaluation with a malfunctioning hearing aid.

Options for dealing with hearing aid malfunction will vary depending on the setting in which you work. If you work with an audiologist, you may be able to obtain a loaner hearing aid of the same make and model that the child wears. If you are doing end-of-the-year assessment in a school system, you may be able to juggle your schedule and work with a child whose hearing aids are functioning properly. In some instances, you may decide to proceed under less than ideal conditions such as having a child who uses two hearing aids wear only one. Be sure to document such situations in your report.

Children often use personal FM amplification systems, sometimes called auditory trainers, in their classrooms. Such devices are used to combat the problems created by distance between the student and teacher, noise, and reverberation. When using these devices, the teacher wears a microphone and transmitter that sends her voice via radio waves to a receiver contained in the student's hearing aid or worn on the student's belt. If the receiver is worn on a belt, one of a variety of schemes can be used to route the signal to the child's ear. While it is important to know whether such equipment is used in the classroom, it is not necessary to use FM transmission during an evaluation that is conducted in the type of environment described earlier. An exception to this would be a child who uses an FM system rather than a hearing aid as primary amplification.

> Beware! If someone swallows a hearing aid battery, call for help from the 24-hour Battery Ingestion Hotline: 202-625-3333.

> Investigate other types of classroom amplification such as sound field amplification systems and large-area loop systems.

Communication Modality

Although most children who are described as hard of hearing use speech as their primary means of communication, there are other possibilities. A girl who has a moderate hearing loss and lives with parents who are Deaf may use American Sign Language (ASL) as her first language. A boy who has a moderate hearing loss and severe dysarthria may use speech for receptive communication and a language board or other assistive technology to express himself.

Cultural Factors

As noted elsewhere in this book, especially in Chapter 2, clinicians must be sensitive to cultural differences among the families with whom they work. Language differences are particularly important. A growing body of evidence indicates that children and adults for whom English is a second language often demonstrate greater speech perception difficulties in adverse listening conditions (e.g., poor signal-to-noise ratio) than do native speakers of English. Clinicians need to remember that such problems can compound the impact of the speech perception deficits associated with hearing loss.

Members of different cultural groups may have markedly different views about the causes of disabilities and the nature of appropriate treatment procedures. These must be understood before we can help the family make plans for diagnosis and treatment.

Children who are hard of hearing may have a strong link to the Deaf culture if their parents identify themselves as Deaf. Although the hearing culture and many of the parents with whom we work view hearing loss as a disability, some parents, especially those who are Deaf, do not.

Many clinicians are familiar with manually coded English (MCE) systems such as Signed English (Bornstein, Saulnier, & Hamilton, 1983) and Signing Exact English (Gustason, Pfetzing, & Zawolkow, 1980). When working with families who communicate using ASL, it is important to remember that ASL and English are different languages. Although it is possible to adapt MCE skills for some social interactions, an interpreter is needed for information exchange.

Test Administration Procedures

The child who is hard of hearing presents a unique combination of communication needs and experiences that will likely require some adaptation of test administration. First, the child needs time to scan the pictures or other materials before auditory stimuli are presented. You do not want the child's attention divided between your face and the tabletop. Second, the child who has a hearing loss may be more alert to visual cues than a child who has normal hearing. Be careful not to provide subtle cues such as glancing at the correct response after stimulus presentation. Third, children who are hard of hearing often misunderstand or are misunderstood. If you request repetition, the child may interpret this as a need to change his response. Be prepared to score the child's first response. Fourth, hearing loss can affect the child's perception of test stimuli. Unless you are measuring auditory perception, you will probably want to select instruments that permit repetition. You may also elect to modify standard administration procedures. If you choose the latter option, be sure to document the modification and weigh its impact as you interpret the data.

Assessment Battery

Much of the information covered in the previous chapters of this book is directly applicable to work with a child who is hard of hearing. You need to devise a combination of evaluation strategies that will provide data to answer the specific diagnostic questions that you identify for each child.

Parent Interview

Parents are not just history providers. Their questions and concerns will guide the diagnostic process. The basic framework for the interview will be the same as for your other clients.

A few special considerations are worthy of note. Questions such as those about previous/current treatment approaches that have been used, types of classroom placement, names of clinicians and teachers, and progress seen by the parents all provide important information. You may find that the school and the parents employ different approaches to communication. Perhaps a child is in a preschool program that focuses on audition without speechreading but uses audition plus speechreading at home. A child whose family has moved often may have been exposed to a wide range of approaches.

You will need to add questions that give you information about the hearing loss, such as etiology (if known), age at identification, any changes in the hearing loss, names of the physician and audiologist who are following the child, and the date and results of the last audiologic evaluation. Information is also needed about any amplification used. For example, you will want to know the age at which the child was first aided, the type of amplification used at home, the type of amplification used at school, and the name of the audiologist or hearing aid dealer who fit the device(s). These data will help you determine what sort of speech signal the child has received in the past and is currently receiving.

As you gather case history information, remember that hearing loss can be caused by genetic factors, environmental factors (e.g., infection, drugs), or a combination of both. Current estimates are that half of all congenital hearing loss is inherited (Jacobson, 1995). It is not your job to determine the etiology of the hearing loss; however, you may well be the one to suggest a referral to a geneticist. Ask whether other family members have hearing losses that were first identified in childhood. Consider cousins as well as the immediate family. As you evaluate the child, be alert for problems other than hearing loss. Approximately one third of genetic hearing loss is associated with syndromic abnormalities (Jacobson, 1995).

A syndrome is a pattern of anomalies with the same specific cause.

Child Interview

Children are often the best sources of information about their communication skills and deficits. Not only can they pinpoint specific problem areas, they can also identify those that they would most like to change. When we work with young children, it is possible to motivate change with praise or tangible reinforcement. As age increases, it becomes more and more important that children work to make changes because they value them.

Depending on your relationship with the child, you may choose to begin the assessment with a formal interview or elect to wait until

...ed rapport through play or other activities. One of the ...aches is simply to ask the child questions about whether ... problems being understood or understanding others, when ...se situations occur, how she feels in these situations, what she feels the causal factors are, and what she does when she encounters communication breakdown. Children who are hard of hearing are usually quite candid about the impact of communication skill deficits on classroom, family, and social interactions.

An example of a guidesheet for assessing students' understanding of classroom interactions is shown in Figure 17–5. Similar sorts of

---

A Guidesheet to Assess Student's Knowledge of Classroom Interaction

Instructions: You know all about our class by now, but a new student might need some help. Please answer the following questions. We will use your answers to help new students learn about our class.

1. Write down exactly what happens in this class on most days. Be sure to explain what happens first, second, next, and so on.

2. Write down the important rules in this class and explain WHY we have each rule.

3. Describe your teacher. Tell what your teacher is like so the new student will get to know this person.

4. Tell WHERE the teacher usually stands when he or she wants everyone to pay attention. Tell WHAT the teacher usually says or does first to get the students' attention.

5. Tell what makes the teacher mad so the new student will not get into trouble with the teacher.

6. Explain the homework system. This will be helpful to the new student:
   (a) How do you find out what the homework is?
   (b) How do you remember what books or papers to take home?
   (c) How do you remember to bring your homework back to school?

7. Tell what is hardest for you in this class. (It might be hard for the new student also.)

8. Tell what YOU do when you do not understand something in this class.

9. How is reading group different from whole class discussion? Tell as many differences as you can.

10. Can you think of anything else the new student should know about this class?

Figure 17–5. A guidesheet for assessing students' knowledge of classroom interaction. (Reprinted with permission from "Assessment Issues for Three Aspects of School Communication," by S. Tattershall, S. Kretschmer, and R. Kretschmer, 1988, Table 1. *Journal of the Academy of Rehabilitation Audiology, 21*(Suppl.). 173–197.)

questions can be asked about a child's interactions at the dinner table or a scout troop meeting.

Auditory Perception

Audiologists are often responsible for determining what information a child can obtain from a speech signal presented without visual cues. Speech-language pathologists may assist in test selection and/or administer some tests themselves.

When these tests are conducted in sound booths, the level of the test signal can be closely monitored and it is an easy matter to eliminate visual cues. However, when auditory perception is assessed via live voice in a treatment room, a different approach must be taken. If you ask the child to turn away from you, the microphone on his hearing aid will also move, thus creating a shadow effect that will reduce the intensity of your voice. The solution is to cover your face. This is best done with a speaker mesh screen of the type shown in Figure 17–6. Using a book or a piece of cardboard will likely reduce the high-frequency components of your speech and confound your data (Niday & Elfenbein, 1991).

When selecting instruments to assess auditory perception, it is important to keep other aspects of the child's communication skills in

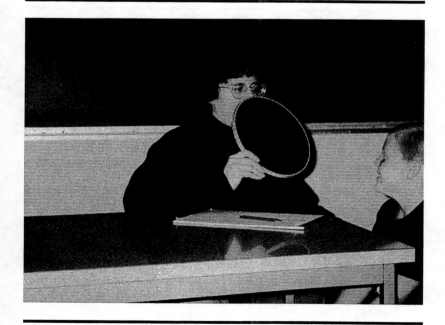

Figure 17–6. Assessment of auditory perception using a speaker-mesh screen to mask speechreading cues.

...bulary and syntax levels of test items are too difficult ...it will not be possible to determine whether errors reflect ...perceptual abilities or language skills or some combination ...two. The child's speech skills also need to be considered. Some auditory perceptual tasks require that the child repeat stimulus items. If the child is not able to say the test items, you will not know if they were heard correctly. For example, if a child often deletes /t/ in the word final position and the stimulus item is "meat," does the response "me" indicate that he didn't hear the final /t/?

An example of an instrument that can provide you with data about a wide range of auditory perceptual skills is the Test of Auditory Comprehension (TAC). Its ten subtests, outlined in Figure 17–7, provide tasks as basic as categorization of sounds as speech or nonspeech and tasks as complex as comprehending a story told in background noise. Because normative data are provided by age and degree of hearing loss, it is possible not only to determine a child's strengths and weaknesses but also to compare the child to age peers with the same degree of loss.

Oral Mechanism

It is easy for clinicians to see a child with a hearing loss as a set of ears and attribute all of the child's communication problems to the

Subtests of the Test of Auditory Comprehension	
Subtest	**Description**
One	Discriminates between linguistic and nonlinguistic sounds
Two	Discriminates between linguistic, human nonlinguistic, and environmental sounds
Three	Discriminates between stereotypic messages
Four	Discriminates between single-element core-noun vocabulary presented in a sentence
Five	Recalls two critical elements from a sentence
Six	Recalls four critical elements from a sentence
Seven	Sequences three events from a story
Eight	Recalls five details from a story
Nine	Sequences three events from a story presented with a competing message
Ten	Recalls five details from a story presented with a competing message

Figure 17–7. Subtests from the *Test of Auditory Comprehension* (Adapted from *The Test of Audiotyr Comprehension*, by J. Trammell et al., 1976. North Hollywood, CA: Foreworks, Inc.)

hearing loss. Be sure to consider all possibilities. The child could have mild craniofacial anomalies that have not yet been detected or could be in need of referral for dental care.

Speech Production

Children who are hard of hearing often demonstrate speech articulation skills that reflect the acoustic signal they receive. Table 17–1 shows data by manner of production for three groups of children ages 5–18 years who have different degrees of bilateral sensorineural hearing loss. Beyond the normal developmental patterns of speech sound acquisition, these children demonstrate the greatest problem with fricatives and affricates. This is consistent with the nature of the speech signals that they hear. Substitutions and oral distortions are the most common errors with the numbers of omissions increasing as hearing loss increases. Errors in the production of vowels are not expected.

Children who are hard of hearing may present with some hoarseness, pharyngeal resonance, and hyper- or hyponasality. They typically do not demonstrate the severe problems with phonation, resonance, speech rate, intelligibility, pitch control, and vocal quality demonstrated by children who are deaf.

Speech production is typically assessed with the same speech articulation tests used with children who have normal hearing. However, some sets of target words and elicitation phrases may contain vocabulary items or syntactic structures that are too difficult for some children. One common solution is to attempt to elicit the target through imitation. This may be effective in some instances, but there is also a possibility that children will have difficulty hearing the phonemes that you are asking them to imitate. An alternative is to substitute a word or elicitation phrase that is appropriate to the child's language skill level.

As is often the case with children who hear normally, a child's speech skills at the word level may be quite different from those in conversational speech. If the measure used includes only word or sentence level tasks, it is important to obtain a conversational sample for comparison.

Sit in on a class discussion or an indoor recess period to obtain a sample of typical communication patterns.

Language Skills

The language skills of children who are hard of hearing also reflect the deficits that exist in the acoustic input they receive (Davis, Elfenbein, Schum, & Bentler, 1986; Elfenbein, Hardin-Jones & Davis, 1994). For example, children with unilateral sensorineural hearing losses have skills that approximate those of their normally hearing peers. Children who have bilateral mild, moderate, or severe sensorineural hearing losses often demonstrate vocabulary skills that lag behind

Table 17–1. Articulation test performance (% correct) of three groups of children who are hard of hearing.[a]

Group[b]	Nasals		Stops		Glides		Affricates		Fricatives	
	Mean	SD	Mean	SD	Mean	SD	Mean	SD	Mean	SD
<45 dB HL	98.07	6.93	93.58	12.59	96.15	9.38	91.02	8.64	77.92	17.61
45–60 dB HL	96.87	7.21	96.52	7.28	89.84	14.59	73.95	27.86	73.09	20.83
61–88 dB HL	98.86	3.76	96.96	5.75	82.62	14.24	68.18	26.30	73.27	13.38

[a] Adapted from "Oral Communication Skills of Hard of Hearing Children," by J. Elfenbein, M. Hardin-Jones, and J. Davis, 1994. *Journal of Speech and Hearing Research, 37,* 216–225.

[b] Pure-tone-average for the better ear.

Professionals disagree about the effects of fluctuating conductive hearing loss on communication skill development. Watch for research reports on this topic.

those of their normally hearing peers. Idioms and words that have multiple meanings are particularly difficult. These children also have difficulty learning the use of morphological endings and complex syntax structures—tasks that require information coded in high-frequency and/or unstressed components of the English language. They do not, however, typically demonstrate the severe receptive and expressive language skill deficits often demonstrated by children who are deaf.

As with the assessment of speech skills, instruments used with children who have normal hearing are used with children who are hard of hearing. In most cases these are appropriate. However, you need to consider how the type of task can affect the child's performance. For example, imitation tasks combine perception and production. You may want to combine the two, or you may not. If you want to evaluate production without the influence of perception, select a different approach.

Be wary of instruments that average normative data from a sample of children who demonstrate a broad range of degrees of hearing loss and provide little or no information about the presence of additional disabilities. There is little to be gained by comparing a child's performance to data from such a heterogeneous group.

Language is the key to academic success.

To gain a clear understanding of the child's communication skills, you may need to use a variety of language sampling techniques. Chapter 10 provides direction on incorporating teachers and classroom settings into the process. Parents can provide information about both general developmental patterns and language skill development in particular. *The MacArthur Communicative Development Inventories* (Fenson et al., 1993), described in Chapter 14, and the *Minnesota Child Development Inventory* (Ireton & Thwing, 1974) are examples of tools useful in gathering this type of input.

As you develop your own collection of assessment tools, you may want to borrow from other disciplines. For example, the *KeyMath Re-*

vised (Connolly, 1997), an inventory of mathematical concepts and skills, is useful in evaluating a child's ability to apply language skills to an academic task. The same basic math concepts are evaluated both in simple computation problems and in word problems. A child who can perform a basic computation process, but cannot interpret a word problem well enough to set up the computation, is demonstrating the effect of language skill deficits. Data such as these can be helpful in explaining the impact of language skill deficits to educators, parents, and the children themselves.

Speechreading

For the child who is hard of hearing, speechreading is considered to be a supplement to audition, not a substitute. Traditional speechreading tests for children were not developed from this perspective. In light of this, clinicians who gather information about speechreading often design their own bisensory evaluations. For example, some compare message comprehension when both auditory and visual cues are available to message comprehension when only auditory cues are available. Others vary environmental factors such as background noise to simulate different real-world listening situations.

If you choose to design your own task, you will need to use the child's language skills as a guide for devising test messages. Language skills are a key factor in the top-down processing required to speechread. As you analyze your data, do not focus simply on the number of words the child can correctly identify. Determining whether the child can gather the gist of the message and what types of strategies she employs when she does not understand may provide a better idea of how speechreading affects the child's daily interaction. For example, does she ask for repetition, change position to improve angle for speechreading, or turn down background noise?

INTERPRETING FINDINGS

Analyzing Your Data

In most instances, you will be using instruments that provide normative data only for normally hearing children. This is certainly a relevant comparison group since children who are hard of hearing must function in classroom and social situations geared to the skill levels of their normally hearing peers. For example, a child whose vocabulary is 2 years behind that of his classmates is going to be at a marked disadvantage in a class discussion.

When you use instruments that provide normative data delineated by age and degree of hearing loss, take advantage of the opportunity to put the child's performance in perspective relative to peers with similar hearing losses. For example, the data may show that, although the child's skills are poorer than those of children with normal hearing, his skills are average relative to children with the same degree of hearing loss.

There may be situations in which you choose not to focus on comparison to normative data. When a child is known to be performing far behind his normally hearing peers, it may be more helpful both to you and the parents to analyze the child's performance in terms of developmental patterns seen in his skills rather than in terms of percentile rank relative to his age group. It is also helpful to compare a child's communication skills to his performance on academic achievement measures. Communication skill strengths and weaknesses sometimes explain patterns of strength and weakness in academic performance. For example, data that show differences in a child's auditory perception in quiet and in noise can help to explain differences between a child's ability to communicate one-on-one with the teacher at her desk and to participate in group discussions while seated next to a cage full of gerbils racing their exercise wheels.

> Children who have unilateral sensorineural hearing losses, particularly those with severe-to-profound losses, are at high risk for academic deficits.

Data From Other Team Members

Data from other specialists may be shared in many ways. If a matter of weeks elapses between evaluations, you may receive formal written reports. When a child is evaluated by several individuals on the same day, information may be exchanged informally as it is gathered, or at a formal staffing. Whatever the format of the discussion, speech-language pathologists need to be familiar with the terminology and procedures used by their colleagues.

> Take advantage of the resources around you. Ask other professionals about the work they do.

Remember that each team member holds pieces of the puzzle that you are trying to solve together. Otologists can provide information about the medical status of the auditory system and any medical treatment planned. Psychologists and teachers can provide information about cognitive abilities, learning patterns, academic achievement, and psychosocial skills. With the addition of data from the speech-language pathologist and the audiologist, the big picture will begin to form.

Parent Conference

The primary focus of the parent conference is to discuss how the information you gathered answers the questions that led to the evaluation. Our role is to sort through the data and develop a description of the problem. This must then be presented to the parents along with options for dealing with the problem. The goal is to provide them with the foundation they need to make informed decisions. Note that, although you should enter the conference ready to share your conclusions and recommendations, you must remember that a final plan of action cannot take shape until the views of each of the other professionals and the parents have been considered.

It is important to remember that diagnosis of hearing loss and associated communication problems can trigger a variety of emotions in family members. Anxiety is common. It is not enough to be able to identify the emotions. Clinicians need to develop strategies for helping clients deal with them. For example, if parents are anxious about their abilities to meet the challenges of raising a child who is hard of hearing, we can start by reassuring them that we are there to help and that we have suggestions for how to begin (Schum, 1986).

> Monograph No. 9 in the NSSLHA series is a good resource for information about counseling (Schum, 1986).

When counseling families about a child's progress in treatment, it is easy to slip into a pattern of reporting a series of percentile ranks and age-equivalents that indicate that the child who is hard of hearing is behind age peers. If the question was "Is continued treatment necessary?" such data may support the answer. However, if the gap between what is expected and what the child is doing persists, it will be more productive to focus on progress made, indicators of the next step to be taken, and the relationships that exist between communication skills, psychosocial development, and academic achievement. In either case, it is important to discuss both the child's strengths and limitations.

Child Conference

Whether the child participates in the discussion of assessment findings generally depends on age. School-aged children should receive direct feedback about the session. Although parents may discuss your findings with their child, the child also needs the opportunity to discuss the results directly with you.

One of the topics often discussed by parents and clinicians is the need to foster independence in children with hearing losses. A clinician-child conference helps the child take an active role in the treatment process. It also provides for information transfer through a neutral party. A child may view parents' concerns about her communication skills the same way she views their concerns about her bedroom cleaning habits.

In some instances you will find a need to meet with the parents and the child separately or meet with the parents first and then invite the child to join you. In others, the entire conference can be conducted with the family as a whole. The information that you gather during the evaluation process will help you determine the need for private meetings.

SUMMARY

Most children who are hard of hearing develop communication skills more like those of peers who have hearing within normal limits than those peers who are deaf. As a result, the approach taken to assess-

to assessment of communication skill development is much like that used with children who have normal hearing. This chapter provided general guidelines for making decisions about the types of skills to assess and ways to modify standard evaluation procedures to limit the impact of the hearing loss on the evaluation process. Clinicians will need to adapt these guidelines to the needs of the individual child. For each child, factors such as age of onset of the hearing loss, degree of the hearing loss, history of (re)habilitative services, the presence of additional disabilities, and family support will combine to affect the development of communication skills.

OTHER RESOURCES

Student clinicians interested in working with children who have hearing losses will find that information on this topic is available from a wide variety of sources. The additional readings section at the end of this chapter provides a list of selected books, journals, and organizations that will be useful as you explore rehabilitative audiology. Although many of the titles include only the word "deaf," you will find that they also have information to offer about the child who is hard of hearing.

A Comment About Adults Who Become Hard of Hearing

This book does not include a chapter about adults who acquire hearing losses. It is important to note, however, that most of the approximately 28 million Americans who have hearing losses acquired those hearing losses as adults (NIDCD, 1994). What this means to you is that clients who come to you with aphasia, motor speech disorders, voice disorders, or fluency problems may also be hard of hearing. Indeed, it is estimated that at least a third of adults over the age of 65 years have significant hearing losses.

As the authors of other chapters have noted, it is important to know how well your clients hear. If you do not know whether your clients can hear your test stimuli, how will you be able to interpret any errors made? Find out whether your clients have hearing losses. Determine whether they use amplification. If they do, be prepared to do a quick listening check to be sure that hearing aids are functioning properly before you do your evaluation. Someone who has had a stroke may no longer be able to take care of this task alone. Also remember that individuals with hearing losses demonstrate poorer ability to cope with background noise than do individuals who have hearing within normal limits. Fans, bedside equipment, or other noise sources may create problems for the client even when they do not cause you difficulty.

Finally, it is important to consider the responses that people have to acquired hearing loss. For example, a client who stutters and has acquired a hearing loss might find group communication difficult not only because of the demands placed on his expressive abilities, but also because he cannot follow rapid changes in topic and is embarrassed to ask people to repeat what they've just said. You will learn more about the impact of hearing loss and strategies for coping with hearing loss when you take your first course in rehabilitative audiology. The message here is to take a client-centered approach to diagnosis in which you examine the broad spectrum of factors that might be contributing to the communication problems with which your clients present.

REFERENCES

Bornstein, H., Saulnier, K., & Hamilton, L. (1983). *The comprehensive signed English dictionary*. Washington, DC: Gallaudet University Press.

Connolly, A. (1997). *KeyMath Revised: A Diagnostic Inventory of Essential Mathematics*. Circle Pines, MN: American Guidance Service.

Davis, J., Elfenbein, J., Schum, R., & Bentler, R. (1986). Effects of mild and moderate hearing impairments on language, educational, and psycho-social behavior of children. *Journal of Speech and Hearing Disorders, 51*, 53–62.

Elfenbein, J., Bentler, R., Davis, J., & Niebuhr, D. (1988). Status of school children's hearing aids relative to monitoring practices. *Ear and Hearing, 9*, 212–217.

Elfenbein, J., Hardin-Jones, M., and Davis, J. (1994). Oral communication skills of hard of hearing children. *Journal of Speech and Hearing Research, 37*, 216–225.

Fenson, L., Dale, P. S., Reznick, J. S., Thal, D., Bates, E., Hartung, J. P., Pethick, S., & Reilly, J. S. (1993). *MacArthur Communicative Development Inventories*. San Diego, CA: Singular Publishing Group.

Finitzo-Hieber, T., & Tillman, T. (1978). Room acoustics effects on monosyllabic word discrimination ability for normal and hearing-impaired children. *Journal of Speech and Hearing Research, 21*, 440–458.

Ireton, H., & Thwing, E. (1974). *Minnesota Child Development Inventory*. Minneapolis: Behavioral Science Systems.

Gallaudet University Center for Assessment and Demographic Studies. (1992). *1991–1992 Annual survey of hearing-impaired children and youth*. Washington, DC: Gallaudet University.

Gustason, G., Pfetzing, D., & Zawolkow, E. (1980). *Signing exact English*. Los Alamitos, CA: Modern Sign Press.

Hawkins, D. (1988). Options in classroom amplification. In F. Bess (Ed.), *Hearing impairment in children* (pp. 253–265). Parkton, MD: York Press.

Humphries, T. (1993). Deaf cultures and culture. In K. Christensen & G. Delgado (Eds.), *Multicultural issues in deafness*. White Plains, NY: Longman Publishing Group.

Jacobson, J. T. (1995). Nosology of deafness. *Journal of the American Academy of Audiology, 6*, 15–27.

Joint Committee of the American Speech-Language-Hearing Association and the Council on Education of the Deaf. (1998). Hearing loss: Terminology and classification position statement and technical report. *Asha, 40*(Suppl. 18), pp. 22–23.

Madell, J. R. (1990). Audiological evaluation of the mainstreamed hearing–impaired child. In M. Ross (Ed.), *Hearing-impaired children in the mainstream* (pp. 27–44). Parkton, MD: York Press.

Niday, K., & Elfenbein, J. (1991). The effects of visual barriers used during auditory training on sound transmission. *Journal of Speech and Hearing Research, 34*, 694–696.

Ross, M. (1990). Definitions and descriptions. In J. Davis (Ed.), *Our forgotten children: Hard of hearing pupils in the schools*. Washington, DC: Self Help for Hard of Hearing People, Inc.

Ross, M., Brackett, D., & Maxon, A. (1991). *Assessment and management of mainstreamed hearing-impaired children*. Austin, TX: Pro-Ed.

Roush, J., & Matkin, N. D. (1994). *Infants and toddlers with hearing loss: Family–centered assessment and intervention*. Baltimore, MD: York Press.

Schum, R. (1986). In E. Cooper (Ed.), *Counseling in speech and hearing practice (Clinical Series 9)*. (Available from National Student Speech-Language and Hearing Association: 10801 Rockville Pike, Rockville, MD.)

Tattershall, S., Kretschmer, L., & Kretschmer, R. (1988). Assessment issues for three aspects of school communication. In R. Kretschmer & L. Kretschmer (Eds.), Communication assessment of hearing impaired children from conversation to classroom. *Journal of the Academy of Rehabilitative Audiology, 21*(Suppl.), 173–197.

Trammell, J., Farrar, C., Francis, J., Owens, S., Shepard, D., Thies, T., Witlin, R., & Faist, L. (1976). *Test of auditory comprehension*. North Hollywood, CA: Foreworks.

RECOMMENDED READINGS

Books and Journal Articles

Carney, A. E., & Moeller, M. P. (1998). Treatment efficacy: Hearing loss in children. *Journal of Speech and Hearing Research, 41*, S61–S84.

Christensen, K. M., & Delgado, G. L. (1993). *Multicultural issues in deafness*. White Plains, NY: Longman Publishing Group.

Davis, J. (1990). *Our forgotten children: Hard-of-hearing pupils in the schools*. Washington, DC: Self Help for Hard of Hearing People, Inc.

DeConde Johnson, C., Benson, P. V., & Seaton, J. B. (1997). *Educational audiology handbook*. San Diego, CA: Singular Publishing Group.

Krestchmer, R. R., & Krestchmer, L. W. (1988). Communication assessment of hearing-impaired children: From conversation to classroom. *Academy of Rehabilitative Audiology, 21*(Suppl).

Ross, M., Brackett, D., & Maxon, A. B. (1991). *Assessment and management of mainstreamed hearing-impaired children: Principles and practices*. Austin TX: Pro-Ed.

Seewald, R. C., Moodie, S. K., Sinclair, S. T., & Cornelisse, L. E. (1996). Traditional and theoretical approaches to selecting amplification for infants and young children. In F. Bess, J. Gravel, & A. Tharpe (Eds.), *Amplification for children with auditory deficits*. Nashville, TN: Bill Wilkerson Center Press.

Tye-Murray, N. (1998). *Foundations of aural rehabilitation: Children, adults, and their family members*. San Diego, CA: Singular Publishing Group.

Journals

American Annals of the Deaf

American Journal of Audiology

Ear and Hearing

Journal of the American Academy of Audiology

Journal of the Academy of Rehabilitative Audiology

Journal of Communication Disorders

Journal of Educational Audiology

Journal of Speech and Hearing Disorders

Journal of Speech, Language, and Hearing Research

Language, Speech, and Hearing Services in the Schools

Seminars in Hearing

Seminars in Speech and Language

Topics in Language Disorders

Trends in Amplification

Volta Review

Organizations

Academy of Rehabilitative
Audiology
P.O. Box 26532
Minneapolis, MN 55426

Alexander Graham Bell
Association for the Deaf
3417 Volta Place, NW
Washington, D.C. 20007-2778
http://www.agbell.org

American
Speech-Language-Hearing
Association
10801 Rockville Pike
Rockville, MD 20852
http://www.asha.org

American Academy of
Audiology
8201 Greensboro Drive
Suite 300
McClean, VA 22102
http://www.audiology.com

Educational Audiology
Association
4319 Ehrlich Road
Tampa, FL 33624
*http://www.audiology.com/edaud/
eaafram.htm*

Marion Downs National Center
for Infant Hearing
University of Colorado at
Boulder
Department of Speech,
Language, and Hearing Science
Campus Box 409
Boulder, CO 80309-0409
http://www.colorado.edu/slhs/mdnc

National Information Center on
Deafness
Gallaudet University
800 Florida Avenue, NE
Washington, D.C. 20002-3695
http://www.gallaudet.edu/~nicd

National Institute on Deafness
and Other Communication
Disorders
Information Clearinghouse
1 Communication Avenue
Bethesda, MD 20892
http://www.nih.gov/nidcd

Self Help for Hard of Hearing
People, Inc.
7910 Woodmont Avenue
Suite 1200
Bethesda, MD 20814
http://www.shhh.org

18

The Child Who Has Severe or Profound Hearing Loss

Nancy Tye-Murray, Ph.D.

Severe and profound hearing loss has many far reaching consequences for children. Not only may they not hear themselves or others speak, but also their language and speech acquisition is likely to be delayed in comparison with their normally hearing aged-matched peers. The purpose of this chapter is to review their speech and language development and to consider the role of a speech and language professional in their intervention plans. We will also consider speech production, language, and auditory training curriculums designed for children who have severe or profound hearing loss. A parallel discussion about children who are hard of hearing is presented in Chapter 17 (Elfenbein).

Recently, many investigations have focused on deaf children who use cochlear implants as opposed to hearing aids. In the upcoming years, more and more of these children, who have severe and profound hearing loss, will use cochlear implants rather than hearing aids, and so a portion of this discussion will consider how this treat-

Over 1 million children in the United States have a hearing loss. Eighty-three out of every 1,000 children have what may be called an educationally significant hearing loss (U.S. Public Health Service, 1990).

ment method may change the prognosis of speech and language development in these children.

Before we begin, a few terms must be defined. A child who has a *severe* hearing impairment cannot hear sounds presented at a level softer than 70 dB HL. A child with a *profound* hearing impairment cannot hear sounds presented at a level softer than 90 dB HL. Persons who are *prelingually* hearing-impaired had their hearing impairment when they were learning language and speech. They may have been born hearing impaired (in which case they have a *congenital* hearing impairment) or they may have lost their hearing early in life, perhaps as a result of meningitis, high fever, or head trauma. These persons often require assistance from a speech-language pathologist. Persons who have *postlingual* hearing loss had normal or nearly normal hearing when they were learning language and speech. They then lost their hearing in late childhood or in adulthood. Typically, these people speak intelligibly and have normal language patterns, especially if they incurred their hearing loss as adults. Most persons with postlingual hearing loss will not seek your services. In this chapter, we will be concerned with only prelingual hearing losses.

HEARING AND SPEECH RECOGNITION SKILLS

By understanding what a child with severe or profound hearing impairment can recognize of the speech signal, you can better select appropriate therapy objectives and teaching methods. For example, if you know that a child cannot hear you or herself speak, you will probably rely more on visual and tactile aids to teach articulation and less on auditory modeling.

As Figure 18–1 illustrates, many different audiometric configurations fall under the rubric of severe and profound hearing impairment. For instance, Child A has a severe hearing loss. He has some hearing across a wide range of frequencies (250 Hz to 8000 Hz). With appropriate amplification, he may recognize some speech auditorialy and may be able to speechread (i.e., recognize speech when using hearing and vision simultaneously) very well. He may also hear many of his own speech sounds while he talks, such as the vowel segments (which tend to be louder than consonants) and consonants that have high amplitude, such as the nasals /m/ and /n/. He will likely hear the rhythm and prosody of his own speech.

Children who have severe and profound hearing impairments are a heterogeneous group: they vary widely in their receptive and expressive communication skills.

Child B has a profound hearing impairment. Like many people with profound impairments, she is not completely deaf. She has some measurable hearing in the low frequencies (250 and 500 Hz). This child will probably not recognize any speech auditorily. She may or may not be a good speechreader. Her speechreading skill will depend on a number of factors. For example, visual speech recognition is determined in part by innate talent, and she may be either a naturally good or a naturally poor speechreader. Using her residual hearing,

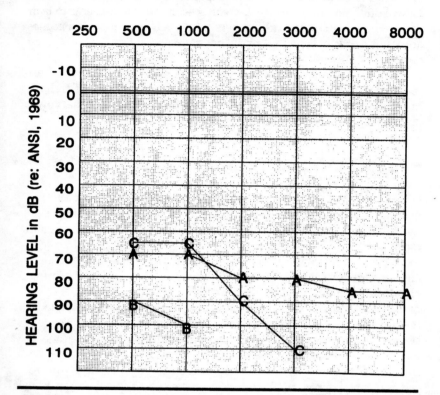

Figure 18–1. Audiometric configurations for three different types of hearing impairments. Letters indicate the level at which a threshold was obtained. Person A has a severe hearing impairment, Person B has a profound impairment, and Person C has a severe-to-profound impairment.

she might listen to prosodic cues and recognize when one word ends and the next word begins (when speechreading, a little bit of residual hearing can provide a great deal of benefit). Finally, if she has ample vocabulary and knowledge of grammar, she will be able to "fill in" words that she cannot speechread. For instance, if she speechreads the sentence, "The salt and _____ are on the table," she might be able to guess the word, "pepper." Child B will hear little if any of her own speech; she may only hear some rhythmic cues.

Many children have a combined severe and profound hearing impairment. Their hearing is typically better in the low frequencies than in the high frequencies. For example, Child C in Figure 18–1 has a "sloping" hearing impairment. He hears some words auditorily. His listening skills will appear to be more inconsistent than either Child A or B. Since he has some hearing in the low frequencies, he will often detect the presence of speech and recognize some words. However, because much of the acoustic information that distinguishes one word from another is contained in the mid and high frequencies, he will often not discriminate the words even though he seems to hear them. Thus, his family and teachers (and even you) may sometimes accuse him of "not listening" or of "not paying attention." Child C may have reasonably good speechreading skills. He will probably hear the rhythm and prosody of his voice while he speaks. He will not hear many of his own consonant productions, particularly sounds that have high frequency information, such as /s/ or /t/. He may hear his vowel productions, but his vowels may all sound similar to him.

SPEECH CHARACTERISTICS

When describing the speech of children with severe and profound hearing impairment, we usually talk about overall intelligibility, segmental errors (errors in the sounds of speech), and suprasegmental errors (errors in speech rhythm and prosody). Generally, children with more residual hearing will speak better and produce fewer segmental and suprasegmental errors than children with less residual hearing. However, you will find that how well a child speaks also depends on numerous other factors. These factors include the following: the speech therapy the child has received, his or her motivation to speak, the consistency with which he uses appropriate amplification, the age at which the child first received hearing aids, and his or her speech environment. For example, a child who hears speech often and who receives positive reinforcement when he or she tries to speak is more likely to acquire intelligible speech than one who does not.

Overall Intelligibility

Most children who have significant hearing loss are difficult to understand. For example, when conversing with children or adults who have congenital and profound hearing losses, you will rarely identify more than 20% of the words they say.

Segmental Errors

Children who have significant hearing loss produce many segmental errors, both when speaking vowels and diphthongs and when speaking consonants.

Vowels

These children most commonly neutralize vowels, so that the phrase *see you* might sound like "sa ya." They also substitute one vowel for another. Other vowel errors include diphthongization (the word *pot* may sound like "poat"), prolongation, and nasalization. Diphthongs may sound distorted or sound like a single vowel.

Consonants

Characteristic consonantal errors include voiced/voiceless confusions, substitutions, omissions, distortions, and errors in consonant clusters. For example, a deaf child might intend to speak the word *goat*, but actually say "koe." In this production, the child has substituted the voiceless /k/ for the voiced /g/, and omitted the final /t/ sound. Many of these children produce consonants that are visible on the face more accurately than consonants that are not visible. For instance, a child will likely produce the word *pat* correctly more often than the word *cat*. The /p/ entails visible lip closure whereas the tongue dorsum closing gesture for /k/ cannot be seen. Apparently, a child with significant hearing impairment relies heavily on visual information for acquiring speech.

Suprasegmental Errors

Suprasegmental errors are commonplace in the speech of children who have severe and profound hearing loss. It is not unusual for their speech to sound breathy, labored, staccato, and/or arhythmic.

Stress

Many of these children place equal stress on all syllables, or stress words inappropriately. For instance, a child may speak the word *paper* as "paPEH."

Speaking Rate

Many children who have significant hearing loss speak very slowly, pausing often. For instance, one scientist found that a group of children with profound hearing loss spoke only 70 words per minute, on average, as compared to 164 words per minute spoken by children who had normal hearing (Voelker, 1938).

Coarticulation

Often these children do not coarticulate sounds in the same way as normally hearing talkers. For instance, a child might say the word *basket* as "ba-a-sa ka-a-ta." In this production, the child has articulated each sound as if it were an isolated unit.

Voice Quality

Sometimes these children have unpleasant voice quality. Their pitch may sound excessively high or variable, or may sound monotone.

Pitch breaks, where pitch abruptly changes from high to low, are common. They may speak too softly or too loudly, and often their intensity will fluctuate inappropriately.

In light of these many segmented and suprasegmental errors, it is not surprising that so many children have extremely poor intelligibility. When these speech problems coexist with language problems, communication becomes difficult if not impossible.

COMMUNICATION MODES AND LANGUAGE SKILLS

Before we consider problems of language, let us consider the four communication modes. The majority of persons who have profound hearing loss use one of four modes to communicate: American Sign Language (ASL), manually coded English, spoken language, or cued speech.

American Sign Language (ASL)

ASL is a manual system of communication. Those who use ASL do not speak while signing because ASL has a different grammar than spoken English. One ASL sign might represent a concept that would require many English words to express.

Currently there is a strong "Deaf Culture" movement. Persons who are a part of this movement advocate that children who have significant hearing impairments use ASL as their primary language, and learn English as a second language.

Facial expressions and body language can impart a variety of meanings to the signs. For example, the word *look* "can be changed to mean *gaze, stare,* and *watch* by making the sign for *look* while moving the hand in a circle, holding it still, or moving it back and forth" (Brownlee, 1989, p. 86). Most deaf adults in the United States utilize primarily ASL.

Manually Coded English

Manually coded English is comprised of manual signs that correspond to the words of English. Words are put together using the same syntactic structures as English. Typically, the person who uses manually coded English speaks simultaneously while signing. For instance, as the deaf child says, "The book is in the car," she signs the article *The,* and then one sign each for *book, is, in, the,* and *car.* The combined use of sign and speech as an educational philosophy is referred to as *total communication* or *simultaneous communication.* The child (or adult) uses every available means to receive a message, including sign, residual hearing, and lipreading.

At present, most children who have a severe or profound hearing loss communicate with simultaneous communication. However, this trend may change in the future. The increased use of cochlear implants may mean that more children use aural/oral communication. On the other hand, a resurgence of deaf pride and interest in Deaf Culture may lead to the choice of ASL.

Aural/Oral Language

Aural/oral language is the same language used by persons who have normal hearing. Children who use aural/oral language speak their messages and use speechreading to receive messages.

Cued Speech

A small number of children (and adults) use cued speech, a communication system that uses phonetically based hand gestures to supplement speechreading. When a communication partner talks to a child, she speaks and simultaneously cues the message. By themselves, the hand signals are meaningless. When coupled with the audiovisual speech signal, speech recognition is enhanced.

In Cued Speech, handshapes are used to distinguish vowels. For example, the consonants /p/ and /b/ appear alike on the mouth. The cue for /p/ is a 1 handshape and the cue for /b/ is a 4 handshape. Thus, if a talker speaks the word *bee*, the individual holds a 4 handshape to the corner of the mouth, because a 4 handshape indicates the phoneme /b/. Placement by the mouth corner corresponds to the /ɪ/ vowel. The word *boo* would be cued by a 4 handshape held to the throat, because a hand placement at the throat corresponds to a /u/ vowel.

Regardless of which communication mode they use most frequently, most children who have severe and profound hearing loss do not learn the English language very well. One way to appreciate how hearing impairment affects language development is to compare normally hearing groups and hearing-impaired groups. Beginning speech-language pathologists often become disheartened when they learn that 8-year-old hearing children have a better knowledge of grammar than do profoundly hearing-impaired adults. Most never acquire a vocabulary that is better than that of a normally hearing fourth grader.

Speech-language pathologists often categorize language difficulties according to whether they are problems of form (syntax and morphology), content (semantics and vocabulary), or pragmatics (use).

Form

The list comprising problems of form is extensive. Children who have significant hearing loss may demonstrate any of the following behaviors:

- overuse nouns and verbs
- rarely use adverbs, prepositions, or pronouns
- omit function words
- produce a preponderance of simple subject-verb-object structure
- speak sentences that have few words when compared to those produced by normally hearing children

Much debate and controversy revolves around the issue of communication mode. Some speech and hearing professionals take firm stands in favor or selecting one mode versus another. Other professionals believe that there is no one right way to go; the best route may be different for different children, depending on such factors as their degree of residual hearing, intelligence, family support, and educational opportunities.

■ rarely create compound or complex sentences
■ omit morphemes that mark plurality or past tense

In telling a story about her cat, one child said, "Socks jump. Cup fall over. Big mess. Mom mad about Socks." In this narrative, the child omitted function words such as *was*, and tense markers such as *–ed*. Her syntactic structures were very simple. Although the listener could probably follow her story, the sentences sounded telegraphic.

Not only do they rarely speak compound or complex sentences, children who have significant hearing loss usually cannot interpret them when they speechread or read. For example, they often interpret sentences in the passive voice (*The cat was chased by the dog*) as though they were in the active tense (*The cat chased the dog*). They might interpret a nominal sentence (*The ending of the school year saddened the teacher*) objectively (*The school year saddened the teacher*).

> Sometimes children order their words incorrectly. A child may say, "Saw cat big," meaning that she saw a big cat.

Content

A common language problem among children who have severe or profound hearing loss is a restricted vocabulary. Children often learn only common everyday words. They may have gaps in their vocabulary, wherein they may not know words relating to an entire concept, such as outer space. Hence, words such as *planet, Martian, star, spaceman,* and *rocket* may all be unfamiliar. They often use words in limited ways. For instance, a deaf child may use a word such as happy as a predicate (e.g., *The boy is happy*) but not as a modifier (e.g., *The happy boy is here*). Most such children cannot identify synonyms and antonyms, or understand idioms such as *She was mad as a hornet.*

Pragmatics

> Literacy is an issue closely related to language development and is typically indexed by a child's performance on reading and writing measures. Most children who have significant hearing loss are greatly delayed in reading and writing skills. For instance, the average reading and writing level of deaf high school students is at a third or fourth grade level, which is not surprising in light of their restricted language skills.

Many children who have significant hearing loss experience difficulty in using language appropriately in everyday conversation. For example, some may not know how to initiate or maintain a conversation, nor know how to repair breakdowns in communication (under such circumstances, the child might nod and bluff, and pretend to understand something). Some children may also not know how to take turns while conversing, how to acknowledge that a message was recognized, and how to change the topic of conversation. In sum, many children may not use language functionally as well as their normally hearing peers.

There are at least three reasons why some children do not learn conversational pragmatics very well. First, they do not receive extensive practice in using language. This is because their unfamiliarity with many language structures and their reduced vocabulary limit their ability to converse. Moreover, if they use a communication mode that incorporates sign, they have fewer conversational partners to interact with because few normally hearing persons know simultaneous communication or ASL.

The second reason is that children with significant hearing loss cannot overhear their parents or other people talking. Thus, they do not receive the everyday, incidental models of how to use language.

Finally, hearing-impaired children do not receive the same formal instruction as normally hearing children. For instance, a mother may carefully explain the rules of politeness to her normally hearing child (do not interrupt; say "thank you"; let someone else say something). She may not explain the rules to her child who has hearing loss, either because of the child's limited language or because of her own limited skill in using simultaneous communication or ASL.

CHILDREN WHO USE COCHLEAR IMPLANTS

Now let us consider children who have severe and profound hearing losses but who use cochlear implants rather than hearing aids. This relatively new group of children performs more similarly to children who have better hearing than to children who have profound and sometimes even severe hearing loss, but who have not been treated by cochlear implant.

The Food and Drug Administration approved implantation of children with multichannel cochlear implants in 1990. At that time, children had to be at least 2 years of age and have no usable hearing. Currently, children as young as 18 months may receive these devices, and they may even have a modicum of residual hearing.

Children who use cochlear implants tend to speak more intelligibly than children who use hearing aids, on average, and there seems to be a wider variability in performance, with some children speaking with 100% intelligibility and others speaking with less than 20% of their words recognizable.

Both vowel and consonant production seems to be better as a result of cochlear implant use. For instance, one study suggests that after 5 or 6 years of cochlear implant use, children may, on average, produce vowels with about 80% accuracy and consonants with an accuracy level of about 70% (Tye-Murray, Tomblin, & Spencer, 1997). Similar scores for young hearing-aid users are 44% for vowels and 28% for consonants (Markides, 1970). Perhaps one of the more interesting outcomes related to consonant production is that many children learn to produce such fricative sounds as /s/ and /z/. Rarely do children with similar hearing losses who use hearing aids produce such sounds accurately and consistently.

Cochlear-implant use also affects suprasegmental speech production. For example, voice quality may be more normal, and speech patterns more melodic.

Cochlear implants appear to affect not only speech acquisition, but language development as well. Initial research suggests that children who receive cochlear implants demonstrate vocabularies with greater

Preliminary research suggests that children who use cochlear implants show greater improvements in their literacy skills than children who use hearing aids. This is probably due, at least in part, to their superior language skills.

number of words and acquire more complex grammatical structures (Tomblin, Spencer, Flock, Tyler, & Gantz, in press).

THE ROLE OF THE SPEECH-LANGUAGE PATHOLOGIST

Now that we have considered the speech and language characteristics of children who have significant hearing loss, let us turn our attention to the responsibilities of the speech-language pathologist: speech and language evaluation, speech-language therapy, auditory training, and consultation.

Evaluation

The evaluation protocol for these children is the same as for all children who are eligible for speech and language therapy: to determine treatment and treatment success. There are sometimes special objectives, such as using the test results to help the team decide whether the child should be placed in a mainstream classroom with a sign interpreter, or a self–contained classroom with other hearing-impaired children, or whether therapy outside the educational setting is needed.

There are five general principles to keep in mind when assessing speech and language skills of children with severe or profound hearing impairment. First, as with children with other disorders, we must remember that these children often use speech and language differently in one setting than another, and they perform differently on varying tasks. For instance, they are more likely to produce a sound correctly when they are imitating the speech-language pathologist than when they are telling a story to their classmates. For this reason, it is desirable to construct a profile of the child's speech and language proficiency from numerous measures that are both formal and informal, for example, an imitated speech sample consisting of isolated words and sentences, a citation speech sample ("Tell me the name of this picture"), and a spontaneous sample of continuous speech. We also need to observe the child informally in therapy, in the classroom, and on the playground. By using a variety of speech tasks, you can determine how robust certain skills are and whether or not they have generalized to real-world settings. This information will help you to plan therapy objectives and evaluate progress.

The second principle to remember is that the speech-language evaluation should be performed with the child's preferred mode of communication (ASL, simultaneous communication, cued speech, etc.). If you do not know the child's sign system, get an interpreter. Children must understand the tasks and the test items if an accurate reflection of their speech and language skills is to be obtained.

Third, again, as with children with other disorders, we must establish satisfactory rapport with children before beginning the evalua-

Historically, children with severe and profound hearing loss ten attended residential schools. Since the 1970s, more of these children remain in their home communities for their education.

tion. Many of these children are shy about using their voice, especially around strangers. If the child does not feel comfortable in your presence, she may not provide speech or language samples that represent her skills.

Fourth, select specific test procedures that are appropriate for the child's age and language. For example, if an articulation test has picture cards, the child must have the vocabulary necessary to name the pictures.

Finally, try to use tests that have been developed for children who are severely hearing impaired (see Figure 18–2). The findings from other tests will be difficult to interpret.

Evaluation of Speech Production

Standard evaluation procedures can be used for these children, with some adaptation to special needs.

Measures of speech intelligibility

Two methods have conventionally been used for obtaining a speech sample for intelligibility assessment. The first method is to obtain a measure from a connected language sample. A clinician can audio or video record a spontaneous conversation with the child and/or can engage the child in a story retelling activity in which the child retells a story that you have just told. The second method is to obtain a citation sample. The child can read a list of sentences or a paragraph.

The intelligibility of a sample can be evaluated in two different ways as well. First, the recordings can be played to a group of listeners. They can assign each sample a value from a rating scale. (See also Chapter 7.) For example, a "1" from a 5-point scale might correspond to "I understood none of the child's message" while a "5" might correspond to "I understood all of the child's message." The listeners might also estimate how much of the speech they understood, such as 10% of the words, 20%, and so forth. The second way to evaluate a speech sample is to transcribe the spoken message (and the signed message when the sample is spontaneous speech) and reference the spoken transcription to the printed text or signed transcription. You then can determine what percentage of the words or sounds were spoken correctly.

Measures of speech intelligibility vary as a function of several different variables. For instance, children will be more intelligible when they read a paragraph than a list of unrelated sentences. Listeners will understand more of a speech sample if they have heard the speech of other children who have significant hearing loss before, instead of never having heard it. Listeners will also recognize less speech if they can only hear as opposed to hear and see the talker speak. When recording intelligibility scores, it is wise to comment on these variables, especially if a child's progress is to be monitored over time.

FORM
Rhode Island Test of Language Structure (RITLS)* (Engen & Engen, 1983)
Grammatical Analysis of Elicited Language (GAEL)* (Moog & Geers, 1975)
Grammatical Analysis of Elicited Language (Presentence Level) (GAEL-p)* (Moog, Kozak, & Geers, 1983)
Test of Syntactic Ability (TSA)* (Quigley, Monranelli, & Wilbur, 1976)
Written Language Syntax Test (WLST)* (Berry, 1981)
Berko Morphology Test (Berko, 1958)
Test for Auditory Comprehension of Language (TACL) (Carrow, 1973)
Developmental Sentence Analysis (DSS) (Lee, 1974)

CONTENT
Semantic Content Analysis* (Kretschmer & Kretschmer, 1978)
Peabody Picture Vocabulary Test—revised form (Dunn & Dunn, 1981)
Reynell Developmental Language Scales (Reynell, 1977)

FUNCTION
Pragmatic Content Analysis* (Kretschmer & Kretschmer, 1978)
Performative Content Analysis (Hasenstab & Tobey, 1991, see their Table 1)

Figure 18- Examples of language that assess form, content, and pragmatics. Assessment designed specifically for hearing-impaired children and teenagers are denoted with an asterisk (*).

Otherwise, the child's intelligibility score might improve as a result of a change in an extraneous variable. This may be misinterpreted as a change denoting an improvement in the child's speaking proficiency.

Segmental Speech Testing

Segmental speech testing determines which sounds the child can articulate and which sounds he cannot. Variables to consider when selecting test procedures include the context and the methods for eliciting sound productions. Segmental speech production may be evaluated by using a choice of contexts, including nonsense syllables, isolated words, sentences, and spontaneous speech. Methodologically, the child might imitate a clinician or might produce the sounds by naming picture cards or reading printed words aloud, or by speaking spontaneously. Conventional articulation tests may be used to assess segmental speech skills, such as the *Goldman-Fristoe Test of Articulation* (Goldman & Fristoe, 1969) and the *Test of Minimal Articulation Competence* (T–MAC; Secord, 1981).

Suprasegmental Speech Testing

Suprasegmental speech skills can be evaluated by rating the child's spontaneous speech such as the method described by Subtelny, Orlando, and Whitehead (1981) or by asking the child to perform specific speech tasks. For instance, a clinician might determine whether or not the child can sustain the vowel /a/ for 5 seconds (to assess breath management) or whether he can speak two-syllable phrases with correct stress and pitch variation (to assess his ability to imitate stress patterns) (Levitt, 1987).

Language Assessment

Figure 18–2 presents examples of language tests that are sometimes used with children with hearing loss. They are organized according to whether they primarily assess form, content, or pragmatics.

Assessment procedures can generally be classified as checklists (example: Moog & Geers, 1975), tests (example: Quigley, Monranelli, & Wilbur, 1976), or language sample analyses (example: Kretschmer & Kretschmer, 1978). In compiling a checklist, the clinician checks whether or not a particular behavior is present. For example, we might check *yes* or *no* for the statement, *The child recognizes the meaning of subject-verb-object sentences.* Tests contain items that formally assess the child's ability to use language structures. If negation is assessed, the child might be asked to change the sentence, *He will go* to *He will not go.* Language sample analyses are usually performed on samples of both the child's receptive and expressive language. The analysis might yield a description of semantic classes that the child uses and recognizes, the child's complex sentence productions, and the child's communication competence.

> Allow plenty of time for language testing. You may need to extend testing over several days. It can be exhausting for both you and the child.

SPEECH-LANGUAGE THERAPY

A second role of a speech-language pathologist in assisting children with severe and profound hearing loss is to provide speech and language therapy. Although this chapter and this text focus on diagnosis, information about treatment is useful as it serves to direct our attention in diagnostic procedures. Here, we briefly review goals and types of curricula that might be considered in therapy.

Speech Production

Goals for a comprehensive speech-language program may include any of the following, depending upon the deaf child's age and stage of development (Carney & Moeller, 1998, p. S62):

- Increase vocalizations that have appropriate timing characteristics and that require numerous vocal tract movements
- Expand phonetic and phonemic repertoires
- Establish a link between audition and speech production
- Increase speech intelligibility

Results from the speech evaluation will guide selection of therapy goals. For example, a clinician might analyze phonetic transcriptions of a child's elicited and spontaneous error patterns and compile an inventory of sounds that the child can produce. A catalogue of the child's deletions, substitutions, and distortions might be made. Therapy goals may then focus on increasing a child's phonetic repertoire and on reducing phonological process errors.

There are many speech therapy curricula designed for children who have significant hearing loss. One way the curricula differ is according to the way speech is presented to the child and how feedback is provided. For example, in an *auditory approach,* instruction and correction about a child's speech are provided primarily via the auditory modality. In a more *visual approach,* we supplement the auditory signal with visual cues, and may even use mirrors, cued speech, or graphic symbols that are paired with specific speech gestures.

Language

We choose goals for language therapy, again, based on the child's age and level of development (Carney & Moeller, 1998):

- Increase communication between parent and child
- Promote an understanding of complex concepts and discourse units
- Enhance vocabulary growth
- Increase world knowledge
- Enhance self-expressions
- Enhance growth in use of language syntax and pragmatics
- Develop narrative skills

The evaluation results will help to indicate whether and how we focus on the development of content, form, and pragmatics. For instance, if a child is very young, with a minimal vocabulary, we likely will provide as much stimulation as possible for the development of nouns, pronouns, and verbs. On the other hand, if the child is in elementary school and has a robust vocabulary, we might devote more time to the development of syntax and semantics.

A number of different curricula have been developed for promoting language growth. One way to differentiate between curricula is by whether they are more structured or more naturalistic. *Structured curricula* may utilize word cards, drills, and instruction while *naturalistic curricula* tend to incorporate language learning into more relevant, everyday experiences. Most modern curricula incorporate more naturalistic elements.

AUDITORY TRAINING

A third role for the speech-language pathologist concerns training in speech perception. Children with significant hearing loss usually receive formal auditory training from their speech-language patholo-gist, although the child's classroom teacher or audiologist occasional-ly provides this training also. *Auditory training* develops the child's ability to recognize speech using only audition. In this section, we will consider two parameters of auditory training: skill level and task type. Appendix 18A presents a list of commercially available audito-ry training curricula.

Skill Level

Most auditory training curricula identify auditory training objectives for the child with significant hearing loss according to four hierarchial skill levels (Erber, 1982; Stout & Windle, 1986; Tramwell & Owens, 1977): awareness, discrimination, identification, and comprehension.

Sound Awareness

A child who demonstrates a skill level of awareness is able to detect the presence or absence of sound. For a child who has not attained this level, an auditory training objective may be to have the child indicate by a hand gesture every time he or she hears his or her name spoken.

Discrimination

A child with skills characteristic of the second level, *discrimination,* can make gross discriminations between two items. An auditory train-

Auditory-verbal educational programs strongly emphasize auditory training in their curricula. In auditory-verbal programs, children are taught to rely on their residual hearing; sign language is usually not permitted.

ing objective at this level may be to ask the child to distinguish between a loud versus a soft sound, or a one-syllable word versus a two-syllable word.

Identification

A child who is performing at the *identification level* can label a word or phrase after hearing it. A child who has just entered this level may perform an auditory training activity in which he or she must listen to a word, and then choose an appropriate response from a closed set of choices (Figure 18–3).

Comprehension

In the final level, *comprehension*, a child demonstrates speech comprehension. During an auditory training session, a youngster at this level might listen to a one-paragraph story, and then answer questions about it.

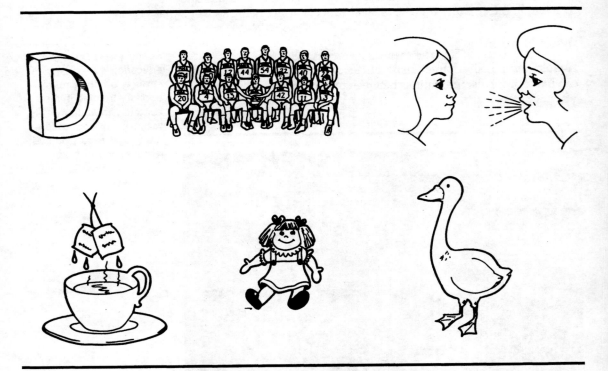

Figure 18–3. Example of a response set that can be used during an auditory training activity at the identification level. The target sounds in this exercise are /t/ and /d/. The speech-language pathologist might say "Show me the team." or "Show me the D." The child then must point to the corresponding picture. (Reprinted with permission from *Communication Training for Hearing-impaired Children and Teenagers: Speechreading, Listening, and Repair Strategies*, by N. Tye-Murray, 1992, p. 48. Austin, TX: Pro-Ed.)

For all four levels, auditory training objectives typically are selected that advance the child from his current skill level (e.g., he currently can identify monosyllabic words when the choices are limited to four) toward the next level (practice identifying words when his choices are limited to six).

Task Type

Two types of training tasks are usually included in an auditory training program, although there is not clear demarcation between the two types. One type is called *analytic training*, in which the child's attention is focused on identifying individual speech sounds. Another is *synthetic training*, in which the child's attention is focused on understanding the gist of a spoken message, and not necessarily every word.

In analytic training, nonsense syllables (such as *pa, ba, ma*) and rhyming words may be presented during analytic listening practice. Figure 18–4 presents an example of an activity that provides practice in syllable recognition. For this activity, the clinician says one of the

Formal auditory training objectives should be pursued informally throughout the day. When the opportunity arises during conversation or class time, a child can be presented with listening tasks that reinforce the auditory training objectives that are being pursued during formal instruction.

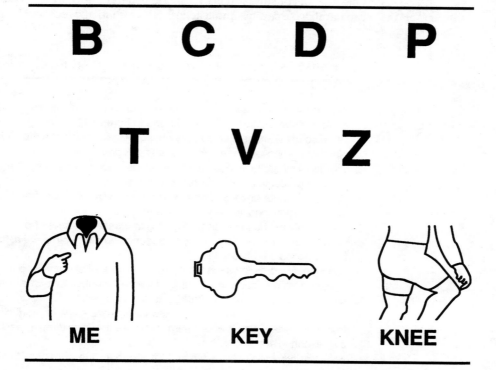

Figure 18–4. Example of a test that can be used during analytic auditory training. The syllables rhyme, so the child must hear the first sound of a word in order to identify it correctly. (Reprinted with permission from *Audiovisual Feature Test for Young Children*, by R. S. Tyler, H. Fryauf-Bertschy, and D. Kelsay, 1991. Iowa City: The University of Iowa.)

training items and the child points to the picture that corresponds to what he or she heard. Table 18–1 presents an example of a hierarchy of analytic training objectives for developing consonant recognition skills. A similar hierarchy can be designed for developing vowel recognition (Tye-Murray, 1998).

Figure 18–5 presents an example of a synthetic auditory training activity. For this activity, the clinician speaks a sentence and the child points to the picture that illustrates it. The child need not recognize every word to perform the task correctly. If the youngster performs well on this task, the clinician may move onto activities wherein the child must paraphrase sentences and then repeat them verbatim, without the assistance of picture cues. Table 18–2 presents a sample of synthetic auditory training objectives, arranged in ascending order of difficulty.

CONSULTATION

The final role we will consider is consultation. The speech-language pathologist frequently consults with a child's parents, teachers, audiologists, and other members of the child's educational planning team. One goal of consultation is to provide general information. A clinician can familiarize parents and teachers with a child's speech and language

Table 18–1. A sample hierarchy of consonant auditory training objectives.

The student:

1. Will discriminate nasal versus nonnasal unvoiced consonants that differ in place of production; for example, *mean* from *teen.*
2. Will discriminate nasal versus nonnasal voiced consonants that differ in place of production; for example, *map* from *gap.*
3. Will discriminate unvoiced fricatives versus voiced stops that differ in place of production; for example, *son* from *gun.*
4. Will discriminate unvoiced fricatives versus unvoiced stops that differ in place of production; for example, *sea* from *key.*
5. Will identify words in which the consonants share manner of production from a four-item and then six-item response set; for example, *sat* from the response set of: *sat, fat, shot,* and *van.*
6. Will identify words in which the consonants are all either voiced or unvoiced from a four-item and then six-item response set; for example, *cat* from the response set of: *cat, pat, tap,* and *sack.*
7. Will identify words in which the consonants share place of production from a four–item and then six-item response set; for example, *pat* from the response set of: *pat, mat, bat,* and *fat.*
8. Will identify words in an open-set format, where the words are familiar vocabulary words.

Source: Reprinted with permission from *Foundations of Aural Rehabilitation: Children, Adults, and Their Family Members*, by N. Tye-Murray, 1998, p. 178. San Diego, CA: Singular Publishing Group.

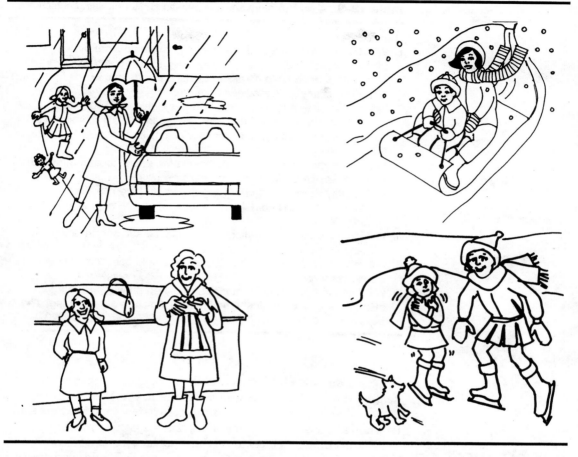

Figure 18–5. Example of a response set that can be used during synthetic auditory training. The speech-language pathologist might recite the sentence, *The woman holds the new dress.* The child then must point to the corresponding picture. (Reprinted with permission from *Communication Training for Hearing-impaired Children and Teenagers: Speechreading, Listening, and Repair Strategies,* by N. Tye-Murray, 1992, p. 50. Austin, TX: Pro-Ed.)

skills, and how the child's skills compare to those of other children. We also can describe how speech and language skills typically progress in normally hearing and hearing-impaired children, and factors that may accelerate progress. This information will help those who know the child to develop appropriate expectations. It may also provide them with ideas about how best to nurture their child's development.

A speech-language pathologist can help parents and teachers learn to speak and sign complete sentences. Many parents and teachers do not match their words to their signs when they use simultaneous communication. A mother might say, "John, get in the car," and simultaneously sign the word "John" and then "car," without signing the verb and connecting words. This presents a poor language model. The child may only receive the message, "John car."

You might recommend that parents and teachers whose children use a communication mode that incorporates sign view commercially available sign language video cassettes, participate in a weekly "sign group," and attend sign language classes.

Table 18–2. A sample hierarchy of synthetic auditory training objectives.

The student:

1. Will discriminate multiword utterances from single-word utterances, using a closed response set; for example, *How are you today?* From *Hi!* Later he or she can be asked to discriminate long words from short words; for example, *Halloween* from *cat.*
2. Will discriminate a spondee from a one-syllable word; for example, ice cream from shoe. Later, he or she can be asked to discriminate a spondee from a two-syllable word; for example, *There's a toothbrush* from *There's a pony.*
3. Will discriminate between words having the same number of syllables; for example, *That's my cat* from *That's my dog.*
4. Will identify simple words from a four-item and then six-item response set; for example, *cat* from the response set of: *cat, dog, elephant,* and *camel.*
5. Will identify picture illustrations from a closed set, after hearing one-sentence descriptions.
6. Will follow simple directions and answer simple questions, using a closed response set.
7. Will listen to two related sentences, and then draw a picture about them; for example, he or she might draw a picture after hearing, *The boy is playing. He has a ball.*

Often, the speech-language pathologist also suggests ways for helping the child to generalize what she has learned in therapy to more real-world settings by informing the parents and teachers about the child's current therapy objectives and suggesting practice materials. For example, a clinician might send home a list of vocabulary words. A parent can practice the words with the child, perhaps in a flashcard game format. The clinician can also observe the child in the classroom and then suggest ways in which the classroom teacher can integrate speech and language practice into the daily routine.

Finally, the speech-language pathologist often provides information to the school audiologist. For instance, if your test results from a speech and language evaluation indicate that the child has an extremely limited vocabulary, the audiologist will not evaluate the child's speech perception skills with recorded sentence lists.

Parents who have difficulty in accepting their child's significant hearing loss may show indications of denial, grief, and anger before they accept the reality of the situation. One role of the speech-language pathologist is to help these parents to interact efficiently with their child and to make important decisions about their child's educational plans.

SUMMARY

Children who have severe and profound hearing impairments typically develop deviant speech and language patterns. Your role as a speech-language pathologist is to assess their speech and language skills, provide speech and language therapy, and consult with their parents and other professionals who work with them. You probably will provide speechreading and auditory training to the children as well. In this chapter, we considered the hearing capabilities of children who have severe and profound hearing impairments, and their characteristic speech and language problems. We then considered the four roles of the speech-language pathologist: evaluation, provision of speech and language therapy, provision of auditory training, and consultation.

REFERENCES

Berko, J. (1958). The child's learning of English morphology. *Word, 14*, 150–177.

Berry, S. (1981). *Written Language Syntax Test*. Washington, DC: Gallaudet College Press.

Brownlee, S. (1989). The signs of silence: A deaf child's brain is primed to learn sign language easily. *U.S. News & World Report, 16*, 86–88.

Carney, A., & Moeller, M. P. (1998). Treatment efficacy: Hearing loss in children. *Journal of Speech, Language, and Hearing Research, 41*(Suppl.), S61–S84.

Carrow, E. (1973). *Test for Auditory Comprehension of Language*. Lamar, TX: Learning Concepts.

Dunn, L., & Dunn, L. (1981). *Peabody Picture Vocabulary Test—Revised*. Circle Pines, MN: American Guidance Service.

Engen, E., & Engen, T. (1983). *Rhode Island Test of Language Structure Manual*. Baltimore, MD: University Park Press.

Erber, N. P. (1982). *Auditory training*. Washington, DC: A. G. Bell Association for the Deaf.

Goldman, R., & Fristoe, M. (1969). *Test of Articulation*. Circle Pines, MN: American Guidance Service.

Hasenstab, M. S., & Tobey, E. A. (1991). Language development in children receiving Nucleus multichannel cochlear implants. *Ear and Hearing, 12*(4), 55S–65S.

Kretschmer, R., & Kretschmer, L. (1978). *Language development and intervention with the hearing impaired*. Baltimore, MD: University Park Press.

Lee, L. (1974). *Developmental sentence analysis*. Evanston, IL: Northwestern University Press.

Levitt, H. (1987). *Fundamental Speech Skills Test*. New York: City University of New York.

Ling, D. (1976). *Speech and the hearing-impaired child: Theory and practice*. Washington, DC: A. G. Bell Association for the Deaf.

Markides, A. (1970). The speech of deaf and partially hearing children with special reference to factors affecting intelligibility. *British Journal of Disordered Communication, 5*, 126–140.

Moog, J. S., & Geers, A. E. (1975). *Scales of early communication skills for hearing impaired children*. St. Louis, MO: Central Institute for the Deaf Press.

Moog, J. S., Kozak, V. J., & Geers, A. (1983). *Grammatical analysis of elicited language (GAEL-p)*. St. Louis, MO: Central Institute for the Deaf Press.

Quigley, S. P., Monranelli, D. S., & Wilbur, R. B. (1976). Some aspects of the verb system in the language of deaf students. *Journal of Speech and Hearing Research, 19*, 536–550.

Reynell, J. K. (1977). *Reynell Development Language Scale*. Windsor, Ontario, Canada: NFER Publishing.

Secord, W. (1981). *T-MAC: Test of Minimal Articulation Competence*. Columbus, OH: Charles E. Merrill.

Stout, C. G., & Windle, J. V. E. (1986). *The developmental approach to successful listening* (DASL). Houston: Stout & Windle.

Subtelny, J. D., Orlando, N. A., & Whitehead, R. L. (1981). *Speech and voice characteristics of the deaf*. Washington, DC: A. G. Bell Association for the Deaf.

Tomblin, B. J., Spencer, L., Flock, S., Tyler, R. S., & Gantz, B. (in press). Language achievement in prelingually deaf children using cochlear implants or hearing aids. *Journal of Speech, Language, and Hearing Research*.

Tramwell, J., & Owens, S. (1977, November). *The test of auditory comprehension (TAC)*. Paper presented at the annual convention of the American Speech-Language-Hearing Association, Chicago.

Tye-Murray, N., Tomblin, B., & Spencer, L. (1997, November). *Speech and language acquisition over time in children with cochlear implants*. Paper presented at the Annual Convention of the American Speech-Language-Hearing Association, Boston, MA.

Tye-Murray, N. (1992). *Communication training for hearing-impaired children and teenagers: Speechreading, listening, and using repair strategies*. Austin, TX: Pro-Ed.

Tye-Murray, N. (1998). *Foundations of aural rehabilitation: Children, adults, and their family members*. San Diego, CA: Singular Publishing Group.

Tyler, R. S., Fryauf-Bertschy, H., & Kelsay, D. (1991). *Audiovisual feature test for young children*. Iowa City: The University of Iowa.

Voelker, C. (1938). An experimental study of the comparative rate of utterances of deaf and normal-hearing speakers. *American Annals of the Deaf, 83*, 274–284.

RECOMMENDED READINGS

Ling, D. (1976). *Speech and the hearing-impaired child: Theory and practice*. Washington, DC: The Alexander Graham Bell Association for the Deaf.

Nevins, M. E., & Chute, P. M. (1996). *Children with cochlear implants in educational settings*. San Diego, CA: Singular Publishing Group.

Quigley, S. P., & Paul, P. V. (1984). *Language and deafness*. San Diego, CA: College-Hill Press.

Tye-Murray, N. (1998). *Foundations of aural rehabilitation: Children, adults, and their family members*. San Diego, CA: Singular Publishing Group.

APPENDIX 18A

AUDITORY TRAINING CURRICULA

A. Clarke School Personnel. (1990). Auditory enhancement guide. Northhampton, MA: Clarke School for the Deaf

B. Erber, N. P. (1982). *Auditory Training*. Washington, DC: The Alexander Graham Bell Association for the Deaf.

C. Moog, J., Biedenstein, J., & Davidson, L. (1995). Speech perception instructional curriculum and evaluation (SPICE). St. Louis, MO: Central Institute for the Deaf.

D. Stout, G. G., & Windle, J. V. (1992). *The developmental approach to successful listening II (DASL)* (2nd ed.). Englewood, CO: Resource Point, Inc.

E. Tye-Murray, N. (1993). *Communication training for hearing-impaired children and teenagers: Speechreading, listening, and using repair strategies*. Austin, TX: Pro-Ed.

F. Vergara, K. S., & Miskiel, L. W. (1994). *CHATS: The Miami cochlear implant auditory and tactile skills curriculum*. Miami, FL: Intelligent Hearing Systems.

Index

A

AAC (alternative/augmentative communication), 177, 432–433. *See also* Mental retardation, adult
  electronic communication devices, 442
AbleNet, 442
Accelerometry, 390
Accuracy, false positive/false negative, 27
Acute Aphasia Screening Protocol (AASP), 326
African Americans, 37
  CVA (cerebrovascular accident), 38
  dialect, phonological/syntactic variations, 46, 47
  learning styles, 42
  oral/speech mechanism assessment, 118–119
  and pseudoquestions, 43–44
Aging process, 164–165
  and voice disorder, 270
Alcohol consumption, 238, 246, 250
Alzheimer's type dementia, 330
American Association of Mental Retardation (AAMR), 428
American Cancer Society (ACS), 367–368
Aneurism, 318
Anoxia, 189
Aphasia, 143
  aneurism, 318
  arteriovenous malformation (AVM), 318
  attitudes, patient, 327–328
  Broca's, 146
  and cancer, 319
  concomitant problems, 328
  CVA (cerebrovascular accident), 318, 319, 331
  defined, 315, 317

  dementia, 330–331
  and dementia, 319
  determination of complaint, 317–320
  dissection, traumatically induced, 318
  and family, 327–328
  inflammatory processes, 318
  motor, transcortical, 146
  or dementia?, 133
  and paralysis, 11
  paraphasia
    neologistic, 145, 322
    phonemic, 322
    semantic, 322
  prognosis, 12–13
    determining, 331–332
  related language disorders, 328–331
  right hemisphere damage (RHD), 329–330
  testing
    auditory comprehension, 321–322
    functional communication, 326–327
    in-depth, 325–326
    oral motor system control, 323
    reading, 323–324
    screening, 325, 326
    verbal expression, 322–323
    writing, 323–324
  traumatic brain injury (TBI), 318, 328–329
  treatment factors, 332
Aphasia Language Performance Scales (ALPS), 326
Aphonia, 249
Apraxia
  AOS (apraxia of speech), 187, 349
  of speech, 187
  verbal, 176, 186, 187, 196